METHODS OF CARIES PREDICTION

(A Special Supplement to Microbiology Abstracts — Bacteriology)

Epidemiology, diet, oral biology as indicators of future caries. Caries models and new detection techniques.

The correct manner in which to refer to a paper from this publication is as follows:

Authors of paper, title of paper.

Proceedings "Methods of Caries Prediction".

Eds. Bibby and Shern. Sp. Supp. Microbiology Abstracts.
pp _ – _ –, 1978.

METHODS OF CARIES PREDICTION

(A Special Supplement to Microbiology Abstracts — Bacteriology)

Proceedings of a workshop conference on methods of caries prediction

October 3–5, 1977
Niagara Falls, N.Y.

Edited by
Basil G. Bibby
Roald J. Shern

Sponsored by
National Caries Program
National Institute of Dental Research
National Institutes of Health

Information Retrieval Inc.
Washington DC and London.

International Standard Book Number 0-917000-04-8
Library of Congress Catalog Card Number 78-50300

Published as a Special Supplement to:
Microbiology Abstracts : Bacteriology
published monthly by Information Retrieval Limited, London

Published by Information Retrieval Inc.
1911 Jefferson Davis Highway, Arlington, VA 22202
Printed in the United States of America

Contents

Contents (continued)

Organizing Committee

Basil G. Bibby
Dept. of Caries Research
Eastman Dental Center
800 Main Street East
Rochester, N.Y. 14603

Stanley B. Heifetz
National Caries Program
National Institute of Dental Research
National Institutes of Health
Bethesda, MD. 20014

Roald J. Shern
National Caries Program
National Institute of Dental Research
National Institutes of Health
Bethesda, MD. 20014

Opening statements and orientation

James P. Carlos

National Institute of Dental Research, Westwood Building, Bethesda, Maryland 20014

My function today is to do two things, and to do them quickly. First, to welcome all of you to this workshop, which I do with great pleasure, and second, to make some preliminary remarks as background for the discussions which are to follow.

The list of workshops and conferences which have been sponsored by the National Caries Program over the past several years is growing rather long, but none of them has addressed a topic so broad and so complex as the one before us. Because early attempts to devise useful caries predictive tests were rather disappointing, and because very little systematic research on the subject has been carried out recently, there seem to be few clear guidelines on how best to proceed to develop such techniques. The major purpose of this workshop is to attempt to establish some guidelines.

It is important to understand that we are not so naive as to think that the workshop will conclude with a caries predictive test or tests, neatly packaged and broadly agreed to. That is obviously an impossible goal. What we do hope to accomplish is a summary of the best expert judgement on which parameters are most likely to have the best potential for use in predicting caries susceptibility. The soundness of those judgements must then be confirmed by subsequent clinical research.

The desirability of better techniques for the *a priori* measurement of caries susceptibility hardly needs to be argued, since they would be useful in so many areas of dentistry. The cost of caries prevention activities could be greatly reduced and their efficiency sharply increased if the practitioner or public health administrator were able to identify, in advance, those subjects at greatest risk of developing caries. This is in contrast to most present programs which deliver preventive regimens to all subjects equally, whether they need them or not.

Great benefits could occur in clinical research as well. If it can be shown that a certain variable is very highly correlated with the subsequent appearance of clinical caries, then the end point of clinical trials might be the effect of the test agent on that variable, rather than the number of carious lesions which eventually appear. It does not seem wildly optimistic to suppose that trials which now require two or more years could thus be concluded in months -- or even weeks.

Finally, the clinical trial design itself could be made many times more sensitive, in a statistical sense, were it possible to assign subjects to test and control groups on the basis of some characteristic, or set of characteristics, known to be highly predictive of caries susceptibility. No doubt other reasons for attempting to develop caries prediction tests can be put forth, but those I've mentioned are more than sufficient to make the effort worthwhile.

Now it seems necessary to ask, "How will we decide whether a potential caries predictive test is a good one? What do we, in fact, mean by a 'good' test?" There are many answers to these questions, but I wish to propose that any such test, to be useful, must be shown to possess at least three characteristics. These are:

Validity
Reliability
Feasibility

These are basic concepts, but it is surprising how often they have been ignored in the past when various screening tests have been proposed. A few remarks about each of these characteristics may prove helpful to our discussions during this workshop.

Validity

By validity I simply mean that a test must measure what it purports to measure. In the case of caries susceptibility tests, we will mostly be concerned with what is called "predictive validity". Predictive validity is most easily explained by a simple example of how it might be measured. One first applies the proposed susceptibility test to a group of subjects and categorizes them as "positive" or "negative" on the basis of their test responses. One must then follow these subjects for some period of time, say 1-2 years, to record the occurrence of clinical caries. If a high percentage of positive test responders subsequently develop caries, we may conclude that validity is demonstrated. (How high that percentage must be depends upon how many false-positive or false-negative test responses can be tolerated in a given program or research situation, something which is difficult to discuss in generalities). Low predictive validity is, of course, a major shortcoming of most caries susceptibility tests which have previously been proposed.

Reliability

A second essential test characteristic is reliability, a word which I intend to be synonymous with reproductibility. It must be demonstrated that there is a high correlation between test results when the test is applied to the same subjects by different investigators, or by the same investigator on different occasions. The kinds of data which must be collected to establish reliability are fairly obvious, and several straightforward and well-known statistical techniques are available to analyze such data.

Feasibility

Finally, a useful test must be feasible for application to the population of interest, and under the conditions likely to prevail. One does not intend to rule out in advance caries predictive tests which may require costly equipment and sophisticated techniques of application, or even which involve slight hazards, but the utility of such tests might be sharply limited in public health programs or large clinical trials. Certainly, given a choice, a test which is inexpensive, non-invasive and easy to use by semi-skilled personnel is to be preferred.

I do not wish to imply that the characteristics of validity, reliability and feasibility are exhaustive of those which a good caries susceptibility test must have, but certainly they are a necessary minimum. I hope that we shall keep them in mind as we proceed to examine the many possible variables and combinations of variables which may be useful to predict the future onset of caries.

On behalf of the NIDR and the National Caries Program, I extend sincere thanks to Basil Bibby, Roald Shern and the others who have helped to organize this excellent program, and I repeat our warm welcome to each of you.

TOPIC I

BACKGROUND ON CARIES PREDICTION TESTS

Moderator:

Herschel S. Horowitz
National Institute of Dental Research
Westwood Building
Bethesda, Maryland 20014

Previous caries prediction tests

Frederick M. Parkins

Department of Pedodontics, College of Dentistry, University of Iowa, Iowa City, Iowa 52242

Widely recognized variations in the caries experiences of different individuals has led clinicians and investigators to seek methods for the early identification of those persons more likely to be severely affected. Susceptibility predictions necessarily involve an appreciation of the causative factors leading to dental caries. G.V. Black and W.D. Miller were probably not the first to attempt the proof of cariogenic mechanisms by seeking a correlation between caries incidence and a variable associated with their theory. Other investigators have selected subjects with very low caries activity and have sought to determine their unique characteristics.

The search for useful laboratory tests which would predict caries activity began before the turn of the century (Miller, 1890). The procedures evaluated have paralleled the evolving theories about the mechanism of caries causation. However, basic criteria for determining the value of a caries prediction test have remained relatively consistent. Those proposed by Snyder (1951) and represented by subsequent authors (Rapp 1962, Socransky 1968, Ellen 1976) are:

1. Maximal correlation with the clinical status of the patient.
2. Maximal correlation with caries increments.
3. Accurate reproducibility of results.
4. Ease of performance, requiring little technical skill.
5. Inexpensive procedures and equipment.
6. Achievement of rapid results.
7. Measurement of factors involved in the caries process.

The further criterion of a 0.9 correlation coefficient between the test and caries increments has been offered as the criterion of usefulness on an individual basis (Snyder, et al 1963).

Socransky (1968) defined caries activity as "The increment of caries, either new lesions or progress of old ones, which occurs in a finite period of time". Most clinical evaluations of caries activity tests have compared the test output to the subjects' total prior caries experience. Only a few investigations have been carried out with longitudinal studies of caries increments. Since the progress of caries is known to vary during different periods of life only the recording of increments which follow a caries activity test is a satisfactory basis for evaluating the test's diagnostic value as a predictor of future caries experiences. Published reviews of caries activity tests are notable for the number of concerns expressed about their limited value. In the opinion of Socransky 1968, Bowen 1969, and Ellen 1976, a test which meets all the criteria for clinical usefulness has not yet been reported.

The tests which have been documented can be grouped according to their methodology. The constant exposure of the teeth to saliva is an obvious factor in test rationales. The ease of collection of saliva and readily available techniques for chemical or bacterial determinations have caused it to become the sample material of choice. The types of tests using saliva can be grouped as follows:

Biochemical Analyses
- pH determinations
- Titratable acidity measurements
- Enzyme assays
- Fluoride determinations

Bacteriological Procedures
- Bacterial counts
- Acid production - saliva
- Acid production - plaque
- Oxidation - reduction potentials

Of the biochemical tests that have been used to indicate caries activity, Socransky (1968) lists measurements of saliva pH, buffering capacity and oxidation-reduction potential as unsatisfactory, and tests of oxygen uptake as over-difficult and of questionable value. Of the enzyme tests he finds the results with alpha amylase unsatisfactory, with urease limited and not encouraging and with hyalouronidase without correlation to caries.

In respect to tests on the bacterial constituents of saliva, lactobacillus counts and the rezasurin test of Rapp (1962) are unsatisfactory and Streptococcus mutans and Bacillus aerogenes counts are untested. Acid production by salivary bacteria has been measured in several ways by a number of investigators, but as indicated in the accompanying table (Table 1) their value is questionable.

Table 1

RELATION OF ACIDOGENIC POTENTIAL OF SALIVARY CONSTITUENTS TO CARIES ACTIVITY

Test	Indicator	Current Evaluation
Davies, *et al*	Acidogenic bacteria per ml.	Unsatisfactory
Dewar	pH	Unsatisfactory
Fosdick	Enamel dissolution	Unsatisfactory
Rickles	Double color indicator	Unsatisfactory
Snyder	Color indicator	Group Correlation
Wach	pH and titratable acidity	Unsatisfactory
Methyl Red	Methyl Red	Unsatisfactory
Alban	Color indicator	Unsatisfactory

(adapted from Socransky, S. 1968)

The recent theory that a special type of 'odontopathic' plaque is responsible for caries has stimulated tests that use samples of plaque as test material. A summary of such plaque tests is offered as Table 2.

Table 2 Relation of Tests on Plaque Constituents of Caries Activity

Test	Indicator	Current Evaluation
Grainger Swab	pH	Unsatisfactory
Woods	S. mutans	Unsatisfactory
Spot Plate	Methyl Red	Unsatisfactory

Enamel fluoride concentration has been measured by micro-sampling techniques. Many investigators have used these methods to study fluoride uptake after fluoride treatments. The assumption has been prevalent that caries susceptibility is directly related to enamel fluoride concentrations. The studies of this hypothesis have generally failed to support the premise. For instance Poulsen and Larsen (1975) could find no statistically significant relationship between caries incidence over a three year period and the fluoride content of the surface enamel of children.

Enamel surface characteristics have more recently become a focus of attention. Methods to detect alterations at the surface which preceed cavitation have been considered. Refraction of ultra-violet light from partially demineralized areas has been tested (Hefferen et al, 1971). Since the surface zone of newly forming lesions remains highly mineralized until more advanced states of enamel destruction (Silverstone, 1977), the value of this approach is questionable. The penetration of marker dyes or other substances which would selectively enter the partially demineralized surface and provide diagnostic value remains a possibliity (Rawls et al, 1975). The worth of such approaches as prediction methods is questioned. However, to the extent that a developing carious lesion can be reversed there may be a rationale for techniques which reveal such beginning destruction.

A further criterion for evaluation of caries activity tests is that they should be sensitive enough to respond to alterations in the patients' caries susceptibility status. While the potential of a valid and reliable caries activity test to anticipate future caries increments is of obvious value, it was pointed out by Jay et al (1933, 1938) that modification of factors in caries etiology could be helpful in the clinical management of the susceptible patient. He advocated the lactobacillus count as a method of monitoring changes in patient eating habits. A fall in the lactobacillus count from an original baseline in association with diet modification and a reduction in refined sugar intake has been shown by Featherstone (1959, 1960 A and B) and Bowen (1967).

Usually, research with caries activity tests has compared a single variable to past caries experience. In a few instances a single variable has been compared in longitudinal studies to caries increments. More recently, two longitudinal studies have compared several simultaneously determined variables with caries increments, thus, taking advantage of the promise that multi-variant analyses should offer. In comparisons of Strepococcus mutans and lactobacillus counts in a longitudinal study employing caries increments, Woods (1971) was unable to demonstrate a significant correlation between the measured numbers of the two different organisms. Marlay (1970) was able to show a "close similarity", but lower correlations between lactobacillus counts and the colormetric results of the Snyder Test, than had previous studies (Dewar, 1950). The relationship of both to the caries increments was also in accordance with previous observations. That is, the tests were only able to assign the subjects into groups of severe, moderate and mild levels. An inverse relationship between DMFS increments and salivary buffer capacity was also obtained at an unacceptable correlation level. A comparison of buffer capacity and lactobacillus numbers was not determined.

Recognition of the role of Strep mutans and plaque in caries suggested to us the possibility of improved caries prediction tests. Wei et al (1972), Wei et al (1973) and Parkins et al (1975) used a selection of tests in a two-year investigation on 206 children, ages 3 to 13. The tests were adapted from those described in test-books and research papers and included an oral hygiene index, a micro-sampling of enamel fluoride and three microbiological culture techniques on samples of plaque collected at the time of clinical examination. All tests were rapid, inexpensive, conveniently performed and easily taught.

Statistical comparisons of the values obtained from the tests and the caries increments were carried out. The readings at different periods from the same test were statistically compared. The reliability of all tests found acceptable ($4.25 < F > 10.55$, $.001 < P > .025$, $.103 < R > .591$). However, an acceptable correlation with caries increments was not obtained with any test, nor was there a correlation coefficient > 0.35 obtained between any of the different tests, while coefficients of 0.7 were obtained when comparing initial and final caries status. (Table 3). Forcing the data by grouping high and low readings, eliminating occlusal surfaces and expressing caries increments as percentages of available surfaces did not appreciably improve the strength of the correlations. (Table 4).

The advent of computer assisted statistical interpretations has made multi-variant analyses practical. A correlation of 0.9 which has been suggested for the criteria of usefulness of a caries activity test on an individual basis is apparently difficult to achieve. The correlations of those tests which <u>have</u> evidenced a relationship between the test results and caries status/increments are not high enough for any of those tests to be useful on an individual basis.

Because dental caries is a disease with multiple etiologic factors, the finding of correlations between more than one caries activity test would probably mean that they were relating to the same causative factor. If a comparison of the results did not correlate highly between tests then the possibility of combining simultaneous measurement of different causative factors exists. Multiple regression analyses with the results of tests which measure different variables might improve the level of correlation. Should the individual tests be of sufficient validity in measuring multiple causative factors, a correlation coefficient of > 0.9 might be achieved.

As a final statistical manipulation the data from the five tests were compared to the caries increments. The correlation coefficient from the multiple regression analysis was 0.26. This value was not higher than the coefficient of the individual test with the highest correlation. That observation indicates the additional tests did not improve predictive value of the individual test.

<u>Table 3</u> Correlation Matrix - Four Surfaces

	OHI	SPOT	COLOR	TURBT	FCONC	DMFT1	DMFS1	DMFT4	DMFT4	PDMFT	PDMFS
OHI	1.000	.347**	.034	-.055	.219*	.099	.127	.162	.162	.055	.001
SPOT		1.000	.298**	.035	.180*	.078	.065	-.001	-.010	-.027	-.043
COLOR			1.000	.093	-.064	.148	.146	-.018	.010	-.032	-.005
TURBT				1.000	.259**	.031	.010	.053	.111	.015	.012
FCONC					1.000	-.162	-.137	-.082	.011	.087	.027
DMFT1						1.000	.948**	.721**	.663**	.289	.258
DMFS1							1.000	.695**	.694**	.316**	.280**
DMFT4								1.000	.852**	.467**	.399**
DMFS4									1.000	.572**	.613**
PDMFT			(*P < .05)							1.000	.096**
PDMFS			(**P < .01)								1.000

Table 4

Correlation Matrix - Occlusal Surfaces Omitted

	OHI	SPOT	COLOR	TURBT	FCONC	DMFT1	DMFS1	DMFT4	DMFS4	PDMFT	PDMFS
OHI	1.000	.347**	.034	-.055	.219*	.151	.160	.168	.136	.071	.004
SPOT		1.000	.298**	.035	.180*	.126	.080	.065	.001	-.008	-.029
COLOR			1.000	.093	-.064	.183	.138	.028	.025	-.021	-.001
TURBT				1.000	.259**	.059	.017	.142	.133	.045	.019
FCONC					1.000	-.072	-.064	.047	.062	.081	.030
DMFT1						1.000	.958**	.788**	.657**	.439**	.364**
DMFS1							1.000	.742**	.679**	.462**	.402**
DMFT4								1.000	.894**	.625**	.567**
DMFS4									1.000	.664**	.703**
PDMFT										1.000	.919**
PDMFS											1.000

(*P < .05)
(**P < .01)

DISCUSSION

Well over three-quarters of a century of continued investigation has been documented. Over these years the new insights into the mechanism of caries development have been used to formulate additional caries activity tests.

Of the seven criteria recommended at the beginning of this report for acceptable caries activity tests, the five relating to reliability/reproducibility and convenience are met by many of the procedures. The two criteria requiring maximal correlations with 1) the patient's clinical status, and 2) caries increments have been approached. The suggested requirements for a correlation coefficient of 0.9 for a test to be valid on an individual basis has not been met. The highest coefficient claimed by any author was 0.7 (Snyder 1960).

The possibility that aggregated results from more than one type of test on the same patients would produce a higher correlation was considered by several investigators. The variability between the tests was notable. The relatively low correlations of individual tests with clinical and/or increments were disappointing. The results when data from different tests on the same patient population were combined indicated correlations which were not appreciably higher than the individual test with the highest coefficient.

The populations under longitudinal study in these investigations evidenced a useful variability in caries increments providing an experimentally adequate range for data comparisons. The variability of test results was notable. The low correlations between caries increments and test results suggest that the tests are not directly measuring fluctuations in the factors causing the caries increments.

Caries activity tests appear to have three fundamental benefits. Initially their development aids in the investigation and conceptualization of mechanisms responsible for dental caries. Secondly, they could provide a means of identifying those patients who require particular attention with respect to prevention. Also, the use of techniques which reveal positive changes as a result of preventive treatments would make it possible to assess the value of those preventive programs. This is relevant to the advent of third party payments, where opportunity to assess measurable changes could answer questions regarding the use of funds for particular preventive activities.

An associated requirement of a maximally useful caries activity test should be the response of the test to changes in patient susceptibility brought about through clinical and behavioral modifications. Those tests related to organism counts, especially lactobacillus counts, have been found to respond to improvements in the patient's oral hygiene status in addition to diet modifications. A more direct correlation with the factors of caries etiology would be desirable. Further evaluations of tests should probably also be expected to demonstrate responses to changes in patient status.

To date the emphasis has been on tests which are convenient, inexpensive and easily taught. The investigations with this type of test have been disappointing. Perhaps the emphasis should shift to those criteria which have remained unmet, i.e. maximal correlation with clinical status/ caries increments. This approach probably will require laboratory tests with more sophisticated techniques. Such an approach would be practical if samples from patients were submitted to a clinical laboratory. The precedent for this is obvious.

Until the advent of new tests, the initial caries status of a patient and the findings in frequent and careful clinical examinations may be the most accurate predictors.

LITERATURE CITED

1. Alban, A. 1970. An improved Snyder Test. J. Dent. Res. 49:641.

2. Birkeland, J.M., Broach, L. and Jorkjend, L. 1976. Caries experience as predictor for caries incidence. Community Dent. Oral Epidemiol. 4:66.

3. Black, G.V. 1899. Susceptibility and immunity to dental caries. Dent. Cosmos 41:826.

4. Bowen, W.H. 1967. The lactobacilli in the saliva plaque and carious dentin in Macaca irus. J. Path. & Bact. 94:55.

5. Bowen, W.H. 1969. Caries activity tests. Internat. Dent. J. 19:267.

6. Dewar, M.R. 1950. Laboratory methods for assessing susceptibility to dental caries. Part II. Correlation of results obtained by clinical examination and by standardized models. Dent. J. Aust. 22:24.

7. Ellen, R.P. 1976. Microbiological assays for dental caries and periodontal disease susceptibility. Oral Sci. Rev. 8:3.

8. Featherstone, J.L. 1959. The oral lactobacilli of Central Australian aborigines. Aust. Dent. J. 4:39.

9. Featherstone, J.L. 1960a. A study of oral strains of Lactobacillus spp. The effects of diet upon indigenous and implanted strains. Aust. Dent. J. 5:149.

10. Featherstone, J.L. 1960b. The oral lactobacilli of Central Australian aborigines III species isolated from nomads in Arnham Land. Aust. Dent. J. 5:204.

11. Grainger, R.M., Jarrett, T.M. and Honey, F.S.L. 1965. Swab test for dental caries activity: and epidemiological survey. J. Canad. Dent. Assn. 31:515.

12. Hefferren, J.J., Cooley, R.O., Hall, J.B., Olsen, N.H. and Lyon, H.W. 1970. Use of ultraviolet illumination in oral diagnosis. J. Amer. Dent. Assn. 82:1353.

13. Jay, P., Crowley, M., Hadley, F.P. and Bunting, R.W. 1933. Bacteriologic and immunologic studies on dental caries. J. Amer. Dent. Assn. 29:2130.

14. Jay, P. 1938. Lactobacillus acidophilus and dental caries. Am. J. Pub. Health 28:759.

15. Marlay, E. 1970. The relationship between dental caries and salivary properties at adolescence. Aust. Dent. J. 15:412.

16. Miller, W.D. 1890. Microorganisms of the Human Mouth, S.S. White Dental Mfg. Co., Philadelphia, p. 364.

17. Parkins, F.M., Wei, S.H.Y., Pinkham, J. and Henderson, W. 1975. Relationships of caries susceptibility tests to caries increments. Proc. Am. Assn. Dent. Res. Abst. #441.

18. Poulsen, S., Larsen, M. 1975. Dental caries in relation to fluoride content of enamel in the primary dentition. Caries Res. 9:59.

19. Rapp, G.W. 1962. Fifteen minute caries test. Ill. Dent. J. 31:290.

20. Rawls, H.R., Robert, U.Q. and Owen, W.D. 1975. Fluorescent caries-disclosing fluids for early diagnosis of incipient lesions. Proc. Internat. Assn. Dent. Res. Abst. #L416.

21. Silverstone, L.M. 1977. Remineralization Phenomena. Caries Res. (Sup.1) 59.

22. Snyder, M.L. 1951. Laboratory methods in the clinical evaluation of caries activity. J. Amer. Dent. Assn. 42:400.

23. Snyder, M.L., Porter, D.R., Claycomb, C.K., Sims, W. and Macho, F.R. 1963. Evaluation of laboratory tests for the estimation of caries activity. Archs oral Biol. 8:541.

24. Socransky, S.S. 1968. Caries-susceptibility tests. Ann. N.Y. Acad. Sci. 153:137.

25. Wei, S.H.Y., Parkins, F.M. and Dwa, W. 1972. Plaque activity tests. Proc. Internat. Assn. Dent. Res. Abst. #831.

26. Wei, S.H.Y., Parkins, F.M., Kwa, W. and Henderson, W. 1973. Caries activity tests. Proc. Internat. Assn. Dent. Res. Abst. #839.

27. Woods, R.A. 1971. A dental caries susceptibility test based on the occurrence of Streptococcus mutans in plaque material. Aust. Dent. J. 16:116.

Discussion of previous caries prediction tests

Carl A. Ostrom

Institute of Dental Research, University of Alabama, Birmingham, Alabama 35294

Dr. Parkins has pointed out that to date the emphasis has been on tests that are convenient, easy and inexpensive. He concluded that studies with the established tests have been disappointing. His own studies indicated that even a battery of tests was not reliable for prediction of caries increments. He suggested that until new, more sophisticated laboratory tests are developed, the most accurate predictor probably is frequent clinical examination.

Since the existing methods are not useful at a practical level, they do not serve as caries prediction tests. Instead they are single function tests that apply only to different cariogenic factors of a multifactorial disease, namely, microbial ecology and substrate availability. They do not reflect caries resistance factors such as original enamel composition, saliva and plaque physiology, immunology, enamel maturation, and enamel adaptation to challenge. When the resistance to caries is low, caries is apt to occur even with a moderate cariogenic attack. Therefore, it is not surprising that it has been unproductive to use tests of the cariogenic factors to distinguish between subjects of high versus moderate future caries increment. It is conceivable that measurements of the resistance factors may provide more useful predictive values than the current tests of cariogenic factors. However, the currently available tests for caries resistance factors, e.g. salivary flow and plaque buffer capacity give low predictive values. Therefore, to serve the objectives of this workshop, it would seem logical to intensify efforts toward development of tests of other resistance factors.

Further development of correlations between past and present caries activity and changes in the anti-body titer of serum and saliva may lead to effective caries resistance tests.[4] Studies on salivary agglutination titers suggest that a rapid, simple test may be helpful in identifying subjects who are high or low risks for future caries increment.[5,6]

Recent reports suggest that caries resistance tests may lie in measurement of the calcium, phosphorus or fluoride content of plaque. In 11 to 12 year old male subjects, the calcium and phosphorus levels in mature plaque were inversely related to the 2 year caries increment.[1] At pH 6 and above, most of the fluoride in plaque is in bound form, but reduction of the plaque pH showed a linear relation to the release of fluoride ion.[2,3]

Perhaps enamel maturation and adaptation to challenge are phases of the same caries resistance factor. We know that enamel of newly erupted teeth is more porous and contains a higher proportion of imperfect hydroxyapatite crystals than the enamel of teeth that has been exposed to the oral fluids. People who have lived in an area with sub-optimally fluoridated water require up to 20 years to reach the same enamel fluoride level that is present at the time of tooth eruption in subjects who have lived in an optimally fluoridated area.[7] Work in Dr. Koulourides' laboratory supports the interpretation that periodic caries attack in the presence of fluoride results in cumulative deposition of insoluble fluoride salts of calcium and phosphate within the microscopic carious lesion. This renders the lesion increasingly resistant to future demineralization episodes. The degree of such fluoride uptake is related to individual patient's caries experience.[8-10] This suggests that comparison of biopsies from normal enamel and from clinical white spot lesions of a given subject might offer a useful caries prediction test for that subject.

To Dr. Parkins' suggestion that frequent clinical examination remains the most effective basis for future caries prediction should be added that the patient's history has predictive value. A person who has always lived in an optimally fluoridated community should have a lower than average caries increment. A person who received fluoride in semi-annual topical application or in a daily mouthwash should have a low caries increment. One who displayed buccal Class V white spot lesions or inter-proximal radiolucencies that did not increase between semi-annual examinations has probably experienced both enamel maturation and adaptation to challenge. This should be predictive of a low caries increment. For a patient's history to have this type of predictive value, the keeping of accurate records becomes important.

A dentist who influences a patient's dental behavior should be able to predict a low caries increment. At the University of Alabama a 2 year exploratory test of a Preventive Dentistry Delivery System has indicated (Tables 1 and 2) that those patients who, at semi-annual recall sittings, meet three criteria may anticipate a caries increment that approaches zero, and almost complete arrest of existing minimal caries lesions.[11] The criteria are (a) Snyder test not higher than 2+; (b) gingival index less than 0.6, with no site greater than 1.0; and (c) semi-annual applications of acid-phosphate-fluoride. While these might not predict different degrees of caries increment, they are useful for prediction of an extremely low caries activity.

Table 1. Caries experience of 20 subjects who were 10-20 years of age at initiation of preventive dentistry program.

			Carious Surfaces					
			To Restore			To Observe		
		MF Teeth	PF	S	BL	PF	S	BL
At Orig. Exam	Mode	0-4	0-2	0	0	0	0	0
	High	13	8	11	5	12	6	12
	Mean	3.4	1.9	1.9	0.4	1.3	1.3	1.3
	Total	68	38	37	7	26	25	26
At 24 Month Recall				Progressed		3	1	0
				Percent Arrested		90	96	100
				New Lesions		4	0	0

Surface - PF = Pit or Fissure
S = Proximal Smooth
BL = Bucco or Lingual

Table 2. Caries experience of 33 subjects who were 21-30 years of age at initiation of preventive dentistry program.

			Carious Surfaces					
			To Restore			To Observe		
		MF Teeth	PF	S	BL	PF	S	BL
	Mode	9	0-2	0-2	0-1	0-5	0-4	0-1
At	High	18	6	11	1	5	12	10
Orig.	Mean	11	0.7	2.0	0.1	0.6	2.2	1.4
Exam	Total	354	23	63	4	20	71	51
At 24 Month Recall			Progressed			0	0	0
			Percent arrested			100	100	100
			New Lesions			0	0	0

Surface - PF = Pit or Fissure
S = Proximal Smooth
BL = Bucco or Lingual

LITERATURE CITED

1. Ashley, F.P. 1975. Calcium and phosphorus concentrations of dental plaque related to dental caries in 11- to 14-year old male subjects. Caries Res. 9 :351-362.
2. Birkeland, J.M. and Charlton, G. 1976. Effect of pH on the fluoride ion activity of plaque. Caries Res. 10:72-80.
3. Rolla, G. and Bowen, W.H. 1977. Concentration of fluoride in plaque - a possible mechanism. Scand. J. Dent. Res. 85(2):149-151.
4. Challacombe, S.J. and Lehner, T. 1976. Serum and salivary antibodies to cariogenic bacteria in man. J. Dent. Res. 55 (Special Issue C):C139-C148.
5. Rundegren, J. and Ericson, T. 1974. Bacterial aggregation by stimulated whole saliva. J. Dent. Res. 53 (Suppl. 1), Abst. 25,
6. Magnusson, I. and Ericson, T. 1977. Variability in saliva concentration of the agglutinin specific for serotype C strains of Streptococcus mutans. Caries Res. 11(2):109-113.
7. Brudevold, F. 1966. The role of fluoride in tooth chemistry and in the prevention of dental caries. Pharmacology of Fluorides, Smith, F.A. (sub ed.) New York, Springer-Verlag.
8. Koulourides,T., Phantumvanit, P., Munksgaard, E.C., Housch, T. 1974. An intraoral model used for studies of fluoride incorporation in enamel. J. Oral Path. 3:185-195.
9. Ostrom, C.A. Koulourides, T., Hickman, F., Phantumvanit, P. 1977. Combined effects of sucrose and fluoride on experimental caries and on the associated microbial plaque. J. Dent. Res. 56:212-221.
10. Koulourides, T., Keller, S.E., Lilley, V. (In press) Enhancement of fluoride effectiveness by experimental cariogenic priming of human enamel.
11. Ostrom, C.A. (In press) Effectiveness of a preventive dentistry delivery system.

A comparison of different methods for prediction of caries activity

Björn Klock

Department of Cariology, Faculty of Odontology, University of Göteborg, Göteborg, Sweden

We have studied the increment of caries in relation to different factors in 302 children 9-12 years old. These children constituted the control group in a study which had the objective to select children at a high caries risk for special preventive measures (Klock and Krasse, 1977a and 1977b). The following factors were determined at the start of the study:

- S. mutans/ml saliva
- Lactobacilli/ml saliva
- Buffer capacity (final pH)
- Saliva secretion rate
- Saliva pH
- Smooth surface lesions in the permanent dentition
- Plaque index
- Caries increment after 1 and 2 years

The linear correlations between the various factors examined at the start of the study and the number of new carious lesions during the first and second year were very weak (Table 1.) However, significant correlations could be demonstrated especially between incipient smooth surface lesions and the caries activity. Also the number of S. mutans during the second year was significantly correlated to the caries activity. It should be stressed that the r-values are very low but due to the large number of individuals an r-value above ± 0.157 means a significant correlation.

Table 1. Linear correlations (r) between various factors at the start of the study and new carious lesions.

Factors	1st year	2nd year
Incipient smooth surface lesions	0.311 xx	0.346 xx
S. mutans	0.073	0.209 xx
Lactobacilli	-0.048	0.020
Plaque index	0.087	0.064
Buffer capacity	-0.126	-0.074
Secretion rate	-0.055	0.013
Saliva pH	-0.019	-0.019

xx - Significant correlations ($p < 0.01$) at $r > \pm 0.157$

Table 2 shows the number of new carious lesions in children during the first year in relation to selected thresholds of the various factors examined. For S. mutans the children with more than 10^6 bacteria per milliliter saliva developed significantly more lesions than the children below this value. Also the earlier caries experience expressed as the number of incipient smooth surface lesions gives a significant difference. For lactobacilli, the salivary factors and plaque index no difference in caries activity was found when the chosen threshold values were used. The mean value for new caries for the whole group was 2.0.

During the second year, the results were similar (Table 3.) For S. mutans especially, the threshold value of 10^7 gave a large difference in caries activity between the groups. For the other factors, there were still no significant differences but for both lactobacilli and plaque index the values approached significance. It is evident that the differences between the groups are more pronounced during the second year. The reason for this is probably that the development of the carious lesion is a slow process and that the mean caries activity in the children was higher during the second year than during the first year (3.1 vs 2.0).

Tables 2 & 3. Relation of new caries lesions to various index thresholds.

2. First Year

Index Threshold	S.Mutans 10^6/ml	S.Mutans 10^7/ml	Lactobac. 10^5/ml	Saliva ml/min	Buffer pH 4.3	Saliva pH 6.8	Lesion 11	Plaque 2.0
Children Below Threshold								
No.	169	262	224	86	56	10	203	258
$\bar{x}$ Lesions	1.7	2.0	2.0	1.8	2.4	2.2	1.7	1.9
Children Above Threshold								
No.	110	17	55	193	223	269	76	21
$\bar{x}$ Lesions	2.4	2.4	1.8	2.6	1.9	2.0	2.6	3.0
Significance (Students t-test)	<0.05	<0.01	NS	NS	NS	NS	<0.01	NS

3. Second Year

Index Threshold	S.Mutans 10^6/ml	S.Mutans 10^7/ml	Lactobac. 10^5/ml	Saliva ml/min	Buffer pH 4.3	Saliva pH 6.8	Lesion 11	Plaque 2.0
Children Below Threshold								
No.	163	254	216	82	55	9	199	252
$\bar{x}$ Lesions	2.7	2.9	2.9	3.0	3.5	2.7	2.5	3.0
Children Above Threshold								
No.	108	17	55	189	216	262	72	19
$\bar{x}$ Lesions	2.6	5.1	3.7	3.1	2.9	3.1	4.4	4.4
Significance (Students t-test)	<0.05	<0.01	NS	NS	NS	NS	<0.01	NS

The results in Tables 2 and 3 demonstrate that no single factor can be used to predict a high caries activity. However, it seems probable that a combination of different factors would give a more reliable prediction. With the above results in mind, incipient smooth surface lesions, S. mutans, lactobacilli and plaque index were tested.

Table 4 shows the number of new carious lesions during the second year correlated with different factors - alone or in combination. A very high mean value of new carious lesions was found in the children with a high number of incipient smooth surface lesions at the start of the study in combination with high numbers of S. mutans and lactobacilli. It is difficult to determine how much each factor really represents in this combination but a multiple regression analysis indicates that the smooth surface lesions weigh most, thereafter, S. mutans and finally the lactobacilli.

Table 4. Relation of various factors - alone and combined - to development of new carious lesions during second year.

Factors	No. of Children	New Carious Lesions
S. mutans $>10^6$ Lactobacilli $>10^5$ ISSL* >11	10	8.4
Plaque index 2 ISSL >11	13	7.2
S. mutans 10^6 ISSL >11	22	5.6
ISSL >1	53	5.2
S. mutans $>10^7$	17	5.1

*ISSL - Incipient Smooth Surface Lesions

If S. mutans and lactobacilli are substituted by the plaque index a high mean caries activity is also found. Even here the factor "incipient smooth surface lesions" has the greatest weight.

As shown in Table 4, the two combinations discussed above give definitely higher caries activity than all the other factors or combination of factors. More than five new lesions were found in children with the combination of high numbers of S. mutans and incipient smooth surface lesions, incipient smooth surface lesions alone and extremely high numbers of S. mutans. An interesting fact is that the 30 children with a plaque index <0.2, i.e. extremely clean teeth had the same mean caries activity as the whole group (3.1). Our figures indicate that the combination incipient smooth surface lesion, S. mutans and lactobacilli gives the best prediction of the caries activity. It is difficult to estimate the absolute value of including the lactobacillus count for the prediction of the caries activity but in our opinion, the lactobacillus count is of greater importance in older children than in children with a mixed dentition. In our population, a large number of children was found with open cavities in their deciduous teeth and it seems probable that these harboured a large number of lactobacilli. This assumption is supported by the fact that the number of lactobacilli had dropped significantly after 2 years when most of the deciduous teeth had been exfoliated. This would mean that in a population without a large number of retention sites such as open cavities the best combination for prediction of the caries activity would be the number of lactobacilli, S. mutans and incipient smooth surface lesions. In this combination, the lactobacilli reflect the carbohydrate consumption (Becks et al.,1944, Jay, 1940), S. mutans - the risk for initial carious lesions (Ikeda et al., 1973, Loesche et al., 1975), and the presence of incipient smooth surface lesions - the caries susceptibility of the individual (Koch, 1970).

CONCLUSIONS

The practical conclusions of our findings are that teenagers with a high number of incipient smooth surface lesions should be examined with regard to S. mutans and lactobacilli. If the number of these bacteria are high, the individual runs a high caries risk and should be given adequate preventive measures.

LITERATURE CITED

1. Becks, H., Jensen, A.L. and Millarr,C.B. 1944. Rampant dental caries-prevention and prognosis. J. Am. Dent. Assoc. 31:1189-1200.

2. Ikeda, T., Sandham, H.J. and Bradley, E.L. 1973. Changes in *Streptococcus mutans* and lactobacilli in plaque in relation to the initiation of dental caries in Negro children. Archs. Oral Biol. 18:555-566.

3. Jay, P. 1940. The role of sugar in the etiology of dental caries. J. Am. Dent. Assoc. 27:393-396.

4. Klock, B. and Krasse, B. 1977. Microbial and salivary conditions in 9-12-year-old children. Scand. J. Dent. Res. 85:56-63.

5. Klock, B. and Krasse, B. 1977. The effect of caries preventive measures in children with high numbers of *Streptococcus mutans* and lactobacilli. To be published.

6. Koch, G. 1970. Selection and caries prophylaxis of children with high caries activity. Odontol. Revy 21:71-82.

7. Loesche, W.J., Rowan, J., Straffon, L.H. and Loos, P.J. 1975. Association of *Streptococcus mutans* with human dental decay. Infect. Immun. 11:1252-1260.

TOPIC II

EPIDEMIOLOGY AND CARIES PREDICTION

Moderator:

Herschel S. Horowitz
National Institute of Dental Research
Westwood Building
Bethesda, Maryland 20014

The validity and reliability of measurements

Stuart Zimmerman

Anderson Hospital, Department of Biomathematics, Houston, Texas

I. Introduction

Prior to the consideration of the reliability and validity of measurements for predicting dental caries experience, it is important for us to define and agree upon some of the terms involved. First, in this paper, prediction is used in the sense of forecasting as opposed to early detection. Therefore, we will not be discussing many of the precedures such as ultrasound, conductivity measurements, or fluorescence which will be discussed by participants later in this program. Rather, we are talking about the predicting of frank, future dental caries on the basis of current or past predictor variables.

The second concern of any valid system for predicting dental caries must be the purpose or intent of the prediction. Three of the more typical uses are as follows:

1. Prediction in Caries Clinical Trials. In this case the intended use of prediction is usually to gain additional precision so that one can detect a clinically significant difference between therapeutic agents in either a shorter period of time or with a reduced number of subjects or both.
2. Public Health Purposes. In this case one is interested in forecasting of the burden of dental caries in a community or population. Intent is usually to assess the amount of remedial dental care that will be required for the community under investigation so that appropriate resources in terms of personnel and materials can be appropriately planned.
3. Prediction of Individual Caries Experience. This aim is simultaneously the most desirable and the most difficult to achieve. The variance associated with individual predictions is always larger than with group predictions thus resulting in tolerance intervals that sometimes are so large as to render the prediction nearly worthless.

Since a different amount of background information and a different degree of control exists between the three situations, it is not surprising to expect that both the techniques and the results of prediction might differ in the three cases.

II. Predictor Variables.

A large number of variables can be or have been used for the purposes of predicting future dental caries experience. The list that follows is representative, but by no means exhaustive.

1. Deciduous Caries Experience. In this case the rate of caries attack on the deciduous teeth is employed to project what experience might be encountered with the permanent teeth. Difficulties in assessing the caries experience on deciduous teeth which are normally exfoliated have tended to limit the utility of this variable.
2. Current or Baseline DMF. The value of the DMF score (either teeth or

surfaces) at the baseline of a clinical trial or epidemiological investigation is frequently employed to forecast future caries experience. Other related measures such as teeth or surfaces at risk are also often used.

3. Diet: The composition and quantity of foods, particularly with regards to its refined carbohydrate content and physical retentiveness have proven to be important factors for prognostication of future caries experience.

4. Microbiological Data: A large variety of microbiological variables have been used as forecasters of future caries activity. These range from whole measures of lactobacillus scores to the current assessment of Streptococcus mutans and dextran synthetase activity.

5. Genetic Variables: There appears to be some heritable component to dental caries, although the mechanism has by no means been clarified. Thus, it is difficult to quantitatively assess the contribution made by genetic factors.

6. Demographic Variables: Variables such as sex, age (either in years or based upon number of permanent teeth), and race have been of predictive value and of value in stratification in clinical trials.

7. Time: In many cases, particularly in comparative clinical trials where most other features have been matched in individuals randomly assigned to a treatment or control group, time will be the best single predictor value of caries experience. The relationship (see Figure 1 from Steinberg and Zimmerman[8]).

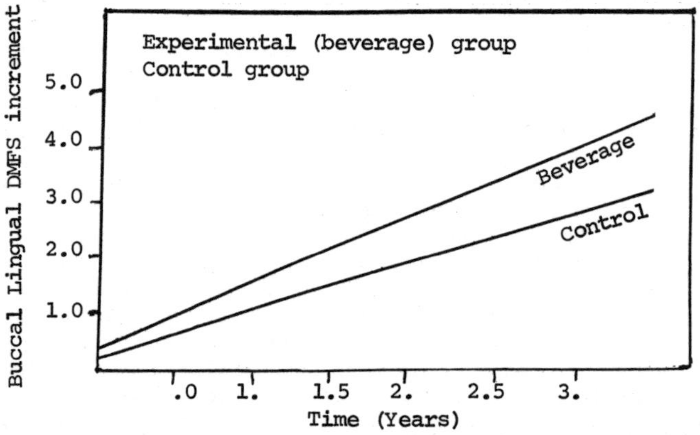

Figure 1: Representation of six-month incremental relationship between time and buccolingual DMFS incremental scores for non-mongloid population LSS.

8. Oral Hygiene: These measures are often combined with microbiological data and usually include measures of plaque, pellicle, and other measures of retained debris.

9. Salivary Chemistry: A variety of salivary chemical measures have been employed that are independent of the microbial flora. These have included such variables as salivary calcium, phosphate, immunoglobulin, titratable acidity, etc.

10. Composition of the Teeth: A chemical composition of the tooth can serve as an important predictor of its future caries experience. There is a considerable variation in the substituent trace minerals both in and absorbed onto the hydroxyapatite lattice as found in different levels of the tooth structure. Fluoride has been demonstrated to have the major caries inhabitory effect and, thus, has the largest overall total literature. Other trace minerals that have been investigated include tin, selenium, molybdenum, and vanadium.

11. Anatomy of the Teeth: Anatomy of the teeth, particularly the configuration of the pits and fissures, can play a role in determining the amount of occlusal caries that will prevail in an individual. Likewise, the contour and spacing of the inter-proximal contacts will have an effect upon the total caries score arising from this region.
12. Therapy: The type and extent of treatment involved can often be one of the most important factors in predicting caries experience. Prophylaxes, topical applications, systemic treatment including water fluoridation are but a few of the treatment modalities that need to be considered.

III. Prediction Methodologies

Several different statistical methods can be used for predicting future caries experience. Among those that will be discussed, in greater detail, are the use of multivariate regression analysis, life table analysis with concomitent variables, and the techniques of time series analysis.
1. Multiple Regression: By the use of multiple regression one can predict a caries increment or procedence as a linear or non-linear function of the independent variables chosen for the purpose of the prediction. Regardless of the functional form of the regression equation in terms of the independent equations, it is desirable that the regression model be linear in the parameter or coefficients of the model. If not, the fitting to the data becomes a numerically much more difficult problem. In particular, one must have reasonable initial estimates of the parameters for the non-linear methods to work, a situation that does not always prevail for caries investigations. For a readable reference on these techniques, the work of Daniel and Wood[5] is suggested. An illustration can be taken from the paper by Chung, Witkop and Henry[3] in which a variety of variables, including some genetic, were used to predict caries scores in an isolated southern Maryland population. The regression equation was of the form

$$Y = A + b_1X_1 + b_2X_2 + b_3X_3 + b_4X_4 + b_5X_5 + b_6X_6 + b_7X_7$$

where Y = def or DMF
X_1 = Sex; 1 = male, 0 = female
X_2 = age in years
X_3 = age^2
X_4 = fluoridation of water; 1 = yes, 0 = no
X_5 = endogamy index; 0, 1, 2, and 3
X_6 = PYC; 1 = taster, 0 = non-taster
X_7 = lactobacillus count; 0, 1, 2, 3, and 4

The same regression equation (with different numerical values of the parameters) was used to fit both the deciduous and permanent caries scores. The variable X_3 (age^2) was included because of a known maximum occurring in the def at about 5-6 years due to exfoliation of the deciduous teeth. Note that the equation is still linear in the coefficients.

For the permanent teeth the analysis revealed the following:

Variable	Mean ± S.E.	Coefficient ± S.E.
DMF	6.39 ± .21	- - - - -
Sex (X_1)	-.429 ± .013	-1.4719 ± .2800*
Age (X_2)	28.67 ± .48	.3496 ± .0272*
Age^2 (X_3)	881.36 ± 33.53	-.0006 ± .0004
Fluoridation (X_4)	.254 ± .012	.5234 ± .3218
Endogamy (X_5)	2.04 ± .03	-.1064 ± .1137
PTC (X_6)	.865 ± .099	.5053 ± .4042
Lactobacillus (X_7)	2.27 ± .042	.7198 ± .0879*
Number	1396	
R^2	.5552	

Three factors (sex, age, and lactobacillus count) were seen to contribute significantly to the regression. From the value of R^2 we can see that 55.5% of the variation in the caries score can be explained by these concomitant variables. An $R^2 > 0.50$ should be considered good for any caries prognostication.

2. Life Table Analysis with Concomitant Variables: The technique of life table or survival analysis[6] is frequently applied in clinical research, particularly in the area of cancer research. Essentially, the proportion of individuals responding in a binary way (death, relapse, etc.) is estimated in each time period. If the exact time is not know, the results are grouped into fixed time intervals and presented in life table form. Corrections are made for subjects lost to follow up or withdrawn alive.

In the case of dental caries, a carious tooth would be considered to be "dead". In certain cases, the scoring could be done by individuals and a subject having one or more carious teeth in a prescribed interval would be considered "affected". (There are certain statistical difficulties with this approach that will be discussed below). Cox[4] developed a method for assessing the effect of concomitant variables in survival analysis. Basically, the logarithm of the hazard function, $\lambda(t)$ (the hazard function represents the probability of dying in an interval between t and t + dt given that one has survived to time t) is regressed against the concomitant variables as

$$\ln \frac{\lambda(t)}{\lambda_0(t)} = \beta_0 + \beta_1 z_1 + \beta_2 z_2 + \dots + \beta_n z_n$$

or in vector notation as

$$\lambda(t;\underline{Z}) = \lambda_0(t) \exp(\underline{Z}\,\underline{\beta})$$

where $\underline{Z}$ is an n-dimensional vector of the concomitant variables, $\underline{\beta}$ is an n-dimensional vector of the unknown parameters to be estimated and $\lambda_0(t)$ is an unknown function giving the hazard function for a standard set of conditions, $\underline{Z}$ =). The Cox method was originally designed for cases in which the survival distribution was computed by the product limit method, which is usually referred to as the Kaplan-Meier estimate of the survival distribution. This method of computing the survival distribution requires knowing the time of "death" (in this case, caries) of each tooth, a goal rarely, if ever, achieved. Holford[7] has extended the procedure to life tables computed by the actuarial method, which would be appropriate to dental data. A typical time period for such a life table would be the interval between dental examinations, i.e. 6 months.

It was mentioned above that the use of this technique in the analysis of dental data violates one of the assumptions of the procedure. This assumption is that the sampling units (individuals, teeth, etc.) be statistically independent. This is not so in the case of teeth, which come conveniently in a cohort ensemble known as the mouth. However, one should note that in the conventional analysis of caries increments we violate several statistical assumptions; to wit, frequency counts are added and the sum treated as a random variable, the distribution of increments is considered to be normal when it is more nearly negative binomial, etc.

Yet, the robustness of the analytical techniques, coupled with the normalizing effects of the Law of Large Numbers for sufficiently large size samples, allows these methods to give valid conclusions. The technique of life-table analysis with concomitant variables should be explored to test its robustness and utility for caries data.

3. Time Series Analyses: This methodology has frequently been employed for forecasting economic trends and in the analysis of industrial control studies. There has been some limited application of these techniques in craniofacial biology growth studies. The limitations of time and space do not permit presentation of the mathematical analyses. For a comprehensive presentation,

the reader is referred to the book of Box and Jenkins[1] .

In the most general case a procedure known as an Auto Regressive Integrated Moving Average (ARIMA) model is used to analyze, and subsequently forecast future values, of a time series. A time series consists of a temporal sequence of measures of a variable; in this case successive values of caries scores would constitute the series. Future values of the series are predicted as a weighted combination of past values plus a random "shock" component.

Some of the advantages are:

a) With an adequate number of successive measurements, a forecast can be developed for an individual without reference to a study population. The parameters of the forecast can be best fit to the individual's own time series.

b) The general ARIMA models have the flexibility to accommodate virtually any combination of changes of level and slope in the data coupled with white noise.

The disadvantages are:

a) A large number of successive observations of the process are needed to develop a reasonable time series analysis. Probably a minimum would be 12 observations, such as six month examinations from age 6 to 12. This limitation would essentially exclude the technique from clinical trials; however, it would still be viable for long term epidemiological studies.

b) Since the ARIMA model uses previous values of the process for the purposes of prediction, one cannot accommodate concomitant variables as readily as either two aforementioned regression procedures. Box and Tiao[2] have recently extended the method through what they call intervention analyses. In this approach, the effect of a concomitant variable on the time series is considered as an impulse function (spike) or as a step function, if the effect is a persistent one. Employing this method, the effect of introduction of fluoride in a community could be assessed through its impact on the time series of caries scores.

IV. Conclusions and Recommendations

1. Representativeness of Group: For any prediction based upon sample data to have any utility, care must be taken that the sample is representative of the population of interest. Preferably, the sample should be a random one. Sometimes this can be obtained by a careful sampling plan and sometimes it can be achieved through the inter-play of other factors. For instance, a military training camp might represent a good opportunity for developing predictors of caries in young males since the recruits would come from nearly every part of the country. While geographic bias is probably avoided in such a group, a socio-economic bias might still exist.

Models developed in fluoridated communities may not perform well in predicting caries activity in non-fluoridated communities. If the extent of fluoride exposure is known for each individual it could be accommodated in the model as in the example in Section III, but all too often this is not the case.

If the sample in the study is all that is available to the investigator, he can develop predictor estimates by "jacknifing" his sample, i.e. the parameters of the model are estimated on a fraction of the population and tested on the remaining $1 - \alpha$ of the population where $0 \leq \alpha \leq 1$. While the estimates can be obtained for the entire sample this leaves no remaining independent group on which to test the predictions.

2. Experience of the Investigator: It is impossible to over-emphasize the role that the knowledge of an experienced investigator plays in the selection of variables for study. While the experimental investigation and its analysis will provide an evaluation of the role played by those variables

that were selected for the study, the experience of the investigator determines which variables were selected for inclusion in the first place.

The inclusions of a large number of variables (some extraneous) in a study can create several difficulties. First, a large sample size is required to estimate the effects of a large number of variables. The analysis becomes more laborious, although with the use of high speed electronic computers this is not prohibitive.

3. Effect of the Design: The design of the study, be it a clinical trial, or an epidemiological field study, can markedly effect both the selection of variables and the contribution each can make for prediction. For example, the cariogenicity of the diet might be a most important predictor variable in a field study. Yet, in a comparative clinical trial of a therapeutic agent in a closed institutionalized population where both the experimental and control groups receive the same diet it would have very little utility.

Likewise, in the comparative trials, randomization prevents bias from occurring amongst concomitant variables that cannot be controlled. Using them as co-variates improves the precision obtained in testing for a therapeutic effect in such a trial and develops estimates of their effects on the caries rate.

4. Validation by the Data: When conducted properly, the analysis of the data should reveal the extent to which each variable contributes, if at all, in predicting caries outcome. Thus, the regression coefficients, or the coefficients of an ARIMA model and their associated variances, or standard errors provide the answer as to whether the variable demonstrates a statistically significant effect and serves to give an estimate of its magnitude. The elimination of spurious variables and the estimation of the effects of those pertinent variables is the goal of the prediction process.

LITERATURE CITED

1. Box, G.E.P., and Jenkins, G.M. 1976. Time Series Analysis: Forecasting and Control. Holden Day, San Francisco.
2. Box, G.E.P., and Tiao, G. C. 1975. Intervention Analysis with Applications to Economic and Environmental Problems. Jour. of Am. Stat. Assoc. 70:70.
3. Chung, C.S., Witkop, C.J., and Henry, J.L. 1964. A Genetic Study of Dental Caries with Special Reference to PTC Test Sensitivity. Am. Jour. of Human Genetics, 16:231-244.
4. Cox, D.R. 1972. Regression and Life Tables. Jour. of the Royal Stat. Soc. (Series B) 34:187-220.
5. Daniel, C. and Wood, F.S. 1971. Fitting Equations to Data. Wiley Interscience, New York.
6. Gehan, E.A. 1975. Statistical Methods for Survival Time Studies. in Cancer Therapy: Prognostic Factors and Criteria of Response, edited by M.J. Staquet, Raven Press, New York.
7. Holford, T.R. 1976. Life Tables with Concomitant Information. Biometrics, 587-598.
8. Steinberg, A., Zimmerman, S., Bramer, M. 1972. The Effect of Acidulated Carbonated Beverages on the Incidence of Dental Caries. JADA 85:81-89.

Discussion of the validity and reliability of measurements

R.M. Grainger

Prescott, Ontario, Canada

General

Now that Dr. Zimmerman has opened up the field so expertly, it only remains for me to add a few points from my personal experience with caries prediction.

First, I agree that there are at least three purposes to be served by this line of research. These I shall re-state.

1. Ability to estimate caries increments provides a considerable improvement in the efficiency of clinical trials through covariance analysis.
2. The process of estimating caries entails the weighing of predictor variables and hence definition of the components of variation between individuals. In simple language, definition of the amount specific variables contribute to the difference in numbers of cavities in individuals. Thus, we are trying to define

$$S_a^2 = s_t^2 + s_r^2 + s_e^2 ,$$

where S^2 is the variance for a frequency distribution of caries increments, s_a^2 is the variation in the attacking mechanism, s_t^2 is the variation in tooth resistance, s_r^2 is the variation in the remineralization mechanism and s_e^2 represents measurement errors plus a probable chance component. Almost everything currently being studied fits into one of these categories and is at the same time an imperfect descriptor.

3. When an equation is available enabling us to account for a practical amount of the variance of a frequency distribution of caries increments -- say eighty to ninety percent, we will have a clinical diagnostic tool.
4. The fourth which Dr. Zimmerman called "Public Health Purposes" is a sociologic or economic application common to many fields.

Predicting or Forecasting

Estimating expected values is a common procedure in a wide variety of sciences such as educational and psychological research, economics, vital statistics, and countless industrial areas. Excellent computer programs are available at most computing facilities for carrying out what we may call "that black box or dirty approach". Usually these programs provide for input of 50 or so predictor variables selected on an intuitive or even empirical basis. The program goes through various combinations of powers, cross-products, etc. by regular or stepwise multiple regression and comes up with the best combination of independent variables for use in prediction. The only criterion of success is that the estimates are sufficiently close for the purpose at hand and no rationalization of the equation is called for.

At the meetings of the Task Force on Design and Analysis of Clinical Trials, Mr. Robert Lehnhoff of the Procter and Gamble Company and I have demonstrated the ability to account for over sixty percent of the variance (i.e. a multiple R close to .8) of a distribution of caries increments by these methods using clinical examinations only. Application of analysis of covariance using the selection variables thus derived can make it possible to run a clinical trial with smaller samples, or else very much improve the sensitivity of a trial. This then is a reality soon to be available for practical application.

It also provides a method for forecasting of resources, etc. required in the public health sense as mentioned by Dr. Zimmerman. Resource studies will no doubt become critically important when the impact of dental research begins to affect dental practice. However, research in this area is very frustrating to the scientist because the best scientific solution is often unacceptable for political reasons. There is no doubt much of the practice of dentistry could be organized more efficiently by re-distribution of tasks to suitable levels of trained personnel, but this would conflict with the traditional interests of the profession. Also, the validity of forecasts can be influenced overnight by new developments. A classic example is the impact of the high speed drill which greatly increased the dentist's output. Long term dental health data sets indicate that the DMF rate is dropping steadily, most likely due to the wide use of fluorides. The effect of this has not been felt in dental practices much yet because of increased demand related to dental insurance and public education. But a cross-over may occur soon forcing us to attempt projections of dental manpower requirements and the number of dental school graduates to be required.

Definition of the Components of Variance

This is really fundamental epidemiology because the goal is to discover and measure the importance of factors influencing the amount of dental caries observed. The importance of any item may vary in degree from that of an essential link (as has been demonstrated for micro-organisms) to that of causing only slight modification in the number of lesions occurring in an individual mouth. In contrast to the "black box" approach to prediction discussed previously, if the object of the analysis is to weigh the true importance of a factor -- i.e. how much caries variation it can account for, more sophisticated applications of multi-variate analysis are required. We cannot go into these at this time, but it needs to be pointed out that when a correlation matrix is the main input to the analysis we must be sure that the true intrinsic relation between each predictor variable and the dependant variable is correctly expressed. By true intrinsic relations we mean the biological relation undistorted by measurement peculiarities. A few illustrations will help. A simple linear product moment correlation co-efficient will under-estimate a relationship that is really curvilinear. Often the biological important changes vary little above a threshold level and the breakpoint may need to be determined. Again, in cases where the scale of measurement is very limited, this coarse grouping will bias the correlation co-efficient downward. When relationships are curvilinear, inter-actions must be anticipated such that the importance of a predictor changes with the magnitude of one or more other predictors.

Actually it is not so much the weight of individual predictors that interest us as it is the strength of the systems in which they play a role. I suggest that the major systems we wish to measure are the attack system, the tooth quality system, and the remineralization system; but this may be right or wrong. The important idea to grasp is that almost all the predictors discussed at this Conference are only partial measures of one or other system. This can be clarified by assigning items Dr. Zimmerman mentioned to a specific system.

Among the items which in some combination should provide a measure of the attack mechanism I would include microbial, diet, plaque, and perhaps oral hygiene data. In most current work the strength of the attack mech -

anism is being extrapolated rom previous caries experience which has obvious limitations. The factors from which we may develop a measure of tooth resistance are less satisfactory, but probably chemical and physical composition of the teeth, morphology and size of teeth, genetic data, and the use of fluorides all should be combined for this purpose. Age is important in that it relates to the number and the types of surfaces at risk, sex to tooth eruption and hence exposure time.

The remineralization system should, I think, be reflected by items such as quantity and quality of saliva, plaque quantity, permeability, etc. and possibly hours per day in which mineralization could occur.

The amount of caries an individual will develop should be some interactive function of these three (and perhaps other) major systems. If this is true, one can see the limitations of predicting caries from a mass of primary and often redundant observations without giving thought to their role in any system.

Clinical Diagnosis

Ability to predict the exact numbers of new cavities to occur may never be achieved because I believe the exact number of cavities may be influenced by chance. That is, after the main factors just reviewed above have been identified and measured, chance (influences similar to those causing variation in the numbers of heads or tails to occur when coins are tossed) will still be there unless the probability of caries occurring is truly zero. Thus, when the probability of caries is low you may still observe some individuals with a few lesions and vice versa by chance alone.

However, in order to diagnose caries and prescribe treatment it may not be necessary to be exact in prediction. Some reliable way of estimating strength of the major systems, the attack, the resistance, and the remineralization may provide a basis for intelligent prescription at an individual level.

Discussion of "The validity and reliability of measurements"

David C. Korts, Ph.D.

Department of Statistics, Mount Sinai School of Medicine, 5th Avenue & 100 Street, New York, New York 10026

In his presentation Dr. Zimmerman has eloquently described many of the aspects and problems of predicting dental caries. In my discussion I would like to expand on several of Dr. Zimmerman's points, specifically: the purpose of caries prediction, the variables considered in this evaluation, and sources of error.

A. Purpose of Caries Prediction

To the list of three purposes for predicting caries, I would like to add a fourth: the identification of variables correlated with caries either on a population or individual basis. While this purpose is implied by Dr. Zimmerman's subsequent statistical analysis, I feel that it is of sufficient importance in itself that it warrants being specifically stated.

The variables so identified fall into one or two categories: Fundamental variables such as microbiological organisms, in either plaque or saliva, diet, oral hygiene, trace element composition of teeth, trace element composition of water supply, or therapy; and Indicator variables such as baseline decay, measures of baseline surfaces at risk, genetic variables and age, sex and race.

The reason for defining variables in this fashion is that our purpose for identifying variables correlated with caries differs for these two classes. The finding that for example, age, or baseline DMFS is related to caries increment does little to help identify the underlying cause or causes of decay, but such a finding does allow for a more appropriate design of caries studies, or help specify sub-population for which more extensive preventive measures could be provided, or to identify sub-populations in which Fundamental variables could be further investigated.

The fundamental variables are of primary importance, because when one of these variables is found to be correlated with the development of caries, research can commence toward development of agents or techniques to alter levels or effects of this variable in individuals, or in communities. Further this variable could be used to identify individuals or populations for more extensive preventive measures.

B. Variables

The list of variables which Dr. Zimmerman has provided is certainly only a partial listing of variables which could be considered as correlates for dental caries, and even within many of these categories more than one variable can be identified as being worthy of further consideration.

To the variables listed I would add the following:

1. While baseline DMFS has been successfully used as a predictor, the number of sound surfaces at baseline, and the product of these two variables could also prove meaningul. Further, the DMFS status of a subset of surfaces, as well as the number of surfaces at risk in this subset, might be stronger

predictors than the overall baseline DMFS and overall baseline surfaces at risk. Subsets which could be considered might include only the first molars, or possibly the first and second molars combined.

2. In addition to sucrose consumption and retention, the frequency of eating given a constant sucrose intake, should be considered.

3. Microbiological data, obtained from plaque samples, are particularly difficult to assess due to the many different organisms which are found, including Strep mutans, Strep mitis, Strep sangui, lactobacilli and others, as well as to the variety of different sites which could be sampled within the individual. Flora obtained by sampling from a carious site can be considerably different than that obtained from sound sites, and even sampling from sound sites on opposite sides of the mouth, or from different types of surfaces can yield considerably different flora. There does not appear to be a clear agreement as to how a single measure can assess oral flora, but it is possible that a combination of these measures could be valuable in predicting caries.

4. Trace elements in sound enamel may ultimately be found to be important predictors of caries, but there is some question whether current enamel biopsy methodology is sufficiently precise to be used for anything but population comparisons.

5. Other variables which might be considered are trace element composition of water supply and possible socio-economic variables.

C. Error

Sources of error in caries studies could be separated into three categories: measurement of caries, evaluation of concomitant variables, and examiner error.

1. Measurement of Caries: the present method of assessing caries by DMFS or DMFT involves the summing over all surfaces or teeth in the mouth to obtain a measure of caries on a per person basis. While this measure may be adequate for our purposes, measures of only a more highly caries prone subset of surfaces as a response variable might prove more sensitive in identifying some predictor variables. We should not feel constrained to only one form of analysis, or only one response variable for a comprehensive evaluation.

2. Evaluating Concomitant Variables: most studies to date have dealt simultaneously with only a few of the variables which Dr. Zimmerman has enumerated. Such studies can fortuitously reveal cariogenic variables, but will not necessarily do so when other cariogenic variables are ignored. On the other hand a high correlation between a variable and caries could only mean that the variable is correlated with an unmeasured cariogenic variable, while the measured variable may have little or no direct relationship to caries. In order to accurately assess caries predictors, variables must be studied jointly.

However, this approach of collecting information on a wide variety of variables and performing, say, a regression analysis, discriminant analysis or survival analysis would require a more comprehensive and costly study than has been accomplished to date. Although the extensive data collection required the need for such a study to be multi-centered, will add to cost it may be that in the long view it may be the quickest and cheapest way to identify cariogenic variables.

The magnitude of the problem is certainly the reason that there has not yet been a study simultaneously encompassing most of these variables, but without such a study inter-relationships of potential caries predictors will not be fully understood.

3. Examiner Error: examiner error is probably the least serious of the errors, various reliability coefficients have been calculated for examiner

error, giving various numerical results. Perhaps the most common reliability coefficient is the intra-class correlation coefficient, which has a meaning similar to the Pearson's product-movement correlation coefficient, and is consequently an intuitively meaningful choice for measuring examiner reliability.

Studies for the prediction of caries are clearly a complicated and costly undertaking, but information obtained through such studies can only bring us closer to the ultimate control of dental caries.

Caries prediction from epidemiologic data

Martin C. Downer

Preventive Dentistry Department, University of Manchester, Manchester, England

The ability to predict future caries activity is of value to the dentist providing care for his individual patient, the administrator planning health services and the research worker alike.

Although this presentation will be concerned with investigations in the field of experimental epidemiology, it is reasonable to assume that the information required by the clinician in deciding whether a patient will be likely to benefit from preventive therapy, or the health service planner in identifying groups of the population at particular risk, will be very similar to that sought by the epidemiologist. However, the epidemiologist will use the information to gain understanding of the natural history of the disease, or will apply it in a practical way to improving the precision or efficiency of caries prophylactic clinical trials. The need in all instances is for knowledge of oral health factors or other characteristics which are useful predictors of a person's future caries experience. The information must be dependable, quantifiable and easily obtained.

The mathematical technique that has been used most frequently in epidemiological studies of caries prediction is correlation because it is concerned with the strength of the relationship between two variables. In this presentation future caries activity will be referred to as the dependent variable while the measurements used as predictors of future caries activity will be referred to as predictor variables.

Examples of measurements of the dependent variables are DMFS increment and the final DMFS score[1]. Predictor variables known to be related to future caries activity include initial caries experience[2,3,4,5,6], and tooth surfaces initially at risk to attack[3,4]. Initial DMFS, which will be designated throughout as IDMFS, refers to known caries experience in the permanent dentition at the beginning of a period for which predictions of future caries activity are being made. Initial surfaces at risk, which will be designated as ISAR, represents a count of surfaces which are sound in teeth erupted at the outset of that period. Previous DMFS increment, a further predictor of possible value, refers to new caries which occurs during some period of time up to the commencement of the period of interest.

The strength of the association between the dependent and each predictor variable may be quantified by a coefficient of correlation. Where the relationship can best be fitted by a straight line and other less important assumptions are satisfied, Pearson's product-moment coefficient of correlation is used. However, the research worker will often wish to know the degree of association between the dependent and two or more predictor variables in combination. This calls for the coefficient of multiple correlation. The contribution of each variable to the coefficient of multiple correlation will depend upon two factors; first, the strength of its own primary association with the dependent variable and secondly, the extent to which it is also correlated with the other predictor variables. In general, the greater the correlation between a predictor and other variables used in the predictive battery, the less its contribution to the coefficient of multiple correlation. For example, there is little merit in using initial measurements of both DMFS and DMFT as predictors for although both are significantly associated with future caries activity, they are, at the same time, highly correlated with one another. Again, by the same reasoning, chronological age is likely to add little to a predictive battery in which IDMFS and ISAR are included.

To confirm the findings of previous studies and investigate caries prediction further, data from control groups in two trials of caries prophylactic agents[7,8] were examined. Both were conducted in non-fluoridated areas of the North West of England over periods of three years using boys and girls aged initially 11 and 12 years. Standardised clinical and radiological examinations were carried out at baseline and each following year, and over 240 subjects in each control group completed the trials.

Table 1.

Correlation between mean three-year DMFS increment and some initial measurements in 244 control subjects in trial A (standard deviations in parenthesis)

	Mean	r
DMFS increment	7.43 (6.07)	--
IDMFS	7.63 (5.34)	0.36*
ISAR	93.53 (20.82)	0.28*
IDMFS X ISAR	724.72 (526.23)	0.41*

* $P < 0.01$

Table 1 shows that in the first trial the value of Pearson's coefficient of correlation between the three-year DMFS increment and initial DMFS was 0.36. This is of the same order as values reported in most previous studies. The correlation between DMFS increment and initial surfaces at risk was 0.28. Initially sex and oral cleanliness were also investigated, but were found to be so weakly related to future caries activity that they were not considered further.

A clinician would foresee both past caries experience and surfaces at risk to attack as influencing future caries activity, yet, as can be seen from the obtained values, neither appeared particularly promising as a predictor when subjected to initial scrutiny. Clinical insight might however, suggest ways in which these predictor variables could be improved and subsequent research proceeded on these lines.

The individual at greatest risk to caries is probably one with a high past experience, but with many tooth surfaces in the mouth as yet unattacked. The product of initial DMFS and surfaces at risk is a mathematical function that would seem to express this risk factor[4,9]. Thus, a subject with very little past caries experience would obtain a low value for the product variable as would a subject with a very high past caries experience and few surfaces remaining unattacked. This is consistent with theory for in neither of these individuals would much new primary caries be expected. On the other hand the peak expectation would be for a subject in whom half the surfaces potentially at risk were already carious and in whom half were still sound. For such an individual the product variable would be at a maximum.

Further analysis of data from the first clinical trial (Table 1) showed that the product of IDMFS and ISAR did indeed produce a higher value of Pearson's r with the three-year increment than either of its two component variables on their own, and might, therefore, be developed as the basis for a better predictor.

A possible way of improving the predictive value of IDMFS X ISAR is to incorporate the total number of erupted surfaces (IDMFS + ISAR) as a divisor. This has the effect of adjusting the product variable for dental age[4]. However, in the present investigation this approach was not pursued. Attention was paid rather to ascertaining how the surfaces at risk measurement could be refined.

One disadvantage of the crude surfaces at risk measurement is that many surfaces, for example linguals of lower incisors are so rarely attacked that they cannot be regarded as truly at risk. Because of this, they probably contribute little predictive information. An examination of individual surface data in both clinical trials disclosed that over 50 percent of the control group increment in fact occurred on only twenty surfaces. In view of this finding some further analyses were performed with the surfaces at risk variable confined to thes surfaces.

The surfaces in which the majority of the increment occurred are represented diagrammatically in the half-mouth chart (Figure 1). It can be seen that they consisted mostly of posterior occlusals. These surfaces will be referred to as "critical surfaces at risk" in further discussion and designated for convenience CSAR.

Figure 1.

CRITICAL SURFACES AT RISK

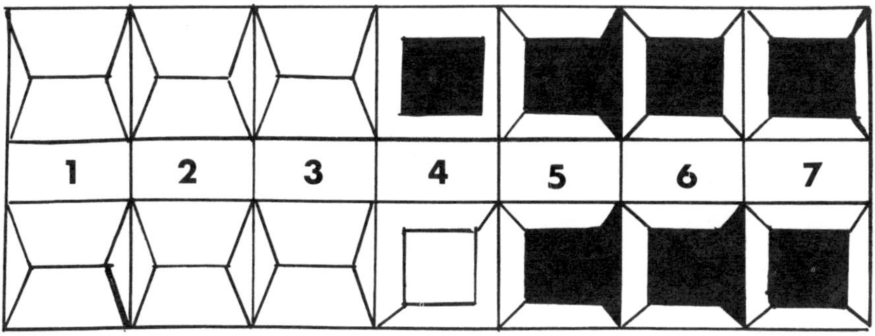

Table 2 shows that in trial A the product of IDMFS and critical surfaces at risk produced a value for Pearson's r of 0.44 with the three-year DMFS increment, compared with the lower value of 0.41 obtained with all sound, erupted surfaces included (Table 1). This tended to support the approach of dropping surfaces with little likelihood of incremental activity from the surfaces at risk variable.

Analysis also showed that in both clinical trials the primary correlation coefficient between DMFS increment and the product of the two predictor variables was slightly higher than the coefficient of multiple correlation (R) with the two variables used independently. This may be attributable in part to the product of IDMFS and CSAR having a more rectilinear relationship with the increment than either of the component variables separately and hence a closer agreement with the assumptions underlying the use of Pearson's r.

Table 2.

Correlation between three-year DMFS increments in two control groups and predictor variables incorporating critical surfaces at risk (CSAR).

	IDMFS and CSAR	IDMFS X CSAR
	R	r
Trial A (n = 244)	0.43	0.44
Trial B (n = 242)	0.47	0.48

It is worth noting here that the inclusion of unerupted critical surfaces in the CSAR variable, which on clinical grounds might be considered an advantage, resulted in a negative correlation coefficient between CSAR and the increment and a diminution in the values of the other correlation coefficients to which it made a contribution. There was nothing gained therefore, from adding unerupted critical surfaces to the predictor.

In these two clinical trials it was found that the majority of the increment occurred during the last two years with little caries activity in the first year of observation. This may be a reflection of the time needed for a lesion to develop to the cavitation stage after a tooth surface has become exposed to the oral environment.

Because of this finding, some further analyses were performed with the DMFS increment for control groups in the final two years of the trials as dependent variable rather than the three-year increment used hitherto. The dependent variable was the DMFS increment which occurred between the first follow-up examination and the end of the trial. Two predictor variables were used. The first was a product variable consisting of DMFS experience at the first follow-up examination and surfaces remaining at risk at that time, while the second was the increment of new DMFS which occurred during the first year.

Table 3.

Correlations between two- and three-year DMFS increments and initial measurements in two control groups.

	Three-year DMFS increment vs IDMFS X CSAR (baseline)	Two-year DMFS increment vs IDMFS X CSAR (first year) and first year DMFS increment
	r	R
Trial A (n = 244)	0.44	0.44
Trial B (n = 242)	0.48	0.52

Table 3 indicates that in trial A, using information available at the end of the first year in this way to predict the increment over the remaining two years, resulted in a coefficient of multiple correlation that did not differ from that between the three-year increment and the product of the two predictor variables at baseline discussed previously. However, in trial B, the coefficient of multiple correlation, using the first year information, attained a value of 0.52 which represented a small improvement.

So far the discussion has been confined to DMFS increment as the dependent variable with the assumption that a simple linear regression exists between this and the predictor variables of initial DMFS or surfaces at risk. Using certain combinations of these predictors a little over 25 percent of incremental variance (calculated by squaring of coefficients of multiple correlation) could be accounted for. However, it has been suggested recently that by fitting more complex curvi-linear regressions to express such relationships far higher coefficients of multiple correlation can be obtained[5]. Provided some biological rationale can be found to explain the nature of these relationships so that they can be generalised to different populations, then extensions of basic research into this area will probably be of value.

As was pointed out at the beginning of this paper, one important purpose of caries prediction is to increase the precision of clinical trials. In connection with this it has recently been suggested that final DMFS scores might be used to evaluate the treatment response rather than incremental measurements[1]. This approach pre-supposes the use of covariance analysis, with initial measurements used as covariables. While it is outside the scope of this paper to argue the relative merits and disadvantages of this technique, it is nevertheless interesting to look at the association between final DMFS and earlier caries experience.

Table 4.

Multiple correlation (R) between Final DMFS and predictor variables of IDMFS at first year and first year DMFS increment.

	R	R^2
Trial A (n = 244)	0.85	0.73
Trial B (n = 242)	0.88	0.77

Examination of the present data showed very high correlations between control group final DMFS scores and measurements of DMFS experience at first year (Table 4). The predictors in this instance were DMFS experience at the first follow-up examination and DMFS increment during the first year of the trials. In the first trial, the value of the coefficient of multiple correlation was 0.85 and in the second 0.88. This meant that over 70 percent of the variance in the final DMFS measurements could be accounted for by DMFS experience two years previously. On reflection, this is perhaps a not unexpected finding since at least half of the final DMFS measurement consists of caries which the subject has already experienced two years previously.

In summary, an attempt has been made to identify variables commonly measured by epidemiologists that may be useful in caries prediction, while focusing attention away from factors that were found to be relatively unimportant. By applying simple linear regression techniques to longitudinal data from two groups of teenage boys and girls, some 25 percent of the variance of their DMFS increment over two years could be accounted for and over 70 percent of the variance of their final DMFS scores.

At the same time, paths along which new research is proceeding have been indicated. Of immediate interest is the extent to which the critical surfaces at risk established in this study also apply in other populations. As regards the mathematical aspects, it is clear that the risk factors pertaining to different types of teeth and surfaces at different periods of development form a complex pattern with future caries activity which cannot be explained adequately by the simple linear regression approach. This is leading research workers in epidemiology to seek other ways of expressing the complicated relationships involved. Elucidation of these relationships will lead to a better understanding of the nature of the disease and its more effective control.

ACKNOWLEDGMENTS

The clinical trials from which the data were obtained were supported by a generous grant from Colgate-Palmolive Limited.

LITERATURE CITED

1. Slakter, M.J. and Juliano, D.B. 1977. The use of analysis of covariance to increase precision with DMFS measures. Community Dent. & Oral Epidem. 5:126-128.

2. Grainger, R.M. 1966. Analysis of caries increments by age and tooth surface in fluoridated and non-fluoridated populations, by electronic computer. In Advances in Fluorine Research and Dental Caries Prevention, ed. James, P.M.C., Konig, J.G. & Held, H.R. Vol. 4 Oxford: Pergammon Press.

3. Cellier, K.M., Fanning, E.A., Gotjamanos, T. and Vowles, N.J. 1968. Some statistical aspects of a clinical study on dental caries in children. Archs. of oral Biol. 13:483-508.

4. Worthington, H.V. 1975. Some Statistical Aspects of Dental Caries Data. Thesis. University of Manchester.

5. Adkins, B.L. 1977. Methodological developments for clinical trials. Jour. of Dent. Rsch. (supplement), in press.

6. Adler, P. 1968. Correlation between dental caries prevalence at different ages. Caries Rsch. 2:79-86.

7. Downer, M.C., Holloway, P.J. and Davies, T.G.H. 1976. Clinical testing of a topical fluoride caries preventive programme. Brit. dent. Jour. 141:242-247.

8. Howat, A.P., Holloway, P.J. and Davies, T.G.H. 1977. Clinical testing of an MFP gel dentifrice. International Assoc. for Dent. Rsch. (British Division), Abst. #96.

9. Lu, K.H. 1966. An experimentally supported "law of tooth decay" and its application. Archs. of oral Biol. 11:757-768.

Discussion of caries prediction from epidemiologic data

Stanley B. Heifetz

National Institute of Dental Research, Westwood Building, Bethesda, Maryland 20014

Dr. Downer's attempt to identify variables that have value in the prediction of future caries experience, by using epidemiologic data from longitudinal clinical trials, is characteristic of the usual approach that has been taken by most other investigators. Of the several variables that he tested for their correlation with three-year DMFS increment, only initial DMFS (IDMFS) and initial surfaces at risk (ISAR) had some predictive value; r was equal to 0.36 and 0.28, respectively.

In an attempt to improve the correlation, Dr. Downer added a few special refinements to the analyses: he reduced the total number of ISAR to 20 of the most critical surfaces at risk (CSAR); multiplied IDMFS by CSAR as another expression of the risk factor; and used the first year's increment as a measure of current caries susceptibility.

Use of CSAR is a valuable technique in partial recording, but it offered only a slight advantage when substituted for ISAR in the product term IDMFS x ISAR, r increased from 0.41 to 0.46 (vide infra). The concept of a product term was proposed by Lu[1] in a 1966 paper describing a model for caries prediction. I am uneasy about the use of this mathematical expression because it does not properly relate past caries experience to a child's dental age. For example, a child with many DMF surfaces, but with few erupted permanent teeth may be scored as having a lower caries risk than another child with only a few DMF surfaces, but with nearly all his permanent teeth erupted. The formula shown in Figure 1, I believe is a more logical expression of caries risk because consideration is given to the total number of surfaces present in the mouth.

Figure 1: Expression of Caries Risk

$$\frac{\text{IDMFS}}{\text{IDMFS + ISAR}} \times \text{ISAR}$$

$$\left[\frac{\text{No. surfaces attacked}}{\text{No. surfaces present in mouth}}\right] \times \left[\text{No. surfaces at risk}\right]$$

Moreover, there appears to be little difference in the value of the simple correlation coefficient and the coefficient of multiple correlation regardless of whether the two variables IDMFS and CSAR are used as a product or additively.

By combining all of the special refinements in the analysis, an R value of only 0.52 was achieved, which means that only about 25 percent of the variability in incremental caries scores could be explained by the best predictive variables and combinations that Dr. Downer could derive -- a disappointing result.

Also included in the paper is a brief discussion of the association found between measurements of DMFS experience at the first year's examination and final DMFS scores two years later. In my opinion, the analyses contribute little information to further our knowledge about caries prediction from epidemiologic data. It is evident that a child's initial DMFS prevalence at age 12 or 13 would be a good predictor of his final DMFS prevalence at age 14 or 15; the two scores are likely to be highly correlated because caries prevalence can only be cumulative with advancing age.

Lastly, I am concerned about what is not included in Dr. Downer's discussion of the findings. His analyses used just two sets of discrete data two limited age groups and incremental caries scores from a specified three-year period of study. Reservations, however, are not expressed about the "generalizability" of the results. It should have been stated that the particular combination of variables determined in these two studies as being best able to predict future caries increment may not prove satisfactory in other studies.

Table 1: Relation between DMF surface increment and selected variables.

Investigator	No. of Children	Initial Age	Months of study	Percent of variance in DMFS increment explained by: All variables*	Initial DMFS
Carlos 1970	281	10-16	21	12	10
	137	11-14	21	25	24
	247	6 and 11	20	[12 14**]	[11 14]
	60	5-8	8	1	0.9
McClendon & Horowitz 1971	124	10 and 11	12		28
			24		35
			36		41
			48	46+	42

* Age, sex, initial DMFS, initial sound surfaces and combinations.
** Includes race.
\+ Age, sex, initial number of teeth, initial DMFT, initial DMFS and combinations.

Work similar to that described by Dr. Downer has been carries out by investigators at NIDR, Table 1 shows the relation between incremental DMFS and selected variables found by Carlos[2] and by McClendon and Horowitz[3]. Carlos analyzed the data of control groups in four clinical trials of caries preventives. Multiple regression techniques were performed using as independent variables age, sex, IDMFS, initially sound surfaces (ISS) or the same as ISAR and IDMFS x ISS as used by Dr. Downer. In three of the trials, the proportion of the variance in caries increment that could be attributed to all the variables combined was 14 percent or less. In the remaining trial, 25 percent of the variance could be explained. Common to all the trials was the finding that IDMFS alone accounted for almost all of what little variance in new DMFS could be explained.

McClendon and Horowitz[3] used one- through four-year incremental data of children of a control group who had participated in a topical fluoride study. They reported that an appreciable proportion, 46 percent of the variance in four-year DMFS increment could be explained by a combination of IDMFS, initial number of erupted permanent teeth, IDMFT, sex and age. However, as was true in the analyses by Carlos[2], practically all of the variability explained in DMFS increment could be uniquely attributed to IDMFS. An additional interesting finding shown in Table 1 was that initial caries prevalence became a stronger predictor of future decay as the time interval from baseline increased.

An examination of the value of the first year's increment as a predictor variable, seen in Dr. Downer's paper, was included in the analyses of McClendon and Horowitz (data not shown)[3]. They found that the correlations between the first-year DMFS increment and DMFS increment for the next one, two and three years were smaller than the correlations between DMFS prevalence at the end of the first year of study and the same one, two and three years of increment.

It can be concluded from the findings in Table 1 that of all the epidemiologic variables tested for caries predictive capability, only initial DMFS prevalence consistently proved useful. However, it was rarely highly correlated with caries incidence. Moreover, the size of the correlation coefficient varied according to the particular data set used. That the findings of Dr. Downer and NIDR investigators are not in complete accord is probably due to this same problem of data-set dependency. Until new epidemiologic variables more closely associated with the development of new decay can be identified, we should not expect complete uniformity in results among the types of studies under discussion.

A few other approaches with potential for caries prediction from epidemiological data deserve comment. Koch[4] grouped 9- and 10-year-old Swedish children into high and low risk groups on the basis of the number of certain restored tooth surfaces:

1. Proximal surfaces of incisors and first molars.
2. Buccal surfaces of upper first molars.
3. Lingual surfaces of lower first molars.

Restored occlusal surfaces were not included because these surfaces had a high frequency of preventive fillings. Children with a score of 4 or more were called the high caries (HC) group and those with a zero score were designated as the low caries (LC) group. After one year, children in the HC group developed an average of 9.5 new DF surfaces compared with an average of 5.3 for their schoolmates in the LC group. The difference between these inordinately large one-year increments was statistically significant. It should be noted, however, that about one third of the children examined could not be classified as to caries risk because their scores fell in between the selected limits. Another drawback of Koch's index may be its suitability only for children that have received a high level of dental care.

Grainger[5] developed a hierarchical method of assessing the pattern of dental caries attack that can be used to measure susceptibility to dental caries. According to which teeth and surfaces are affected by decay, the index categorizes the dentition into five zones that represent increasing severity of caries experience. For example, decay of the proximal surfaces of mandibular anterior teeth is considered the severest type of involvement and carries with it a zone 5 classification. Underlying the validity of the method is the assumption of cumulative zone membership, i.e., if an individual is in zone 5, it can be assumed that he also belongs to all lower severity zones. Evaluations of the index by Poulsen and Horowitz[6] and by Katz and co-workers[7,8] showed that with but a few modifications, the assumption of cumulative membership is upheld. They also found a positive correlation between Grainger's Index and the prevalence of dental caries (DMFS). One of the reports showed correlations as large as 0.74[8].

Taking the lead from these encouraging results, Dr. Kingman of the Biometry Section, NIDR, has tested the potential value of Grainger's Index and modifications thereof in predicting DMFS increment. I hope that Dr. Kingman will have the opportunity to present some of the highlights of his work at this meeting.

LITERATURE CITED

1. Lu, K.H. 1966. An experimentally supported "law of tooth decay" and its application. Archs. oral Biol., 11:757-768.

2. Carlos, J.P. 1970. Some statistical problems in clinical fluoride trials. Presented at ORCA Colloque Odonto-stomatologique Vicheres, Suisse, Sept. (Unpublished).

3. McClendon, J.B. and Horowitz, H.S. 1971. Comparability of study groups in clinical trials. J. Dent. Res., (Annotation) 50:1357.

4. Koch, G. 1970. Selection and caries prophylaxis of children with high caries activity. One-year results. Odont. Revy. 21:71-81.

5. WHO. 1967. International dental epidemiological methods series. Manual No. 3 (first draft). Geneva, Switzerland, 26-29.

6. Poulsen, S. and Horowitz, H.S. 1974. An evaluation of a hierarchical method of describing the pattern of dental caries attack. Comm. Dent. Oral Epidemiol. 2:7-11.

7. Katz, R.V., Radi, W.R. and Barmes, G.P 1976. Evaluation of a simplified caries index for use by the U.S. Army Dental Corps. J. Dent. Res. 55:935-938.

8. Katz, R.V. and Meskin, L.H. 1976. Testing the internal and external validity of a simplified dental caries index on an adult population. Comm. Dent. Oral Epidemiol. 4:227-231.

MODERATOR'S SUMMARY OF DISCUSSION OF TOPIC I AND TOPIC II

It seems essential to define what is a carious lesion before methods for prediction of dental caries are evaluated. Dental caries may be correctly defined as being present anywhere along a spectrum that ranges from the very beginnings of enamel demineralization to frank cavitation, depending upon the interest of and methods of detection available to an investagator. Even with criteria established, interpretation of those criteria are likely to vary from one investigator to another. From a practical standpoint, it is probably suitable to define dental decay as those lesions that are generally repaired by dental practitioners, in other words, those in which there is overt visual-tactile or radiographic evidence of decay. If methods were available for predicting which individuals would develop in the forseeable future lesions with true cavitation, then a valuable diagnostic tool would exist. Dr. Kleinberg correctly pointed out, however, that dental caries is a disease and that a carious lesion or cavitation is a result of that disease.

It has been suggested by Snyder that for a caries predictive test to be meaningful for individuals, the coefficient of correlation (r) should be at least 0.9. Yet, in the papers presented at this Conference, none of the reported correlations approaches a value near 0.9. There was a general consensus that a correlation coefficient of 0.9 was unrealistically high. It was suggested that a correlation of 0.7, which would account for about 50 percent of the variation in the dependent variable, might be a more reasonable target level. It was generally conceded that it is easier to get higher correlations for groups of people than for individuals.

Dr. Ostrom's findings that a patient's history and present clinical status may have predictive value are interesting. For example, the fact that groups of patients with low Snyder test scores, low gingivitis scores and a history of regular topical fluoride applications have a caries increment that approaches zero may indicate that various batteries of tests may be useful for prediction. It is an area of research that deserves further study.

TOPIC III

DIET AND CARIES PREDICTION

Moderator:

Abraham Nizel
Tufts University
School of Dental Medicine
Boston, Massachusetts 02111

Clinical correlations with diet

Bo Krasse

Faculty of Odontology, University of Göteborg, Göteborg, Sweden

The diet is one of the main factors in the host-parasite- environment complex affecting the teeth. However, only a few relationships between certain dietary factors and dental caries in man are incontrovertible. In his introduction to the workshop conference on the role of human foodstuffs and dental caries, Henry Scherp (1970) said: "individual reviews, symposiums and conferences devoted to various aspects of nutrition and caries are quite abundant. I believe I have read the majority of the associated publications and I am left with the dismaying small resultant that controlled intake of fluoride is good, uncontrolled intake of sugar is generally bad, and it is particularly bad when the intake is frequent, there might be protective substances naturally present in some foodstuffs and we need more research".

Even if much research has been done since 1970, Scherp's statement still seems valid. However, it is important to discuss how our meagre knowledge can be used for the prediction of caries in the individual case and in groups of persons.

The relationship between sugar intake and dental caries has been reviewed by Gustafsson (1954) and by Mandel (1970). In 1954 Gustafsson stated that an overwhelming amount of evidence is available in favor of sugar promoting caries, but that clinical studies have given conflicting results. In 1970 Mandel wrote that by using the Vipeholm study as a base apparent contradictions about the relationship between sugar and dental caries can be resolved. He stressed that the Vipeholm study had changed the frame of reference from the exploration of the relation of total intake of sugar to caries to an examination of the effect of the form and frequency of sugar ingestion on caries.

One of the main conclusions of the Vipeholm study was that the risk of sugar increasing caries was greatest if sugar is consumed between the meals and in a form in which the tendency to be retained on the surfaces of the teeth is pronounced, thus giving a transiently high concentration of sugar on these surfaces.

Let us now analyze what happened in the groups which were given sugar in sticky form between the meals. The main diagram (Figure 1) is well known. It clearly demonstrates that the caries activity dramatically increases, and then returns to its original value when the caries accelerating between-meal addition to the diet is withdrawn.

Less well known are the diagrams which illustrate the percentage distribution of patients with a varying number of new carious surfaces (Figure 2) The diagrams show that large variations occur. They also show that in all the dietary groups except one - the female 24 toffee group - 15 to 30 percent of the patients did not get any new carious surfaces at all when sugar

FIGURE 1.

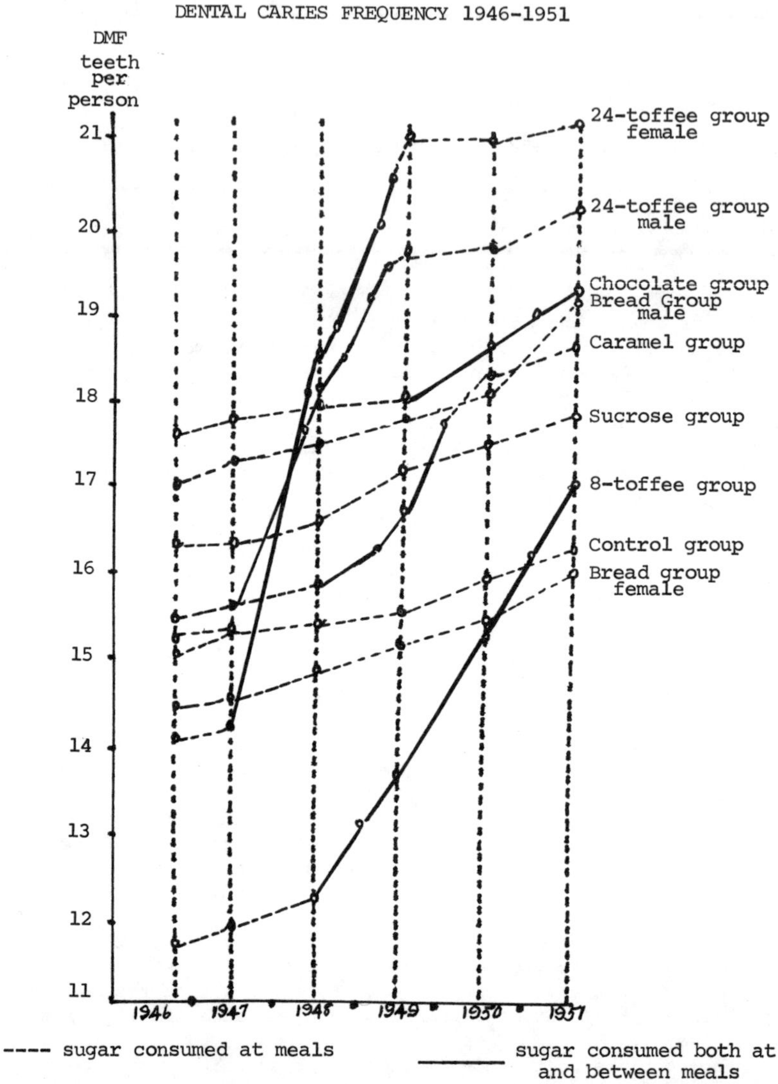

was given in sticky form between the meals. This was the case also in the 8-toffee group when the caries accelerating dietary addition had been given for 3 years. In this group as well as in the others there were patients who did not consume any of the sweets and patients who swallowed the toffees without chewing them. However, the fact remains that some patients did not get any new lesions, although they were eating sweets between the meals for a long time. To a certain extent, this might have been due to the high caries resistance in their teeth. However, a variation in caries activity always exists. It has been observed in animal experiments on programmed

FIGURE 2.

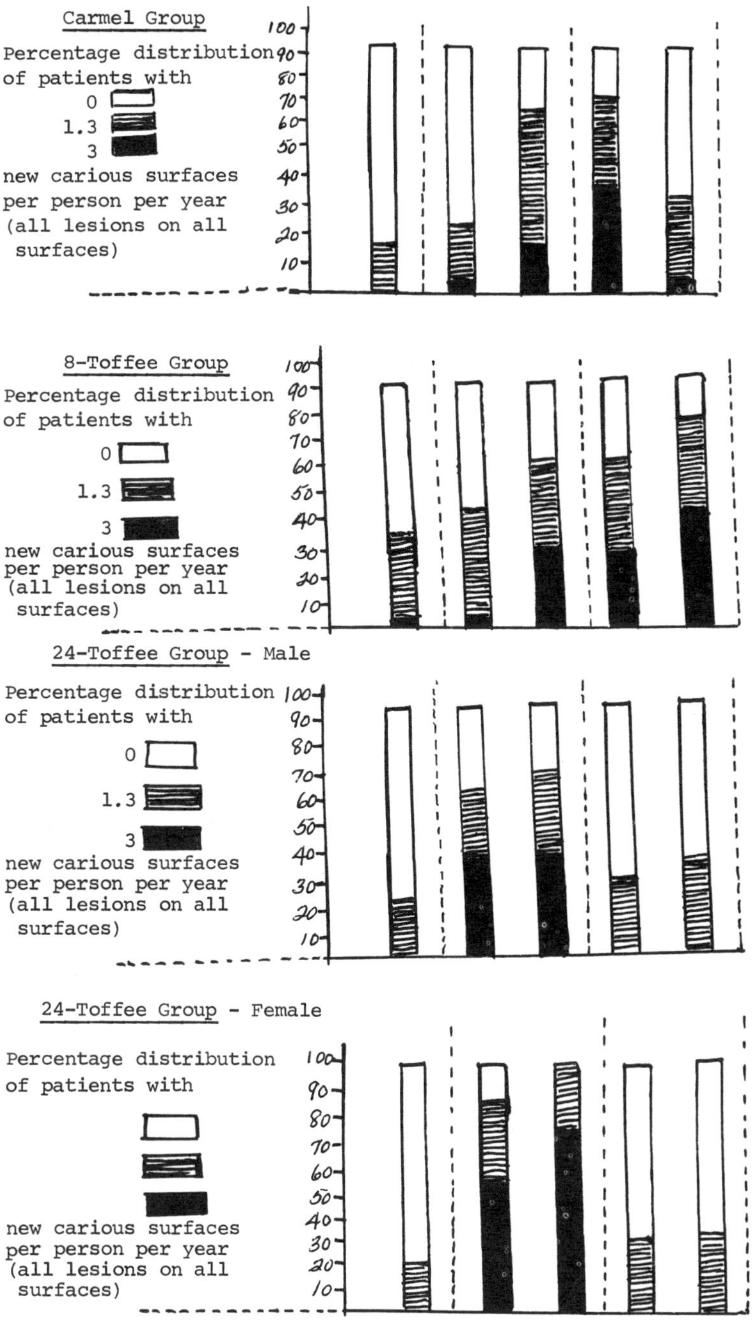
Carmel Group
Percentage distribution of patients with
0
1.3
3
new carious surfaces per person per year (all lesions on all surfaces)
100
90
80
70
60
50
40
30
20
10
8-Toffee Group
Percentage distribution of patients with
0
1.3
3
new carious surfaces per person per year (all lesions on all surfaces)
100
90
80
70
60
50
40
30
20
10
24-Toffee Group - Male
Percentage distribution of patients with
0
1.3
3
new carious surfaces per person per year (all lesions on all surfaces)
100
90
80
70
60
50
40
30
20
10
24-Toffee Group - Female
Percentage distribution of patients with
new carious surfaces per person per year (all lesions on all surfaces)
100
90
80
70
60
50
40
30
20
10

feeding (König, 1970). Also, it is common observation both by laymen and dental practitioners that a high and often repeated consumption of sweets does not always result in caries. From clinical studies it can be assumed that up to 25 percent of the individuals in a group might not get an increased caries activity when eating sucrose in a caries promoting manner. This would mean that in the dental practice, prediction of caries on the basis of the diet alone might be wrong in 1 case out of 4.

In this connection another point ought to be stressed. In the Vipeholm study there were persons in whom active caries was noted while they were on a diet very low in carbohydrate content. This observation suggests the existence of some types of caries in which sugar and other carbohydrates play only a minor role as a causal factor.

Analogous observations as those made with regard to the sugar intake have been made with regard to fluorides. In populations from areas with an optimal concentration of fluoride in the drinking water individuals are always found with a fairly high caries frequency. So for example, in Galesburg where the mean value was 2.0 DMF teeth, 25 percent of the children had $>$ 4, and 13 percent $>$ 5 DMF teeth (Dean, 1940). In a comparable study in Sweden, where the mean value for 13 year old girls was 7 DMF teeth, 20 percent had $>$ 11 DMF teeth (Sellman et al, 1957). It has also been observed in the Swedish school dental service that about 25% of the children develop a high caries activity under the conditions of a strict preventive program containing regular topical fluoride applications (Forsman and Ericsson,1973).

Several other dietary factors than sucrose and fluorides have been associated with the development of caries (for a review see Bibby, 1970). Such factors are for example trace elements, phosphates and fats. In addition it has been suggested that the physical properties of the diet is of importance for its caries producing potential. Generally all these factors show only a weak or possible connection with the caries activity. Some of them might support each other and increase the caries accelerating properties of the diet while others might out-weigh each other. Such interferences might be one explanation for the controversial opinion about the relationship between certain foodstuffs and caries and they ought to be considered when the food intake is examined.

For determining the food intake and food habits different kinds of nutrition analyses are used e.g. balance sheets, weighing methods and interviews. Different kinds of nutrition interviews are most common. The dietary history is a quantitative estimation of the nutrient intake over a period of time either during 3 to 7 days or during the preceding 24 hours, the so called 24 hour recall. The dietary history as a tool in research has been reviewed by Burke (1947), and other interviewing methods by Young (1966). Burke states that as any dietary history cannot be exact there has been a tendency to discredit it in research. However, if it is properly taken and its pitfalls are thoroughly understood the dietary history will furnish as reliable information as is possible. Completed with cross-checking it gives average values in fairly small groups, which are quite reliable. The method is therefore most suitable in large groups of persons. The reliability is reduced to the extent that the number of studied individuals is diminished (Roine and Pekkarinen, 1968). In dental practice a more qualitative type of interview, the food habit inquiry is the method of choice. It gives information on the patients usual eating habits and the kinds of food generally eaten. The food habit inquiry might be completed with the searching interview when one is concerned with knowing more about the patient and his living habits in general. Such a detailed case history is generally necessary as a basis for successfull dietary counselling.

Good interviewing requires skill, time and ability to understand the needs and attitudes of the patient as well as factors in his economic and social background. Food intake and eating habits are among the most complex aspects of human behavior. "Accurate assessment of nutrition needs and deficiences have never been easy" (Davidson and Passmore, 1969), and the fact that sweets, cookies and soft drinks are so called "conflict items" does not make it easier to obtain a reliable basis for caries prediction.

However, a 7-day diet survey in Indiana (Zita et al, 1959) and a 24 hour recall in West Tennessee (Weiss and Thritart, 1960) both disclosed a direct relationship between caries experience and the frequency of eating items of high sugar content or high degree of adhesiveness between meals. These and similar observations from other studies support the general applicability of the main results of the Vipeholm study.

As stated previously a large individual variation in caries activity is observed also in persons living under well controlled dietary conditions. If the diet does not vary the observed variation must primarily be ascribed to differences in the other main factors affecting caries i.e. the host or the micro-flora. Such differences may be related to the diet. Consequently clinical and laboratory examinations ought to be used in addition to the dietary analysis when trying to predict the effect of nutritional factors on the caries susceptibility. At the gross appraisal of the patients such factors as obesity and pregnancy should be noted. Overweight may be due to a high consumption of sugar and sweets, and during pregnancy the pica syndrome may lead to a caries accelerating intake of sweets. Furthermore, it is a common observation that an untidy appearance often is associated with irregular caries accelerating food habits.

Naturally the most important clinical observations with regard to the caries risk are made at the oral examination. Voluminous plaque formation might reveal a high intake of sucrose (Carlsson and Egelberg, 1965) and the localisation, appearance and number of cavities and fillings may disclose a previous or actual high caries activity. Likewise discolorations of the enamel may indicate fluoride intake during the mineralization period. Inspection of the mucous membranes might indicate dryness of the mouth due to reduced saliva secretion, a situation which easily can be confirmed by a simple test. At our institution we determine the saliva secretion rate when chewing on a piece of paraffin wax of a standardized size. The normal secretion rate at this test is 1 to 3 ml per minute and a value of 0.7 ml or less generally means that the patient has subjective discomfort. The case history or the searching interview might disclose factors which promote caries accelerating food habits e.g. stress, irregular working hours, profession, diseases and medication. It ought to be observed that several medicaments contain high amounts of sugar for example cough mistures and laxatives. Place of residence will reveal possible fluoride intake.

The laboratory examination which is most used for evaluation of the food intake and the caries risk is the lactobacillus count. A high lactobacillus count in the saliva is not always associated with a high caries activity, but when eating a caries accelerating diet persons with a high lactobacillus count run a larger risk of developing a higher caries activity than those with low counts. This is illustrated by finding in some of the groups in the Vipeholm study (Krasse, 1954). For instance, in the 8-toffee group, 85 percent of the patients with high lactobacillus counts showed the mean caries activity against zero percent of those with low counts. The patients with a high lactobacillus count in the 8-toffee group developed an average of 7.5 new carious surfaces per year while the corresponding figure among the patients in the control group was 1.1 The test lso showed that 85 percent of the persons with lactobacillus counts developed caries, as against 0 percent of these with low counts. These findings imply that the lactobacilli are involved in the development of caries following the consumption of carbohydrates in a caries-promoting manner.

Table I

Support (+) from Clinical and Laboratory Findings for Dietary Histories

Clinical and Laboratory Data	Dietary Factor: Frequent Sucrose	Fluoride	Other
Host Background			
Age, Residence, Occupation Disease, Pregnancy	+	+	
Teeth			
Caries, Fillings Discoloration	+	+	
Saliva			
Secretion Rate Buffer Capacity	+		+
Microflora			
S. mutans, lactobacilli plaque	+		

Also, the number of Streptococcus mutans in the saliva can be used as a supporting laboratory test. However, while the lactobacilli might reflect the total carbohydrate intake Streptococcus mutans seems to be associated mainly with the sucrose intake. We have found that in most patients these can be reduced by reducing the use of carbohydrates in the diet. However, in one case it was found that a persistent maintenance of a high lactobacillus after dietary restriction was attributable to the thrice daily use of a medicine containing twenty percent of sugar.

Table 1 summarizes the clinical and laboratory examinations which can be used to confirm the dietary history or to disclose digressions from it. A combination of several observations pointing in the same direction increases the chance of predicting a correlation between a dietary factor and caries. For example, no fluoride exposure, high counts of Streptococcus mutans and lactobacilli, low saliva secretion and chalky enamel on buccal surfaces makes a high caries acitvity very likely if there is a frequent sucrose intake. In contrast mottled enamel, low values of Streptococcus mutans and lactobacilli, good saliva secretion and buffer capacity indicate low risk of caries on the same type of diet.

SUMMARY

Although the diet is one of the main components in the complex affecting caries only a few dietary factors are known to be closely associated with caries activity:

1. Between meal eating of sugar in sticky form
2. Intake of fluoride during the formation of teeth.

However, a high and often repeated consumption of sweets is not always associated with caries and, conversly, in areas with an optimal concentration of fluoride in the drinking water persons are sometimes observed with a large number of carious teeth. From different studies it seems as if 20 to 25 percent of the individuals fall into such groups of exceptions.

The determination of the food intake and food habits is difficult. All methods have certain inherent errors. The commonly used interview methods completed with cross-checking give reliable results in fairly small groups, but the reliability is reduced when the number of individuals is diminished.

Due to the individual variation in caries susceptibility and the error in the determination of the food intake, the prediction of caries in the individual case on the basis of diet alone is very uncertain. However, if the dietary analysis is combined with clinical and laboratory examinations the chances of a correct prediction increases. For example, when eating sugar in a caries promoting manner, the caries risk is considerably higher in persons with a high lactobacillus count than in those with a low count.

LITERATURE CITED

Bibby, B.G. 1970. Inferences from natural occurring variations in caries prevalence. J. Dent. Res. 49:1194-1199.

Burke, B.S. 1974. The dietary history as a tool in research. J. Amer. Diet. Assoc. 23:1041-1046.

Carlsson, J. and Egelberg, J. 1965. Effect of diet on early plaque formation in man. 16:112-125.

Davidson, S. and Passmore, R. 1969. The assessment of nutritional status. Human Nutrition and Dietetics. 50:712-730. Edinburgh and London.

Dean, H.T. 1946. Epidemiological studies in the United States. Dental Caries and Fluorine pp. 5-31.

Forsman, B. and Ericsson, Th. 1973. Kariesutveckling vid systematisk tandhälsovård. Undersökning av ett svenskt skolbarnsklientel. Socialmed. tidskr. 5:298-303.

Gustafsson, B.E. 1954. The Vipeholm dental caries study. Survey of the literature on carbohydrates and dental caries. The Vipeholm Dental Caries Study. Acta Odont. Scand. 11:207-231.

Gustafsson, B.E., Quensel, C.E., Swenander-Lanke, L., Lundquist, C., Grahnen, H., Bonow, B.E. and Krasse, B. 1954. The Vipeholm Dental Caries Study. The effect of different levels of carbohydrate intake on caries activity in 436 individuals observed for five years. Acta Odont. Scand. 11:232-364.

Krasse, B. 1954. Relationship between caries activity and the number of lactobacilli in the oral cavity. Acta Odont. Scand. 12:157-172.

König, K.G. 1970. Feeding regimes and caries. J. Dent. Res. 49:1327-1333.

Mandel, I.D. 1970. Effects of dietary modifications on caries in humans. J. Dent. Res. 49:1201-1211.

Roine, P. and Pekkarinen, M. 1968. Metodik vid kostundersökningar. 2. Intervjumetoder. Metodik vid nutritionsundersökningar på homo. Kungälv 30/10-1/11. Lund 1970.

Scherp, H.W. 1970. Introduction: Why another conference? J. Dent. Res. 49:1191.

Sellman, S., Syrrist, A. and Gustaffson, G. 1957. Fluorine and dental health in southern Sweden. An epidemiological study. Odont. Tidskr. 65:61-93.

Weiss, R.L. and Trithart, A.H. 1960. Between-meal eating habits and dental caries experience in preschool children. Am. J. Publ. Health 50:1097-1104.

Young, C.M. 1966. Interviewing and counselling the patient on normal diet and meal planning. In Nizel, A.E. (ed.): The science of nutrition and its application in clinical dentistry. Philadelphia, W.B. Saunders Company.

Zita, A.C., McDonald, R.E. and Andrews, A.L. 1959. Dietary habits and the dental caries experience in 200 children. J. Dent. Res. 38:860-865.

Discussion of clinical correlations with diet

Kenneth O. Madsen

Dental Branch, University of Texas, 6516 John Freeman Avenue, Houston, Texas 77025

Dr. Krasse has described the value of not relying on dietary observations alone for caries prediction. He documented his approach by demonstrating with clinical cases that when measures are taken which control certain caries factors in individuals that caries will predictably decrease.

I suggest, however, that dietary observations alone may be more useful than commonly recognized by clinicians or researchers. As for those individuals who appear resistant to fermentable carbohydrate, I postulate that there are fewer of them in the normal population than indicated by the institutional study at Vipeholm.[1] Dr. Krasse has estimated from the Vipeholm study that in a private practice one would overestimate the number of caries patients by 25% if he accepted a caries-promoting usage of fermentable carbohydrate as the basis for predicting caries development. Since in the U.S., at least, more than 90% of the population has experienced some sort of caries it is reasonable to suppose that they developed caries while using carbohydrate in a caries-promoting fashion so that if the times of frequent carbohydrate usage are carefully determined, one should be able to predict caries more than 90% of the time. Accuracy is imporved, of course, if one studies individuals and observes several factors as Dr. Krasse demonstrated.

The critical times when caries develops need not be long nor present at the time of caries scoring. In the Vipeholm study, for example, nearly twice as much caries developed in only 6 months when caramels were eaten 4 times rather than 2 times between meals. We frequently observe that a specific patient often changes his frequency of fermentable carbohydrate usage, or what I will call the "frequency factor". The carbohydrate items responsible for caries at one time may fade from frequent use and then at a later time be resumed or be replaced by the frequent use of other fermentable items. Many personal factors are responsible for habit changes. It is apparent in our clinical population, for example, that popularity of between meal items varies with age. Dr. Krasse has already commented on the detection of behavioral patterns or changes associated with diet and caries. To the extent that the frequency of carbohydrate usage changes prior to the time that caries is evaluated, the frequency count is in error and its importance will be falsely estimated.

Dr. Nizel and a few others, including ourselves, have for many years now,promoted the importance of actually counting oral carbohydrate exposures when counselling patients for caries prevention. Yet to my knowledge there are no clinical studies in which the frequency factor has been quantitated for a significant number of patients. Several recent inadequate epidemiological surveys have diluted the impact of the Vipeholm study, and the many epidemiological surveys which suggest that the frequency factor is crucial. The study by Weiss and Trithart[2] may represent the best actual measurement of the frequency factor in an epidemiological study. If one counts all meals and snacks as cariogenic and assumes 3 meals per day, then the children in their study showed a direct correlation between frequency and caries when they were exposed to a range of from 3 up to 7 total cariogenic exposures per day. Using similar estimates with the data of Hankin et al[3] indicates a correlation with caries when the frequency ranged from 3 to 8 exposures per day.

It is our clinical impression based upon observing 5-day food records for many years that caries is present or will develop when the frequency factor becomes a constant total of 4-6 exposures per day. When the record, or further probing of habits not shown on the record, shows that a patient's mouth is exposed to 2-3 meals per day that habitually contain fermentable carbohydrates, and when in addition there are 2-3 fermentable items regularly used between meals, we would predict pit and fissure caries within a matter of months followed by smooth surface lesions within a year if the frequency factor remains high. If oral hygiene is good and fluoride benefits are present, this caries rate will be slower, but the constant pressure of such a frequency will nearly always evidence itself in caries.

While one can state such clinical impressions rather boldly, I now invite you to revisit Vipeholm and evaluate my attempts to measure the frequency factor in that study even though actual frequency counts were not made.

The Vipeholm design included 4 meals a day for all groups with superimposed between-meal carbohyrates in the experimental groups. The basic 4 meals caused a low level of caries even when the diet was low enough in carbohydrate (130 grams) to cause some ketosis and even when it contained no added sucrose. When the controls were given a normal carbohydrate diet daily (440 grams) including 70 grams of sucrose added to the 4 meals, there was a small but significant increase in caries. This increase appeared without an apparent increase in the frequency factor. I suggest, however, that the actual frequency count was increased from less than 4 to a count of 4 per day. On the very low carbohydrate regimen with no added sucrose some of the 4 meals may not have been cariogenic since only 15% developed caries. On the high carbohydrate regimen of the control group, all 4 meals were cariogenic and 30% developed caries even though as mentioned the scores were very low.

It may be most difficult of all to predict the spurious, low level of caries that continues to develop when the frequency factor is only 3 or 4. The average age of Vipeholm patients was 32. Younger patients would predictably be more sensitive to low frequency counts. I have estimated the frequency factor in the children in the Hopewood House studies[4] to have been only about 2 or at the most 3 exposures per day although they ate 5 times daily. Under these conditions, including poor oral hygiene as also existed in Vipeholm, about 30% still developed caries. Again, however, the caries scores were very low at these low frequencies.[5] Based upon the discussion thus far, it may be useful to offer a mechanism for the frequency factor and its study. Perhaps it may take a full between interval, or about 3 hours for the tooth to recover from the caries attack produced by a cariogenic meal. This assumes 4 hours between meals with 30 minutes of exposure during eating, and another 30 minutes for plaque pH to recover. In other words, a total of only 2-3 cariogenic exposures as either meals or snacks spread throughout the day may produce little caries. The Hopewood House studies support this idea since caries in the orphanage was very low.

If the interval is shortened by even one between meal exposure, significant caries may develop. This idea is supported by the Vipeholm control group which showed significantly more caries when the frequency factor was increased to 4 with the result that one between meal interval permitted only 1 hour for tooth recovery before the next exposure. Then when both of the two remaining 3-hour between meal intervals in the Vipeholm regimen were shortened by between meal sweets, there was a sharp increase in caries in all cases. That is, the most striking caries effect in the Vipeholm study occurred when the frequency count was increased from 4 to 6 by the addition of 2 between meal sweets. With this regimen no complete tooth recovery could have occurred during the day until after the evening meal. Further caries response was sometimes seen when 2 additional sweets or a total of 4 between meal exposures were given. In the case of the group given toffees, the response to only 2 between meal feedings was very great and was not significantly increased by 4 feedings. In the caramel group, however, the 2 exposures produced significant, but more mild response followed by a further significant response with 4 exposures.

From this examination of the Vipeholm data, the most dramatic caries response was seen when a rather uniform frequency factor of 4 cariogenic meals per day was increased to 6 cariogenic exposures, although a further increase to 8 exposures was shown in some cases to provoke more caries. I have argued that any encroachment upon about a 3-hour tooth recovery period after each cariogenic exposure may be crucial whether it be a meal or between meal occasion.

I am aware that the frequency factor is not new. However, if we are to make any progress in caries prediction, it seems necessary to me that this factor be isolated for study and its quantitative influence measured. In 1935, Dr. Bibby observed that, "Another determinant of the presence of food about the teeth is the frequency. This fact is obvious, but gains significance because it represents one of the greatest differences between the dietetic habits of the relatively caries-immune native races and caries-ravaged civilized peoples."[6] Dr. Bibby has cited as many as 35 epidemiological surveys in which the authors themselves attributed high caries scores to the frequency factor.[7] Nevertheless, the fact remains that the frequency factor has still not been quantitated.

Frequency must be a potent factor since it so readily overrides other factors found to influence caries scores in populations or groups. This is especially noteworthy since in such group studies the frequency factor was detected as important despite the use of prevalence data instead of caries increments associated closely in time with changing dietary habits. Even when caries increments are used, the detection of variables, such as the frequency factor, may be jeopardized if the caries baseline is not held constant. In fact, several speakers at this conference have stated that the initial caries status is the most predictive caries measurement. If so, variations in the caries baseline should overide other variables. Nevertheless, in the Vipeholm study where all experimental groups began with different baseline caries scores, an increase in the frequency count from 4 to 6 determined the caries rate without regard to the initial caries status.

For experimentation I suggest that one could determine the effect on caries increments of eliminating one or more exposures in selected individuals where habitual frequency counts can be established with high reliability. To assess the frequency factor, the best study would require the complete elimination of one or more specific cariogenic exposures so that one or more 3-hour tooth recovery periods are added each day. In other words, eliminating only 1 or 2 exposures during an afternoon of frequent exposures would perhaps be less effective or ineffective compared to providing an additional full 3-hour period between exposures. Intended in this argument is the contention that the substitution of a cariogenic exposure with one considered to be less cariogenic would be relatively ineffective compared to lengthening times between exposures. It would be interesting to see if the salivary microbiological tests suggested by Dr. Krasse today, or the Snyder test, would be suitable for detecting the subtle changes in the frequency factor that I have postulated to affect caries.

It would not seem possible at the present time to be sure that one had reduced the frequency factor by using a wide variety of recommended between meal snacks to replace cariogenic ones since the relative cariogenicity of fermentable carbohydrate items depends upon a host of variables not yet well understood. Alternatively, one could replace cariogenic exposures with "zahnschonend" items which are known to be "safe for teeth" according to Mühlemann's criteria[8], or perhaps one could assure the usage of sugarless gum chewing or uniform vigorous rinsing after the cariogenic exposures.

Incidentally, I am deliberately avoiding the subject of food cariogenicity and am arguing that any generally accepted readily fermentable carbohydrate exposure should be counted in measuring the frequency factor. At the present time it appears that even a low concentration of sugar or a very small amount of fermentable carbohydrate constitutes an exposure that should be counted.[8] All of the Vipeholm sweets were a mixture of fermentable carbohydrates and all contained starch, dextrins, sucrose and at least one other sugar. This uniformity in composition as well as rather uniform stickiness may have favored the isolation of frequency as being of prime importance.

In summary, I have deliberately belabored the matter of measuring only one caries factor, since to date there are no quantitative data in the human. Interestingly enough, there is also very little in the rodent data that would attempt to distinguish between the caries effects over the ranges of from 3 to 8 exposures spaced at strategic intervals comparable to the human experience.

I am sure many of you already agree that we can predict caries with considerable success when we observe several parameters in individual patients over a period of time. It is heroic to depend on only one measure, but of them all, I maintain that the actual counting of frequency may prove to be one of the most predictive. The fact is that it still remains as one of the least used and least studied procedures for predicting caries.

LITERATURE CITED

1. Gustafsson, B.E., Quensel, C.E., Lanke, L.S., Lundquist, C., Grahnen, H., Bonow, B.E. and Krasse, B. 1954. The Vipeholm Dental Caries Study. The effect of different levels of carbohydrate intake on caries activity in 436 individuals observed for five years. Acta Odont. Scand. 11:232-264.

2. Weiss, R.L. and Trithart, A.H. 1960. Between-meal eating habits and dental caries experience in pre-school children. Am. J. Pub. Hlth 50:1097-1104.

3. Hankin, J.H., Chung, C.S. and Kau, M.C.W. 1973. Genetic and Epidemiologic studies of oral characteristics in Hawaii's school children: Dietary patterns and caries prevalence. J. Dent. Res. 52:1079-1104.

4. Gillham, J. and Lennon, D. 1958. The biology of the children of Hopewood House, Bowral, N.S.W. II Observations extending over 5 years (1952-1956 inclusive) 4. Dietary Survey, Austral. Dent. J. 3:378-382.

5. Sullivan, H.R. and Harris, R. 1958. The biology of the children of Hopewood House, Bowral, N.S.W. II Observations extending over 5 years (1952-1956 inclusive) 2. Observation on Oral Concitions Austral. Dent. J. 3:311-317.

6. Bibby, B.G. 1935. Neglected factors in the study of dental caries. J. Am. Dent. Assoc. 22:222-239.

7. Bibby, B.G. 1975. The cariogenicity of snack foods and confections. J. Am. Dent. Assoc. 90:121-132.

8. Imfeld, T. and Mühlemann, H.R. 1977. Evaluation of sugar substitutes in preventive cariology. J. Prev. Dent. 4:8-14.

Cariogenicity and caries prediction

Basil G. Bibby

Eastman Dental Center, 800 Main Street East, Rochester, New York 14605

Caries is a food dependent disease. No serious student of the disease questions that fact. To date no one has been able to demonstrate that any other variable is as closely related to greater or less caries activity in man. Beyond that we can be sure of very little. Our knowledge of the effects of various dietary items is insufficient to permit fuller understanding of what makes foods more or less cariogenic and information on the relative destructiveness of the principal classes of foodstuffs is lacking.

The existing belief in the dominating importance of sucrose seems to have evolved from casual clinical observations and simple laboratory experiments. As far as we can tell it had its origin in the 18th century with Pierre Fauchard's [1] indictment of cane sugar as the "seductive poison"that caused caries. W.D. Miller's[2] conclusion that flour and potatoes were more important than sucrose was never accepted and additional clinical observations reinforced confidence in the importance of sucrose. Noteworthy in this respect was the finding that war time rationing reduced both sugar consumption and caries.[3,4,5] Unfortunately the question of whether sucrose restriction was the sole cause of the observed changes has not been clearly established. Some later investigations, such as the Vipeholm Study,[6] have tended to show that variables other than the total amount of sugar eaten, for instance the frequency of use and the associated substrates play an important part in determing the cariogenicity of foodstuffs. It is the role of these other variables that change the cariogenic potency of foods that has to be better understood before we can build a firm bridge between patients'diets and their present or future caries activity.

Before turning to a consideration of the factors that modify the role of sucrose, note should be made of some reasons why some reservations have developed on the unique importance of sucrose in caries. The first is that the seemingly dominant effect of sucrose may be explained by the fact that it is the fermentable carbohydrate that appears most frequently in the human diet. The second, it is now realized that candies and such like items that contain very high concentrations of sugar may have been blamed unjustly. They are responsible for less than ten percent of the sucrose eaten in the United States and the damage they do to the teeth depend more on their acidity than sucrose content. Three times as much sucrose is used in either beverages or starchy foods which are not usually rated as being highly cariogenic. The third reason is that a lack of consistent parallelism has been noted between sugar consumption and caries prevalence in population groups,[7] between the sugar content of animal diets[8] and the caries produced; and between the sugar levels in foods and the production of bacterial enamel demineralization[9] or *in vitro* caries.[10] Finally, and most importantly, it must be pointed out ~~that sucrose~~ sucrose is almost never used by itself.

Even in beverages and hard candies it is mixed with acids or flavoring agents that can modify its effects. In its other uses, as when mixed with starches, milk products or soup bases, the other ingredients must play a part.

Pointing out that it is an over-simplification to attempt to assess caries activity solely on the basis of the sucrose content of foods and the total sucrose intake would be destructive rather than constructive unless some additional method of assessing the cariogenicity of a diet is used or some improved way of assessing food or sucrose effects is developed. We have been seeking ways of doing this.

If we conclude, as it seems we must, that there is not a simple direct relationship between sugar consumption and the strength of the caries attack, we have perforce to look for some things other than the sugar content of diets as indicators of their cariogenicity or their usefulness for caries prediction in diet analysis. This will, of course, be a summation of the cariogenicity of the individual foods that make up the diet each modified by the frequency of their use. This could be expressed as an equation $P = \sum f_n \times i_n$ (f = frequency: i = index of cariogenicity).

It would be extremely difficult to work out with any degree of accuracy the cariogenic potential for every item that a person eats during a week or even a day. However, it is probable that the desired end could be achieved if we had information on the relative cariogenicity of the four or five most blameworthy foods that were eaten more than a few times a week. If data on the cariogenicity of such foods were known, working out an effective caries prediction score for a patient's diet would be no more difficult than calculating its total sucrose content. At a practical level it might be enough to find out what were a patient's favorite snack foods and the frequency of their use, and then factor each with its cariogenicity index. By totaling the results, a caries prediction index could be obtained.

The disqualifying weakness of the outlined approach to caries prediction is that we do not have information on the relative cariogenicity of individual snack foods and confections. Even more fundamental is the fact that there is no consensus as to how dependable measurements of the cariogenicity of foods can be obtained. It is impractical and almost impossible to carry out the usual type of clinical study on caries initiation with a single food, let alone the wide variety of foods for which cariogenic data is needed. The obvious alternative is the development of a simplified short-term clinical procedure, the use of animals or of *in vitro* methods. Which, if any, of these suggested methods has value has yet to be determined.

Before discussing the various approaches that have been made to the problem, mention should be made of some of the physical and chemical characteristics of foods that complicate the attempts at measuring cariogenicity, and raise doubts as to how the findings should be interpreted. The fact that foods may be dry, moist, liquid, solid, granular, gelantinous or sticky introduces sampling and analytical difficulties. Thus, when quantative comparisons are needed, the methods have to be modified according to the problems involved. The physical properties of some foods interfere with the making of uniform mixtures or separating them by filtration or centrifugation from test materials such as dental enamel. Food colors, natural or artificial, and the opacity of most food mixtures complicate any chemical measurement that depends upon color reactions or light transmission. Further, the wide range in osmolarity has important bearing on any tests that involve bacterial action.

The chemical composition of foods is poorly understood. They are compounded of chemically undefined ingredients to suit the tastes of consumers rather than the convenience of chemists. Even what is known about them is not readily available. Manufacturers withhold such information.

Further, even if the exact chemical composition of a food were known at the time it is mixed, the changes that occur on processing and cooking are unknown and can modify their cariogenicity. Such effects of heat have been shown on the cariogenicity of dried milk in animal diets,[11] on the fermentability of starch by Streptococcus mutans[12] and the greater caries production in rats by gelatinized than raw starches.[13]

The acidity of many foods poses a special set of problems. Many beverages, fruits and candies are highly acid, some having a pH below 3. This means that bacterial fermentation and acid production will be inhibited. It also means that the inherent acid of such foods will demineralize enamel. The effect of fruit juices in producing erosion of the enamel is wellknown, but the relationship of this action to clinical dental caries has yet to be resolved. Obviously a decision on that is needed before the role of food acidity in cariogenicity can be decided.

At different times various properties of foods has been named as of primary importance in determing their cariogenicity. The association between sucrose consumption and caries noted by early dentists seems to be background for the work of Jay[14] who showed a fairly consistent parallelism between the carbohydrate content of diets and caries. However, their work was not extended to show proportionality between the cariogenicity of individual food items and their sucrose content. This is also true of the suggested association between the total carbohydrate content of foods and caries activity.

The first quantitative comparison of the cariogenicity of foods seems to have been made by Miller[2] who measured acid formed on fermentation of foods in saliva, or lactic acid production in bacterial cultures or saliva. Enamel demineralization produced by foods was compared by Osborn et al,[15] to provide an explanation for low caries in natives who ate coarsely refined diets. The amount of food retention on the teeth was also claimed by Miller[2] to be an important determinant of their cariogenicity. More recently the effects of foods on plaque pH and animal caries have been used as indicators of their cariogenicity. One or another of these procedures have been used by a number of modern investigators. However, the usefulness of much of the work is limited because only pure carbohydrates were tested rather than foods of the actual sort that are found in the human diet.

The studies that have examined a sizable group of foods as distinct from laboratory carbohydrates are those of Frostell[16] Edgar et al,[17] and Mühlemann[18] on acid formation in plaque; of Lundquist,[15] Bibby et al[20] and Swenander Lanke[21] on food retention, of Stephan[22] and Konig[23] on animal caries and of Bibby and Mundorff [9] on enamel demineralization.

None of the above measurements of cariogenicity has gained any measure of acceptance in the United States although the situation is different in Switzerland where the in vivo plaque pH methods of Mühlemann and associates[24] for assessing the cariogenicity of foods has been officially accepted for classification of foods. The validity of this test remains to be decided. While the pH findings in a sense combine the effects of acid production from a food with its retention on the teeth, their significance suffers because of the fact that the amount of acid produced does not parallel the amount of enamel dissolved[9] and hence the cariogenicity.

We have used all of the above methods. The reason for using all of them is basically that we are not satisfied that any one of them, alone, gives a reliable index of cariogenicity. It was reasoned that if we obtained results by a variety of methods we should be able to find supportive correlations between some of them, and that such a finding would justify placing increased confidence in the results of those particular tests. This

Table 1.

CARIES PRODUCTION BY BREAKFAST CEREALS
WITH DIFFERENT SUGAR CONTENTS

	Sugar Content %	Caries Teeth	Sugar[1] Daily	Enamel[2] Dissolved	Plaque pH
Corn Flakes (100%)	8	11.3	0.24	6.76	4.5
Captain Crunch (100%)	43	10.0	1.76	3.73	4.5
Life (100%)	19	5.4	1.20	0.15	4.5
Corn Flakes (64%)	5.2	10.1	0.58		
Captain Crunch (64%)	27.9	9.6	2.90		
Life (64%)	12.3	7.5	1.32		

(1) gms (2) Ratio to 2% Sucrose = 10

would be particularly true if the findings could be confirmed by in vitro methods that duplicate oral conditions or by some type of in vivo test. The improved in vitro method that we developed for the purpose is our Orofax system that provides a flow of biologically active human saliva to tooth surfaces on which test foods are placed. The in vivo systems which we feel will serve our purpose would be modifications of Koulourides' method[21] or our test that holds foods on the surfaces of vital teeth in the mouth. Little information from in vivo tests is yet available. It has yet to be established whether any of these tests give true indications of what will happen in natural caries in the human mouth.

A summation of our findings obtained during the past five or six years with the methods we have used is given as Table 2. The differences in the results are very obvious. However, the wide spread between the high and low values obtained by all of the methods reinforces our contention that there are many factors in foods that influence their cariogenicity. The necessary number of test results obtained under uniform conditions that is

Table 2.

MEASUREMENTS OF CARIOGENIC CHARACTERISTICS OF FOODS

Characteristic	Measurement	No. of Foods	Range of Findings Min. - Max.
Total Carbohydrate	Percent	54	4 - 99
Soluble	Percent	54	4 - 99
Shelf	pH	180	2.65 - 8.47
Inherent Acidity	ml 0.05M NaOH/gm	180	0 - 4.70
Fermentation Acid Formed	ml 0.05M NaOH/gm	180	0 - 3.78
Enamel Dissolved	Ratio: 0.2 Sucrose=10	180	1.2 - 20.0
Food Retained 5 min.	mg CHO	54	3.4 - 49.8
Food Retained 15min.	mg CHO	54	2.4 - 11.6
Food Retained 30min.	mg CHO	54	1.9 - 5.8
Plaque pH	Minimum pH	59	5.22 - 6.82
Plaque pH	Sum of depressions	59	0 - 4.88
In vitro caries (5 day)	Demineralization (μ)	20	10 - 33.3
Rat Caries	No. of lesions	20	8.6 - 38
Rat Caries	Severity Score	20	10.5 - 94

needed to make correlations has not been completed. Two tables (3 & 4) will show about where we are at on that matter at this time. These give some encouraging preliminary evidence of correlations, but at least as many absences of similarities.

The significance of laboratory tests can be questioned because we do not know the relative importance in caries causation of the various parameters they measure, and because findings have not been adequately correlated with clinical caries. Indications of relationships between some food characteristics and clinical caries seem to have been shown in only a few instances. One of these is Jay's[14] demonstration of some parallelism between the carbohydrate content of diets (but not individual foods) and caries increments. Another is Lundquist's[19] finding, made in connection with the Vipeholm study, that in general the diets that showed greatest retention in the mouth also produced more caries. It is unlikely that more definite correlations than these will be forthcoming now that restrictions on research in human subjects seem to prevent the feeding of cariogenic foods.

As an alternative approach to establishing the relationships between the caries causing effects of foods and the results of in vitro cariogenicity tests we are exploring the use of two quasi-clinical methods. One of these is the Koulourides "Intra-oral Caries Test",[25] and the other a new method we have brought to the state of clinical trial.

Table 3.

SOME CARIOGENIC INDICES OF THREE PAIRS OF FOODS

Food	% Sol. CHO	Enamel Demin.(1)	New Acid(2)	Plaque pH(3)	Reten. 15 min.(4)	Caries(5) Orofax	Caries(5) Rats
Graham Crackers	35	1.7	2.04	1.49	9.02	8.4	8.0
Potato Chips	54	5.7	3.78	2.04	4.88	8.9	7.8
Dark Chocolate	61	3.4	0.46	1.98	8.07	4.4	10.4
Light Chocolate	53	2.9	0.92	2.35	6.79	2.2	8.7
White Bread	17	7.4	1.35	1.20	10.00	7.1	---
Whole Whear Bread	10	5.8	2.06	3.68	6.91	4.5	---

(1) Ratio to 2% Sucrose = 10
(2) Fermentation acid, ml 0.05 NaOH/gm
(3) Depressions from start
(4) mgs CHO
(5) Ratio to Diet MIT-200 = 10

Table 4

VARIABLES AMONG FOODS WITH COMPARABLE DEMINERALIZATION

Food	Enamel Demin.(1)	% Sol. CHO	Food pH	New Acid(2)	Plaque pH(3)	CHO Retained(4)
Potato Chips	5.7	54	6.4	3.78	2.04	4.88
Choc. Cake	5.6	52	7.12	1.96	3.66	10.63
Doughnut	5.2	27	7.25	2.21	2.96	7.52
Whole Wheat Bread	5.8	10	6.30	2.06	3.68	6.91
Angel Food Cake	5.8	52	6.34	1.24	--	11.39

1. Ratio to 2% Sucrose = 10
2. Fermentation acid ml 0.05NaOH/gm
3. Depressions from start
4. 15 mins. after eating

The Koulourides test has been described in the literature and will be discussed later in this meeting. It repeatedly exposes enamel blocks mounted on an appliance to cariogens in vitro and estimates changes in hardness in the enamel blocks after they have been worn in the mouth for one week.

Our new method will hold food in removable food holders on vital human teeth. The holders will be removed daily and the enamel surfaces examined by special methods for the first signs of demineralization. The time taken to produce the first signs of 'caries' will serve as a measure of cariogenicity.

We do not anticipate that either of these quasi-clinical methods can be used for testing many foods. The technical complexity and need for test subjects would make that impractical. However, it is our hope that because the methods approach clinical reality they could be used in place of full clinical tests as standards against which the reliability of the indices of cariogenicity given by the simpler in vitro tests could be evaluated. Thereafter the more reliable of the in vitro procedures could be used for screening large numbers of foods.

To accomplish the needed evaluation, the cariogenic indices of foods will need to be determined by all the available methods. Thereafter the relations between the indices given by the various in vitro and the two in vivo methods could be evaluated statistically, by multiple linear regression or other methods, to produce a mathematical equation which will indicate the relationship between the various indices and show which would have the best caries predictive value. By this means it is hoped that one, or perhaps several, of the relatively simple in vitro methods could be used alone, or in combination, to give rapid and reliable indications of how caries conducive foods would be.

SUMMARY

More needs to be known about the caries producing potential of individual foods before information on the frequency of use of foods can be made useful for caries prediction. To obtain the requisite knowledge concerning the wide range of snacks and confections that are available in today's market, it is necessary to have a relatively simple way for obtaining trustworthy assessment of their cariogenicity. It is believe that the most suitable method can be identified by testing the cariogenicity of a series of foods by existing in vitro procedures, such as acid formation, enamel demineralization, food retention, acid formation in plaque, in vitro caries and animal tests, and then determining by statistical means which of these gives results most closely resembling those given by the same foods in the human mouth by two quasi-clinical testing methods.

LITERATURE CITED

1. Fauchard, P. 1746. Le Chirugien Dentiste, Manette, Paris.

2. Miller, W.D. 1898. Microorganisms of the Human Mouth. S.S. White, Philadelphia.

3. Sognnaes, R.F. 1948. Am. J. Dis. Child. 75:792.

4. Toverud, G. 1957. Milbank Mem. Fd. Quarterly Bull. 34:354.

5. Tukeuchi, M. 1960. Bull. Tokyo Dent. Call. 1:58.

6. Gustaffson, B. et al. 1954. Acta Odont. Scand. 11:195.

7. Bibby, B.G. 1975. J. Am. Dent. Assoc. 90:121.

8. Choung, U.B., Bibby, B.G. and Losee, F.L. 1973. J. Dent. Res. 52:504.

9. Bibby, B.G. and Mundorff, S.A. 1975. J. Dent. Res. 54:461.

10. Yaari, et al. 1974. Abst. #609 Proc. Internal Assoc. Dent. Res.

11. McClure, F.J. and Falk, J.E. 1955. J. Nutrition 55:589.

12. Thomson, M.E. and Wills, R.B.H. 1976. Arch Oral Biol. 21:779.

13. Frostell, G. and Baer, P.M. 1971. Acta Odont. Scand. 29:401.

14. Jay, P. 1938. Am. J. Pub. Health 28:759.

15. Osborn, T.W.B. et al. 1937. J. Dent. Res. 16:549.

16. Frostell, G. 1969. Acta Odont. Scand. 27:3.

17. Edgar, M.W. et al. 1975. J. Am. Dent. Assoc. 90:418.

18. Muhlemann, H. et al. 1977. O.R.C.A. Abstracts.

19. Lundquist, C. 1952. Odont Revy. #:Supp. 1.

20. Bibby, B.G. et al. 1951. J. Am. Dent. Assoc. 42:491.

21. Swenander Lanke, L. 1965. Nutrition & Dental Caries. Almquist & Wiksell, Stockholm,

22. Stephan, R.M. 1966. J. Dent. Res. 45:1551.

23. Konig, K.G. 1967. Brit. dent. J. 123:588.

24. Imfeld, T. and Muhleman, H.R. 1977. J. Prev. Dent. 4:8.

25. Koulourides, T. 1976. Caries Res. 10:427.

Discussion of cariogenicity and caries prediction

Simon Katz

Oral Health Research Institute, School of Dentistry, Indiana University, 1121 W. Michigan Street, Indianapolis, Indiana 46202

The message that comes out loud and clear from Dr. Bibby's paper is that concerning diet and caries there is much more that we don't know than there is that we do know. Even what we believe we know, may be questionable. If this is so at a research level, what can be expected at the delivery end of the ladder? How can a clinician attempt to predict dental caries by assessing a patient's diet when research workers don't even know what the cariogenicity of foods depends upon?

While no one will argue that dental caries is a food related disease, or will question the statement that no other variable is as closely related to caries activity in man as food[1]. Although with the possible exception of plaque flora[2-5], perhaps fluorides[6-9] the quality and texture of enamel[10], the flow and composition of saliva[11,12], and God only knows what else, it just might be true.

To emphasize that the assessment of caries activity on the basis of sucrose alone is an over-simplification and a gross one at that.

Until this is clearly understood, it is doubtful that clinicians will look more critically at other possible ways of predicting caries activity. It is also doubtful that dental educators will teach a more realistic approach to diet control for the prevention of dental caries. The traditional position that the cariogenicity of the diet is due to its sugar content[13,14], modified by the adhesiveness of the sugar-containing foods[14], the frequency of ingestion[14,15] and perhaps the time of ingestion[14], may have some merit from a statistical viewpoint. However, it is of little help to the clinician who needs to predict caries activity in a given patient and not in an unidentified and faceless member of a study sample. If we want to provide the clinician with a tool he can use with enough confidence as to warrant his efforts to modify his patients' eating behavior, we must learn a great deal more about the manner in which foods influence dental caries.

Dr. Bibby has pointed out that sucrose is seldom used except as a constituent of foods, and that a number of factors inherent in these foods, and even the manner in which these foods are prepared and the circumstances in which they are ingested are important determinants of their cariogenicity. We have conducted studies with breakfast cereals and other foods which corroborate this view[16,17]. In some cases our results suggest that starchy foods could be as cariogenic or more so than sugar-containing foods[17].

The delusive simplicity of the equation proposed by Dr. Bibby[1] to assess cariogenicity vanishes when one tries to list the components of the second term, i.e., what he calls "index". Perhaps a third term should be added to modify the factor representing frequency by a coefficient expressing the effects of the time at which the cariogenic foods are eaten. But going back to the second term, the "index", it has been traditionally accepted that it comprises such factors as the amount of sugar in the food, adhesiveness of the food, and ability of the food to induce plaque and acid formation by oral micro-organisms. In our studies none of these parameters were correlated with the cariogenic potential of the cereals either in vitro or in animal studies[18-20]. We measured sugar retention on extracted human teeth by having these teeth "chew" mixtures of cereals and milk in an ad hoc chewing machine, and then determining the amount of sugar present in known amounts of distilled water in which the teeth were repeatedly rinsed. We found that sugar retention did not depend upon the sugar content of the cereals (which ranged from 1% to over 40%), but was related to the nature of the cereal and perhaps the manner in which the cereals had been processed. We assessed plaque formation by weighing the amount of plaque accumulated on teeth which, after chewing the cereal-milk mixtures, were incubated with Streptococcus mutans in so called artificial mouths. We assessed in vitro cariogenicity using mouth simulation conditions with teeth which had chewed the cereal-milk mixtures daily. McDonald and Stookey[20] studied the cariogenicity of a variety of these cereals in albino rats. We found that the only characteristic of the cereals which correlated fairly well with their cariogenic potential was their ability to neutralize acids, which for the sake of simplicity we called "buffering capacity"[18,19] We found that some of the cereals released their "buffers" very rapidly when soaked in water. Other cereals retained a large proportion of their buffers even after repeated soakings. Still other cereals were able to release their buffers in a sustained manner through several successive soakings.

Our data suggest that a balance of rapid and sustained release of buffers is necessary to reduce the cariogenic potential of the cereals. It can be hypothesized that a rapid release of buffers is necessary to neutralize the acids formed in the plaque immediately upon ingestion of the cereals, and then a sustained release to protect the teeth throughout the time period the acids may persist in the plaque. At this time this is just a hypothesis, but if it is ever proven correct, then the more adhesive a food with the right balance of buffering characteristics, the greater the caries protection it would provide. The finding by Dr. Bibby's group[21], and our group as well[16,20], that a rather adherent cereal containing more than 20% sugar (Life) was less cariogenic than a cereal which is considerably less adherent, has about 7% sugar and practically no buffering capacity (Corn Flakes) lends support to this hypothesis. Obviously, in this case predicting cariogenicity on the basis of sugar content and adhesiveness would have been tantamount to predicting the wrong way.

Time does not permit presentation in detail of our work suggesting that starchy foods can be as cariogenic as sugary foods, but this is another finding which supports our initial statement that a great deal of knowledge has to be gained before caries prediction on the basis of foods can be successfully attempted. I would like to give another example. A few years ago one of our graduate students found that alkali treated chocolate (so called Dutch chocolate) reduced the growth of, and acid formation by, Strepococcus mutans to a greater extent than American chocolate[22]. He could propose no explanation for his findings. Today we may be tempted to attribute the difference to alkali-soluble components of plant cell walls (including those in cocoa), which we are currently studying[23-28]. These compounds have a remarkable ability to inhibit in vitro plaque formation and, in some instances, acid formation as well. Again, if it can be shown that these plant extracts influence caries formation, then a hitherto unknown manner in which food processing may affect cariogenicity would have come to light.

Dr. Bibby has presented problems related to, and suggested methods for, the assessment of the cariogenic potential of foods. I would like to add that basic studies to unravel the intricacies of the role of foods in caries etiology should be conducted before we can seriously think of predicting caries activity on the basis of foods. This work should comprise, among other things: (1) efforts to determine the role and desirable characteristics of food buffers; (2) the potential effects upon bacterial adherence and glycolytic activity of food components released during processing; (3) the effects of starches upon plaque and caries formation under controlled *in vitro* conditions (if such conditions can ever be obtained); (4) the inter-actions between food components and the balance of the oral flora (not exclusively *Streptococcus mutans*); (5) the inter-action between food components or additives (such as phosphates or trace elements), and cariogenicity; (6) the inter-action between the components of the diet and its overall cariogenicity, etc.

I would like to finish with a few questions. Dr. Bibby proposes his own Orofax method and Dr. Koulourides' method as semi-clinical methods for assessing caries formation. The Orofax is a sophisticated method that measures enamel decalcification. Dr. Koulourides' method measures changes in enamel hardness, again a measure of enamel decalcification. Is it valid to equate clinical caries with enamel dissolution?

From a clinical viewpoint, are we talking of predicting acute (rampant) caries or just average caries, i.e., one or two cavities per year, or are we referring to caries in absolute terms? In this case, how do we define caries? And finally, the most disquieting of my questions is: In view of the many variables which participate in the clinical process of caries formation, will it ever be possible to develop a method to clinically assess the cariogenicity of foods?

LITERATURE CITED

1. Bibby, B.G. 1977. Cariogenicity and caries prediction. Workshop - Conference on Methods of Caries Prediction, Niagara Falls.

2. Orland, R.J., Blayney, R., Harrison, R.W., Reyniers, J.A., Tresler, P.C., Wagner, M., Gordon, H.A. and Luckey, T.D. 1954. The use of the germ free animal technique in the study of experimental dental caries. J. Dent. Res., 33:147.

3. Stephan, R.M. 1953. The dental plaque in relation to the etiology of caries. Int. Dent. J., 4:180.

4. Keyes, P.H. 1960. Infectious and transmissible nature of experimental dental caries - findings and implications. Arch. oral Biol., 1:304.

5. Stiles, H.M., Loesche, W.J., and O'Brien, T.C., Ed. 1976. Microbiological aspects of dental caries (Vols. I, II, and III). Information Retrieval Inc., Washington, D.C. & London.

6. Dean, H.T. 1938. Endemic fluorosis and its relation to dental caries. Public Health Rep., 53:1443.

7. Dean, H.T. 1946. Epidemiological studies in the United States. In dental caries and fluorine, edited by F.R. Moulton. Am. Assoc. Advan. Sci., Washington, D.C.

8. World Health Organization. 1970. Fluorides and human health, W.H.O. Monograph series #59, W.H.O., Geneva.

9. Newbrun, E. 1975. Fluoride and dental caries; Contemporary concepts for practioners and students. Charles C. Thomas, Springfield, Illinois.

10. Katz, S. 1970. Enamel and dental caries. In improving dental practice through preventive measures. 2nd ed., edited by Muhler, J.C. and Bernier, J.C., 4:59 The C.V. Mosby Co., St. Louis.

11. Brown, L.R., Dreizen, S., Handler, S., and Johnston, D.A. 1975. Effect of radiation induced xerostomia on human oral micro-flora. J. Dent Res., 54:740.

12. Ericsson, Y. 1959. Clinical investigation of the salivary buffering action. Acta Odont. Scand., 17:131.

13. Jay, P. 1940. The role of sugar in the etiology of caries. J. Amer. Dent. Assoc., 27:393.

14. Gustafsson, B.E., Quensel, C.E., Lanke, L., Lundquist, C., Grahnen, H., Bonow, B.E., and Krasse, B. 1954. The Vipeholm dental caries study: Effect of different levels of carbohydrate intake on caries activity in 436 individuals observed for five years. Acta Odont. Scand., 11:232.

15. Eeg-Larsen,N. 1965. Caries prevention versus other health and nutrition habits. In Blix, G., ed.: Nutrition and Caries prevention. Swedish Nutrition Foundation, Upsala, pp. 83-94.

16. Katz, S., Olson, B.L., and Park, K.C. 1975. Factors related to the cariogenic potential of breakfast cereals. J. Pharmacol. & Therap. Dent., 2:109.

17. Katz, S., and Park, K.C. Sugar retention and plaque formation on molar teeth after chewing ten different foods. An in vitro study. Unpublished.

18. Katz, S., Olson, B.L., and McDonald, J.L. Jr. 1974. Buffering capacity, sugar retention and cariogenic potential of foods. J. Dent. Res. (Program and Abstracts of Papers) 53 (special issue) :206 Abst. #607.

19. Katz, S., Olson, B.L., and McDonald, J.L. Jr. Buffering behavior, sugar content and cariogenic potential of breakfast cereals. Submitted to J. Pharmacol. Therap. Dent.

20. McDonald, J.L. Jr., and Stookey, G.K. Animal studies concerning the cariogenicity of breadfast cereals. To be published by J. Dent. Res.

21. Choung, U.B., Bibby, B.G., and Losee, F.L. 1973. Some effects of breakfast cereals on caries in rats. J. Dent. Res., 52:504.

22. Liu, K.T. Unpublished data.

23. Katz, S., Park, K.C., and Miller, C.H. 1976. Plaque inhibition by plant cell wall fractions. I.A.D.R. Abst. #827, Miami.

24. Katz, S., Miller, C.H., and Park, K.C. 1976. Plaque inhibition by plant cell wall fractions: Mechanism of action and related factors. I.A.D.R. Abst. #828, Miami.

25. Park, K.C., and Katz, S. 1976. Plaque inhibition by plant cell wall fractions: *In vitro* findings. I.A.D.R. Abst. #829, Miami.

26. Palenik, C.J., Park, K.C., Katz, S., and Stookey, G.K. 1977. Studies of anti-plaque substances derived from cocoa. A.A.D.R. Abst. #272, Las Vegas.

27. Katz, S., Olson, B.L., Park, K.C., and Miller, C.H. 1977. Inhibition of *Streptococcus mutans* plaque formation by modified oat hulls. Submitted to Archs. oral Biol.

28. Katz, S., Park, K.C., and Miller, C.H. 1977. Inhibition of *Streptococcus mutans* plaque formation by alkaline extracts of various plant tissues. Submitted to Archs oral Biol.

MODERATOR'S SUMMARY OF DISCUSSION OF TOPIC III PRESENTATIONS

Dr. Mandel noted that the Bagramian and Russell study of 1975 found no correlation between the frequency of eating sucrose snacks and the number of carious teeth; a finding which the authors thought could be attributed to the fact that sucrose consumption was so high that it obliterated the frequency factor. Dr. Horowitz suggested the failure to show higher caries in users of pre-sweetened cereals could be explained in the same way and should not be interpreted as meaning that such sweetened cereals were more cariogenic than unsweetened cereals.

The importance of collecting dietary data on the frequency of food use was stressed by Dr. Madsen, who was unhappy that the only data that correlates the frequency that patients eat with their caries score is that collected by Weiss and Trithout almost 20 years ago. He felt that information obtained in a searching interview that probed the frequency of use of sugar in medications, antacid chewing gum and laxatives, that are not usually included in a food diary, would be profitable.

Dr. Koulourides pointed out that since caries was a dynamic competition between the forces of demineralization and remineralization, research was needed to classify foods according to their demineralization or remineralization potentials. In respect to the protective effects of foods, Dr. Brudevold suggested the desirability of knowing whether natural foods or eating practices, like eating firm detersive foods at the end of a meal, reduced plaque formation. He felt that if such evidence were forthcoming, dependence on tooth brushing and flossing to remove plaque and food deposits would be lessened.

Dr. Nizel pointed out that the effectiveness of diet counseling was largely dependent upon the patient's personality and behavior. The patient's personality should be classified as rational, rigid or apathetic. His behavior can be determined by finding out when, where, with whom and under what conditions he eats his meals and/or snacks. In other words, to get the desired patient response one has to find out not only 'what' a patient eats but also 'why' he selects certain food and 'why' he eats frequently, in a normal 3 meal pattern or otherwise.

Dr. Mühlemann felt the behavior modification approach, especially with respect to decreasing sweets intake, was too difficult. He suggested that a better approach would be to offer patients food alternatives of lower cariogenicity as indicated by his *in vivo* dental plaque pH telemetry method. While he was not sure that his testing procedure can identify non-cariogenic food items, he was satisfied that foods that do not form significant amounts of acid when they come in contact with the dental plaque would be 'safe' food alternatives.

TOPIC IV

BIOLOGICAL FACTORS AND CARIES PREDICTION

Moderator:

I. Kleinberg
State University of New York
School of Dental Medicine
Stony Brook, New York 11790

Microbial analyses related to caries susceptibility

G.H. Bowden, J.M. Hardie, E.D. Fillery, P.D. Marsh and G.L. Slack

Department of Oral Microbiology and MRC Dental Epidemiology Unit, The London Hospital Medical College, Turner Street, London E1, England

Introduction

The dentist in everyday clinical practice would welcome a reliable test with which to predict caries activity or susceptibility. In the planning of dental care for the individual patient he must at present rely upon a combination of his clinical experience and guesswork. He may know which tooth surfaces are immediately at risk, but he is unable to gauge with accuracy the time, rate, and weight of the caries attack.

It is therefore, important that every method of measurement of caries susceptibility is explored, Hence, the object of this paper is to examine aspects of the microbiology of the mouth which are considered, along with other parameters, as having a possible relationship to caries susceptibility.

Selection of susceptible subjects in diseases involving bacteria is not ususlly based upon microbial detection, but on immunological tests such as the Schick or Mantoux which relate to the potential susceptibility of the subject. Microbiological tests are generally reserved for diagnosis. One of the few examples of prediction by bacterial detection is in meningitis when the numbers of isolations from subjects increases prior to an outbreak of the disease[1].

Is it reasonable, therefore, to expect microbial detection either to predict caries effectively, or to diagnose the disease which already exists? In caries the distinction between prediction and diagnosis is difficult to make. In part this derives from the relative insensitivity of the methods of diagnosis, which can only be made with certainty late in the disease process. Figure 1 shows that prediction and diagnosis could be difficult to separate, although early diagnosis of caries may be an effective screen for a susceptible population.

The proposal that microbiological tests could predict or measure the caries activity of a subject is dependent upon the known involvement of bacteria in the disease process[2,3,4], and as we have seen tests based upon the isolation of specific bacteria Lactobacillus sp. and S. mutans have been employed[5]. In the latter case these organisms are known to have a high cariogenic activity in animals and to be associated with the disease in man[4,6]. The detailed studies on S. mutans involves polymer production[7], adherence[8,9], microbial interaction[10], and metabolic activity[11,12] have served to emphasize the importance of ecological mechanisms in understanding microbial populations.

It is not digressing, therefore, to examine some concepts of ecology and in particular the concept of the ecological niche. This will allow selection of those parameters related to bacterial populations which may be involved in enamel decalcification.

Figure 1.

Prediction and diagnosis of a carious lesion

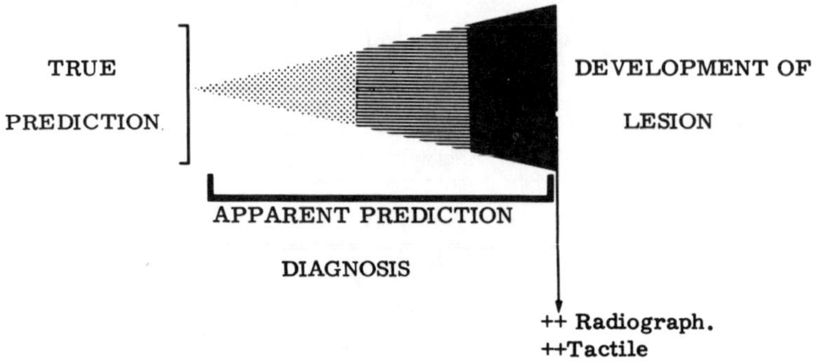

The ecological niche

Ecological considerations applicable to other habitats can be applied to the tooth surface. Within the microbial population of habitat each organism will occupy an ecological niche and the niche occupied will result from its requirements, characteristics and products. Organisms having similar characteristics will compete for the same niche within the population, those which differ in their characteristics will occupy distinct niches without interaction. The concept of a niche set by a variety of parameters has been proposed and ably described by Hutchinson[13]. Organisms may occupy a 'principal niche' which infers lack of reactivity with other bacteria, or a 'realised niche' which results from interrelationships with other members of the population. Figure 2 shows possible niches set by three simple parameters, oxidation/reduction levels, presence of carbohydrate and presence of lactate. In this figure Actinomyces and Streptococcus might be expected to occupy relatively large niches and be in competition. Less competition might occur between Veillonella and Neisseria. Examples of competition for niches are quoted by Hutchinson and one, in particular refers to a small animal, the Pocket Gopher. In this instance, one species of gopher (G. Bursarius) can compete successfully with others under ideal conditions. However, the other species are capable of living in a wider niche, and thus, survive in poorer terrain. So, despite the ability of G. Bursarius to exclude others from a habitat, its niche is circumscribed by the need for optimum conditions. Do these types of relationships operate in dental plaque?

In order to answer this question even in the most general way, it is necessary to have a detailed knowledge of the microbiology of plaque. However, it is essential when looking at the results of all examinations of plaque that the severe limitations of the methods are appreciated[14]. Among the best documented plaque composition is that of the approximal area in children[15-17]. Most of the data quoted here on composition, with the exception of that on plaque development will be based on approximal samples, it must be recognized that tooth fissure, a different habitat, may support a different population[18].

Plaque population and ecology

The development of plaque on a tooth surface provides some evidence that organisms occupy distinct ecological niches in plaque and are able to establish at various times [8,14,19-22]. The concept of bacterial local-

Figure 2.

Ecological niches set by three vectors

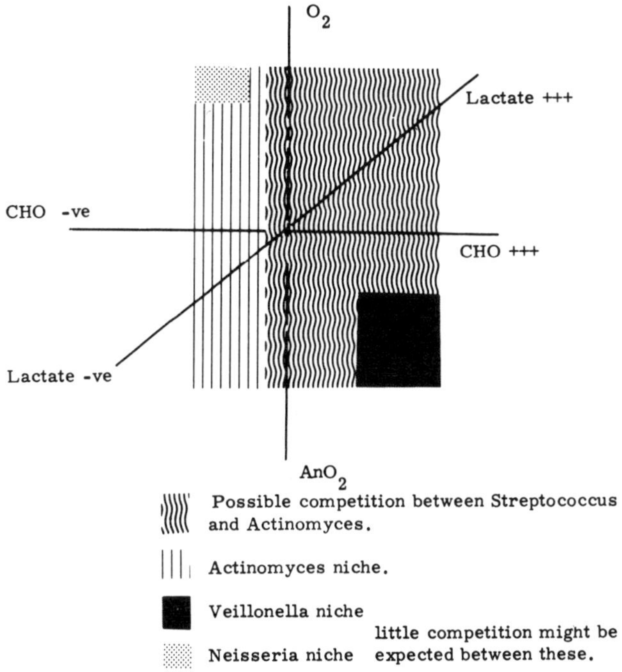

isation on surfaces in the mouth as a result of surface interactions has been recognised as a significant mechanism of oral ecology[23,24]. However, it may be important to differentiate between initial localisation at the tooth surface and the subsequent increase in the bacterial population.

The concept of a 'Basic Plaque'

Organisms which are efficient colonisers of the tooth surface would be expected to be, a) present in 100% of all samples from a site, and b) found in relatively high numbers. Examination of approximal samples in man[16,17], shows that some genera would fall into this category, these are Streptococcus Actinomyces, Veillonella, and perhaps Bacteroides. Species showing this type of distribution include S. sanguis, A. viscosus, A. naeslundii, and V. alcalescens, (Table 1).

Table 1. Quantitive data for some organisms present in approximal plaque

Organisms	Isolation frequency(n60)	Mean[a)]	Modal Range[b)]	Range
Actinomyces	100	49.9	47-58	0.9-86.0
Streptococci	100	14.0	12-16	0.04-61.0
G-ve Rods (AnO2)	98.0	17.0	0-2	0-76.0
Veillonella	98.0	12.0	1-3	0-47.0
S. sanguis	95.0	5.8	0-0.6	0-51.0
S. mutans	62.0	1.8	0	0-13.0
Lactobacilli	47.0	0.2	0	0-1.8
Bacterionema	23.0	0.2	0	0-0.7

a) Expressed as a percentage of the total anaerobic viable count.
b) Closest range to include 25% of the values.

These organisms might be regarded as components of a 'basic plaque' in man. Further indication of the role of Actinomyces and Streptococcus as part of a 'basic plaque' in animals and man can be found by examinations of animal plaque[25,26]. These genera persist in a wide variety of animals (Table 2) and Actinomyces in particular seem to be specifically oral organisms limited to the mouth as a habitat[27,28].

Table 2. Qualitative Composition of Animal Plaque

Animal Species	Action.	Strep.	Veill.	Lacto.	Roth.	B'rema.	Cor'bact.	Sang.	Mutans
Man	+	+	+	+	+	+	-	+	+
Gorilla	+	+	?	-	-	-	-	+	-
Patas Monkey	+	+	+	+	-	+	-	+	+
Spider Monkey	+	+	?	-	-	-	-	+	-
Orang Utan.	+	+	?	-	-	-	+	+	-
Baboon	+	+	?	-	-	-	-	+	-
Marmoset	+	+	+	+	-	-	+	+	+
Slow Loris	+	+	?	-	+	-	-	+	-
Tamarin	+	+	?	-	+	+	-	+	-
Kangaroo	+	+	?	-	-	-	+	-	-
Wallaby	+	+	?	-	-	-	+	-	-
Deer	+	+	?	-	-	-	+	-	-
Bear	+	+	?	+	-	-	-	-	-
Yak	+	+	?	?	-	-	-	-	-
Llama	+	+	?	?	-	-	-	-	-
Spiny Tenrec	?	+	?	?	-	-	-	-	+
Fruit Bat	+	+	+	?	-	-	-	+	+

? = Data not yet available

The composition of plaque is determined by environmental pressures on the organisms and a population equilibrium may never be reached. These conditions will, a) select the species which will grow from the 'basic plaque' e.g. the presence of S. sanguis and S. mutans in the fruit bat could be the result of diet, or b) allow specific bacteria which are less commonly encountered e.g. Lactobacillus, B. meleninogenicus to compete effectively for a niche.

Examination of sequential samples of plaque from approximal areas shows examples of this selection, where a particular species will consistently be found in high numbers[16,17].

Thus, the microbial population of plaque can be related to the environmental conditions of the habitat and changes in these conditions would introduce changes in the microflora. The metabolic activities of plaque would be a direct result of the relationship between the microbial population and the environment, and this activity might lead to the development of a carious lesion. A series of interrelated factors can be proposed to express the microbial population and metabolic activity of plaque, Figure 3.

Prediction of cariogenic potential of plaque

In Figure 3, four areas p1, p2, p3 and p4 are delineated, this subdivision is made to simplify the discussion of those parameters which might be related to caries. Moreover, it should be recognised that the development of a lesion may be an intermittent process, and that the earliest decalcification which is detected by x-ray may reverse. This adds to an already complex situation and serves to emphasise the need to examine many of the characteristics associated with the tooth surface in relation to caries. The consideration of several parameters will be made later as it is

FIGURE 3

Factors involved in determining the population and metabolic expression of dental plaque

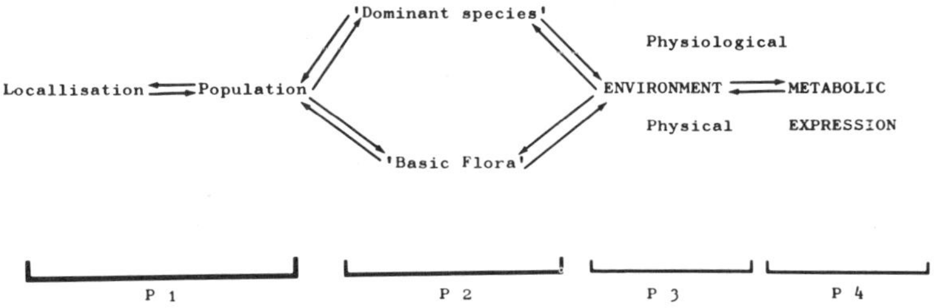

unlikely that any tests limited to a single parameter, be it microbiological or environmental will accurately predict caries susceptibility.

Area P1: The measurement of the numbers of specific organisms in saliva which are thought to be involved in caries has been used as an index of caries activity or susceptibility for several years[5]. The levels of organisms may indicate their degree of colonisation and effective establishment in the mouth and therefore, give a general picture of the oral population.

This type of test is still used and considered valuable in the selection of groups at risk and in dietary control[31,32]. Lactobacillus or S. mutans are usually counted and recently S.mutans has been shown to be related to incipient lesions while lactobacilli showed a relationship to all lesions[31]. One observation which could be made is that the strains of lactobacilli are not identified to species level. Thus, with S. mutans a species is related to the occurrence of caries while the lactobacilli represents a genus. More precision in prediction might be obtained by identifying the Lactobacillus species.

Little modification of the microbial examinations of saliva can be proposed, except to suggest that other organisms could be counted in conjunction with S. mutans and Lactobacillus. Veilonella[10,16,17,35] and A. israelii[35,36] have been associated with carious lesions. A. odontolyticus[33] was originally isolated from carious dentine, but recent studies did not confirm this[34]. Media for such examinations are available[16,37-40] and recently broth media have been developed to determine S. mutans levels[41,42].

Although these tests only provide general observations, they may be among the best that are available at this time, when one considers their ease of application and simplicity. However, their very nature, that is taking saliva as a representative of plaque composition means that their accuracy is unlikely to be increased.

Area P2: Measurement of pooled plaque for specific bacteria, as an indication of caries activity and susceptibility was a logical extension of the examination of saliva. As with saliva however, the results give only a general indication of the levels of organisms in plaque, individual site variations are obliterated[16]. Again, the test is of some value as a group indicator when S. mutans is taken as the specific organism[29,34]. Swenson et al[29] used pooled samples from approximal areas of the first permanent molars to assay for S. mutans. They found that 90% of the children who experienced caries during the two years of the survey had a level of greater than 1% S. mutans in the initial sample. However, the predictive value of a negative test was poor and had little use in selecting low risk subjects. This study highlights two important points, a) samples from known susceptible areas may be suitable as overall indicators of disease, b) the accuracy of the test could be improved by considering other parameters e.g. the data for lactobacilli. Thus, tests of susceptibility could use samples from well defined susceptible areas examined for a range of bacteria together with other parameters e.g. local environmental conditions, diet, and the buffer capacity of saliva.

This leads to the consideration of the microbiology of individual sites known to be highly susceptible to caries. Careful sampling coupled with reasonably detailed bacteriology can be carried out on a field basis[16, 17], and it is possible to assay for the 'basic plaque' components and to monitor the development of any 'dominant species'. However, both occlusal and approximal surfaces are difficult to sample and sequential samples from well defined areas are important in demonstrating the stability and persistence of the bacterial population[16,17]. In addition to this, bacteria may be present on limited areas of the tooth surface and, as Van Houte[8] points out, S. mutans can be localised at 'white spot' lesions. It follows from this that: a) Bacteria may be missed by sampling method, b) They may be inaccurately assessed in terms of their concentration in the sample area. It might be proposed that there is an 'eclipse' phase when the organism enters the decalcified lesion and cannot be detected in plaque samples. If such a phenomenon occurs an organism might only be isolated when and if it increased to a level to grow into plaque overlying a lesion. Loesche and Syed[15] have detected S. mutans in plaque overlying lesions, but the lesions were extensive and may have differed from enamel decalcification. Despite these problems, when an organism is isolated from sequential samples in relatively high numbers it is likely that it has become established at a site. The results of the examination of a sample for specific organisms can show therefore,

a)	Not present	The organism may be absent, not having localised at the tooth surface, it may have been unable to compete for a niche or have been missed in sampling.
b)	Present	The organism localised and grew to a detectable level. Teh level indicates the state of the population at the time of sampling.
c)	Present in significant or relatively high numbers	The organism localised and competed effectively with other members of the population.

In c) S. mutans[16,17], lactobacilli[47] and A. israelii[35,36] are examples of organisms where increases in the population of a site may be associated with caries, Localisation of S. mutans has been demonstrated by several workers[16,17,44-47], and it seems reasonable to suggest that if S. mutans is present as a significant part of the population, its potential activity may be similar to that in experimental animals given suitable environmental conditions. The converse does not hold however. Transient increases in numbers may not be significant, although the period of active growth of the organism necessary to achieve a high level in the population may be important. The levels of other organisms such as Veillonells[10,17, 35] may indicate the metabolic activity in the sample in relation to lactate. High levels of Veillonella have been proposed by Orstavik and Brandzaeg[48] to be a possible cause of the significant negative correlation between serum antibody levels and DMF. Neisseri[49], Bacterionema[50], and Eubacterium[51] also metabolize lactate, but in the first two cases the numbers in the plaque are low and there is little information on the presence of E. alactolyticum in plaque. Strains of this organism have been isolated from carious dentine[34]. The role of other specific bacteria which may reflect the potential metabolic activity of plaque has received little attention.

In b) there is no reason to suppose that a population of organisms in the absence of S. mutans would not be able to decalcify enamel if the conditions permit. Microbiological selection of 'cariogenic plaque' in this case is an exceptionally difficult task as the metabolic activity of plaque is not solely dependent upon the population, but is related to the environment. Analysis of the 'basic plaque' population could be considered as a first stage towards the understanding of plaque metabolism in these cases. The organisms analysed should include Actinomyces viscosus/naeslundii, Actinomyces israelii, Veillonella, Streptococcus mutans, Streptococcus sanguis, Streptococcus mitior, Lactobacillus species and Bacteroides. Selective media are available for most of these organisms[16, 37-41,52,53], and such monitoring might also be undertaken using fluorescence antibody techniques[54]. Together with estimations of the bacterial flora specific characteristics of the organisms which may aid in the effective extension of their population may be detected. Characteristics of this type (e.g. bacteriocin production) will be mentioned in a later paper at this meeting. Environmental conditions which can promote successful growth of an organism in a mixed population can be examined in chemostat[70]. Preliminary results indicate that an increase of dilution rate from 0.5 to 0.2 allows organisms resembling S. sanguis to compete successfully in a mixed population of oral organisms (Ellwood, Bowden and Hunter, unpublished). Thus, the local environment may 'trigger' the increase in population of a specific organism.

Bacteriological examinations of plaque populations provide data which can be included with other non-microbiological parameters in the measurement of susceptibility e.g. a) increase in numbers of a specific organism beyond a 'threshold'

i. S. mutans may aid positive prediction of a lesion.
ii. Lactobacillus may indicate a lesion.
iii. A. israelii may indicate a lesion.
iv. Veillonella - High Veillonella may count against lesion formation.

b) relatively stable population.

The activities of this type of population can only be measured in terms of metabolic expression, see p4. This is an area where more basic research is required.

An important aspect of the possibility of prediction in a) is the setting of a threshold level. Detection of S. mutans for example in approximal areas[16,17,50], or fissures[18,55] does not lead to the production of a lesion in all cases. This is to be expected if the metabolic expression is not entirely dependent upon the bacterial population.

Area P3: The local environment includes factors which contribute to the microbial composition of plaque. The role of saliva in colonisation has been discussed by Van Houte[8], and reduction of saliva flow as a result of irradiation causes changes in the microflora of pooled plaque[31,56,57], although these changes are related to sucrose.

In a recent review Bibby[58] has given details of the evidence for a relationship between diet and plaque microflora. He concluded 'that transient contact with human foods was unlikely to modify the bacterial population in more than the superficial layers of micro-organisms'. When one considers a 'basic plaque' flora found in both man and animals, it is likely that it will be relatively unaffected by dietary changes. However, substrate could control those species of the basic genera which will compete for a niche and modify the environment to produce a unique niche. Bibby[58] suggests that carbohydrate produces a low pH which favours aciduric organisms; this is probably so, but it is not known how sensitive the plaque population in defined areas is to substrate changes. General changes in the oral microflora e.g. increase in lactobacilli[31,32], may indicate a high carbohydrate intake, which relates to a high caries incidence. Measurements of the effect of a local application of substrates for periods of time on the plaque of defined areas would show whether prolonged exposure was necessary to modify the flora. It could also be seen if plaque subjected to a particular substrate always developed in the same way. Examinations of this type on the general effect of carbohydrate on plaque have been made[59,60]. Studies on other substrates with better defined samples and more comprehensive bacteriology are now indicated. These techniques could show whether specific bacterial components in plaque were related to the substrates available.

Area P4: The metabolic expression of plaque represents the final stage of the relationship between flora, environment and substrate and as substrate and environment vary, so might the metabolic products. Thus, plaque of a given microbial population may give different products and plaque of differing microbial population similar products. Demonstration of variation in metabolic products with changes in the environment has been made in chemostat studies on streptococci[61]. There is no knowledge of the relationship between the microbial population and metabolic products in man. Considering such well studied materials as volatile and non-volatile acids[62] we cannot be certain that even large differences in plaque composition will be reflected in the acid profiles. That such variations may exist has been shown by Gilmour *et al*[62] who detected differences between the acids in plaque samples, although these could be ascribed to substrate limitations.

It would seem reasonable that in caries prediction tests some assessment of metabolic activity must be considered in conjunction with the microbial composition. This could be undertaken by measuring the products and substrates in the field phase of well defined areas of plaque. Such studies could reveal, any relationship between *Veillonella* and lactate metabolism, or a specific flora associated with base production[64]. Experimental animal studies along these lines have been made and Minah and Loesche[65] have provided a basis for the examination of human plaque samples. It is essential that such studies are made on plaque *'in vivo'* however, as samples examined *'in vitro'* may reflect the activities of those organisms capable of metabolic activity in the test system. Methods for the determination of acids in small plaque samples are available[62,63], and standard methods for assay of glucose and amino acids are sensitive enough for use.

Such complex tests would be too involved to carry out as a routine clinical measure, but they would provide a basis for the development of more simple tests. One test which could be of immediate value in the field is treatment of the sample with fluorescein labelled acetate. The uptake of this material by bacteria is said to be related to their viability and metabolic activity[66]. This may have some value as a simple estimate of the metabolic activity of a sample by showing the ratio of stained to unstained organisms in a plaque sample.

Possibilities for Microbial Prediction of Caries

The above sections have outlined those microbial parameters which may be related to caries prediction. Some of the tests have been used and their value is well known, others may appear complex, but it would be incorrect to exclude an assay of potential value because it could not be immediately employed in field use. Table 3 summarizes those microbial parameters which could be of some predictive value.

Table 3

Microbial Parameters to be considered in conjunction with others as indicators of caries susceptibility

Sample	Organism	Possible Interpretation
Saliva	S. mutans Lactobacillus sp.[1]	High levels may indicate: 1) High caries risk 2) High carbohydrate consumption 3) Low saliva flow/buffer
	Veillonella	High levels may indicate: 1) Reduced caries risk Low levels may indicate: 1) Low lactate production 2) Reduced capacity to metabolise lactate
Pooled plaque - The results of the examination of pooled plaque can be considered in the same way as those of saliva.		
Sequential samples of plaque from defined susceptible areas	S. mutans	High levels may indicate: 1) High caries risk at site 2) Presence of a lesion 3) Site subjected to high carbohydrate levels
	Lactobacilli	High levels may indicate: 1) Presence of advanced lesion 2) Area of relatively low pH
	Veillonella	High levels may indicate: 1) High capacity to metabolise lactate 2) Reduced caries risk at site Low levels may indicate: 1) Low lactate production 2) Reduced capacity to metabolise lactate
	A. israelii	High levels may indicate: 1) A lesion
	Stable 'basic plaque' [2]	1) Plaque population has been exposed to a stable environment 2) Cariogenicity will depend upon the local conditions of the sample area
	Unstable plaque population[2]	1) Environmental conditions are fluctuating

1) Strains of Lactobacillus should be identified to species level.
2) Basic research is necessary on the relationship of plaque populations to local environment.

Considerations of Several Parameters

From the foregoing it can be seen that the use of a single microbiological parameter is unlikely to provide an accurate measure of caries susceptibility in the individual. Even with well characterized infections the factors which influence the outcome are many[67]. In those cases where assay of a single organism shows some relationship to caries (S. mutans, lactobacilli) they probably are so because the presence of the organism at a detectable level reflects other parameters (carbohydrate consumption, acidicity in plaque, saliva flow, buffer capacity) related to caries.

Therefore, to establish any accuracy in prediction many parameters should be considered and then those most significant to the prediction required selected. This type of analysis has been made by Gyllenberg et al[68] on market milk, when those parameters most related to the keeping qualities were selected. Gyllenberg et al[68] stated 'Accordingly, the conclusion may be drawn that the predisposition for rapid spoilage is rather a result of the simultaneous occurence of several potentially deteriorative organisms than the predominance of only one specific organism'. Caries is a multifactorial disease which might lend itself to this type of analysis. Indeed, we would be isolating those parameters which influenced the microbial population niches to produce a 'cariogenic'

Accordingly a preliminary attempt has been made to obtain a cluster of samples from carious sites by constructing a similarity matrix of seventy-two samples of approximal plaques from children[16]. (Fillery, Bowden, Marsh, and Hardie, unpublished). The characters coded for each sample included numbers and types of organisms, the increase or decrease of each organism in sequential samples, gingival state, radiographic data, racial origin, sex, school, area and local physical condition of the sample area. No definite clusters were produced and samples from lesions seemed to show a random distribution. However, samples from sites which only developed lesions after four sequential samples had been taken clustered closely together. This could suggest a stable situation in terms of population before a lesion develops. Although these early results were not immediately successful in providing clusters of carious samples, they indicate that the technique could be of use in measuring similarities between plaque samples. Data on substrate availability, salivary characteristics metabolic potential and products were absent from the initial analysis, these important parameters should be included. The possibilities for use of this type of analysis are well described by Sneath and Sokal[69].

Attempts to diagnose or predict must be based upon accurate information derived from carefully selected and therefore, relevant parameters. Methods and systems to obtain the information are, in the main, available and prediction of caries susceptibility based upon more than one parameter has been made[29,31,32].

The stimulating paper by Stewart [68] in The Lancet makes it clear that disease is not the inevitable outcome of infection and supports the concept proposed here that many parameters should be considered in relation to susceptibility.

LITERATURE CITED

1. Wilson, G.S. and Miles, A.A. 1975. Topley and Wilsons Principles of Bacteriology, Virology and Immunity, 6th Edition. 2:1882-1885, Edward Arnold, London.

2. Keyes, P.H. 1960. The infectious and transmissible nature of experimental dental caries. Archs. oral Biol. 1:304-320.

3. Fitzgerald, R.J. and Keyes, P.H. 1960. Demonstration of the etiologic role of streptococci in experimental caries in the hamster. Amer. Dent. Assoc. 61:9-19.

4. Gibbons, R.J. and van Houte, J. 1975. Dental Caries. Ann. Rev. Med. 26:121-136.

5. Ellen, R.P. 1976. Microbiological Assays for dental caries and periodontal disease susceptibility. Oral Sciences Rev. 8:3-23.

6. Session IV. 1976. Proceedings 'Microbial Aspects of Dental Caries' Eds. Stiles, Loesche and O'Brien. Sp. Supp. Microbiology Abstracts 185-246.

7. Newbrun, E. 1976. Polysaccharide synthesis in plaque. Proceedings 'Microbial Aspects of Dental Caries'. Ed. Stiles, 649-664.

8. van Houte, J. 1976. Oral bacterial colonisation: mechanica and implications. Proceedings 'Microbial Aspects of Dental Caries'. Ed. Stiles, 3-32

9. Rolla, G. 1976. Inhibition of adsorption - general considerations. Proceedings "microbial Aspects of Dental Caries'. Ed Stiles, 309-324.

10. Mikx, F.H.M., van der Hoeven, J.S. and Walker, G.J. 1976. Microbial symbiosis in dental plaque studied in gnotobiotic rats and in the chemostat. Proceedings 'Microbial Aspects of Dental Caries'. Ed. Stiles, 763-772.

11. Wittenberger, C.L. and Crow, V.L. 1976. Regulation of carbon flow within and between metabolic pathways in certain species of Streptococcus. Proceedings, 'Microbial Aspects of Dental Caries'. Ed. Stiles, 617-630.

12. Hamilton, I.R. 1976. Intracellular polysaccharide synthesis by cariogenic micro-organisms. Proceedings, 'Microbial Aspects of Dental Caries'. Ed. Stiles, 683-702.

13. Hutchinson, G.E. 1965. The Ecological Theater and the Evolutionary play! Chap. 2. The Niche: an abstractly inhabited hyper volume. Yale University Press. New Haven.

14, Hardie, J.M. and Bowden, G.H. 1976. The microbial flora of dental plaque: bacterial succession and isolation considerations. Proceedings 'Microbial Aspects of Dental Caries'. Ed. Stiles, 63-87.

15. Loesche, W.J. and Syed, S.A. 1973. The predominant cultivable flora of carious plaque and carious dentine. Caries Res. 7:201-216.

16. Bowden, G.H., Hardie, J.M. and Slack, G.L. 1975. Microbial variations in approximal dental plaque. Caries Res. 9:253-277.

17. Bowden, G.H., Hardie, J.M., McKee, A.A.S., Marsh, P.D., Fillery, E.D. and Slack, G.L. 1976. The microflora associated with developing carious lesions of the distal surfaces on the upper first premolars in 13-14 year old children. Proceedings, 'Microbial Aspects of Dental Caries'. Ed. Stiles, 223-241.

18. Fejerskov, O., Theilade, E., Karring, T., and Theilade, J. 1977. Plaque and caries development in experimental human fissures. Structural and Microbiological Features. J. dent. Res. Special Issue A, 157.

19. Howell, A. Jr., Rizzo, A. and Paul, F. 1965. Cultivable bacteria in developing and mature human dental calculus. Archs. oral Biol. 10:307-313.

20. Ritz, H.L. 1967. Microbial population shifts in developing human dental plaque. Archs. oral Biol. 12:1561-1568.

21. Slack, G.L. and Bowden, G.H. 1965. Preliminary studies of experimental dental plaque 'in vivo'. Adv. in fluorine Research and Dental Caries. Prevention. 3:193-215.

22. Socransky, S.S., Manganiello, A.D., Propas, D., Oram, V. and van Houte, J. 1977. Bacteriological studies of developing supragingival plaque. J. Periodontal Res. 12:90-196.

23. Gibbons, R.J. and van Houte, J. 1975. Bacterial adherence in oral microbial ecology. Ann. Rev. of Micro 29:19-44.

24. Gibbons, R.J., Spinell, D.M. and Skobe, Z. 1976. Selective adherence as a determinant of the host tropisms of certain indigenous and pathogenic bacteria. Inf. Imm. 13:238-246.

25. Dent, V.E., Hardie, J.M. and Bowden, G.H. 1976. A preliminary study of dental plaque on animal teeth. J. Dent. Res. Special Issue D, 127.

26. Brown, L.R., Handler, S., Allen, S.S., Shea, C., Wheatcroft, M.G. and Frome, W.J. 1973. Oral microbial flora of the Marmoset. J. dent. Res. 52:815-822.

27. Bowden, G.H. and Hardie, J.M. 1973. Commensal and pathogenic actinomyces species in man 'Actinomycetaceae Characteristics and Practical Importance'. Ed. Sykes and Skinner. Soc. App. Bact. Symposium No. 2. Academic Press, London.

28. Slack, J.M. and Gerencser, M.A. 1975. Actinomyces, filamentous bacteria, biology and Pathogenicity. Burgess Publishing Co., Minneapolis, Minnesota.

29. Swenson, J.I., Liljemark, W.F. and Schuman, L.M. 1976. A longitudinal epidemiologic evaluation of the association between the detection of plaque streptococci and development of dental caries in children. Proceedings 'Microbial Aspects of Dental Caries'. Ed. Stiles, 211-222.

30. Svanberg, M. and Loesche, W.J. 1977. Salivary concentrations of S. mutans and S. sanguis and the colonisation of artificial fissures in humans by these organisms. J. dent. Res. Special Issue A, 455.

31. Klock, B. and Krasse, B. 1977. Microbial and salivary correlations in 9-12 year old children. Scand. J. Dent. Res. 85:56-63.

32. Krasse, B. 1976. Approaches to Prevention. Proceedings 'Microbial Aspects of Dental Caries'. Ed. Stiles, 867-876.

33. Batty, I. 1958. Actinomyces odontolyticus a new species of actinomycete, regularly isolated from carious dentine. J. Pathol. Bacteriol. 75:455-459.

34. Edwardsson, S. 1974. Bacteriological studies on deep areas of carious dentine. Odont. Revy. Supp. 32:25.

35. van Palenstem-Helderman, W.H., Sampaio Camorgo, P. and de Stoppelaar, J.D. 1977. The bacterial composition of plaque in caries-free and caries-active military recruits. Abst. Caries Res. 11:119.

36. Howell, A. Jr., Stephan, R.N. and Paul, F. 1962. Prevalence of Actinomyces israelii, A. naeslundii, Bacterionema matruchotii, and Candida albicans in selected areas of the oral cavity and saliva. J. dent. Res. 41:1050-1059.

37. Rogosa, M. 1956. A selective medium for the isolation and enumeration of the Veillonella from the oral cavity. J. Bact. 72:533-536.

38. Korman, K.S. and Loesche, W.J. 1977. A selective medium for the isolation of Actinomyces viscosus and Actinomyces naeslundii from dental plaque. J. dent. Res. Special Issue B, 56:221.

39. Ellen, R.B. and Balcerzak-Raczkowski, J.B. 1975. Differential medium for detecting dental plaque bacteria resembling Actinomyces viscosus and Actinomyces naeslundii. J.clin.Microbiol.2:305-310.

40. Beighton, D. and Colman, G. 1976. A medium for the isolation of enumeration of oral Actinomycetaceae from dental plaque. J. Dent. Res. 55:875-878.

41. Loesche, W.J. and Bhat, M. 1976. Evaluation of diagnostic broths for Streptococcus mutans. Proceedings, 'Microbial Aspects of Dental Caries'. Ed. Stiles, 291-301.

42. Loesche, W.J. and Straffon, L.H. 1977. Longitudinal studies of Streptococcus mutans colonisation of human caries-free fissures. J. Dent. Res. Special Issue B. 56. 356.

43. Loesche,W.J.,Rowan,J., Straffon, L.H. and Loos, P.J. 1975. Association of Streptococcus mutans with human dental decay. Inf. and Imm. 11:1252-1260.

44. Gibbons, R.J., DePaola, P.F., Spinell, D.M. and Skobe, Z. 1974. Interdental localisation of Streptococcus mutans as related to dental caries experience. Inf. and Imm. 9:481-488.

45. Ikeda, T., Sandham, H.J. and Bradley, E.L. Jr. 1973. Changes in Streptococcus mutans and lactobacilli in plaque in relation to the initiation of dental caries in negro children. Archs. oral Biol. 18:555-566.

46. Mikkelsen, L. and Poulsen, S. 1976. Microbiological studies on plaque in relation to development of dental caries in man. Caries Res. 10:178-188.

47. Hardie, J.M., Thomson, P.L., South, R.J., Marsh, P.D., Bowden, G.H., McKee, A.S., Fillery, E.D. and Slack, G.L. 1977. A longitudinal epidemiological study on dental plaque and the development of dental caries - interim results after 2 years. International Conference on Oral Biology, Copenhagen. (in press).

48. Orstavik, D. and Brandtzaeg, P. 1977. Serum antibodies to plaque bacteria in subjects with dental caries and gingivitis. Scand. J. Dent. Res. 85:106-113.

49. Hoshino, E., Yamada, T. and Arata, S. 1976. Lactate degradation by strain of Neisseria isolated from human dental plaque. Archs. oral Biol. 21:677-683.

50. Iwami, Y., Higuchi, M., Yamada, T. and Araya, S. 1972. Degradation of lactate by Bacterionema matruchotii under arobic and anaerobic conditions. J. Dent. Res. 51:1683.

51. Holdeman, L.V. and Moore, W.E.C. 1972. Anaerobe laboratory manual. Anaerobe laboratory, Virginia Polytechnique Institute and State University, Blackburg, Va. p. 43.

52. Emilson, C.G. and Brathall, D. 1976. Growth of Streptococcus mutans on various selective media. J. Clin. Micro. 4:95-98.

53. Rogosa, M., Mitchell, J.A. and Wiseman, R.F. 1951. A selective medium for the isolation and enumeration of oral bactobacilli. J. Dent. Res. 30:682-689.

54. Identification of Cariogenic Bacteria by fluorescent antibody and other techniques. Ed. Bleiweis. 1976. J. Dent. Res. 55 Special Issue A.

55. Loesche, W.J. and Straffon, L.H. 1977. Longitudinal studies of Streptococcus mutans colonisation of human caries-free fissures. J. Dent. Res. 56, Special Issue B.

56. Brown, L.R., Dreizen, S. and Handler, S. 1976. Effects of selected caries preventive regimens on microbial changes following irradiation induced xerostomia in cancer patients. Proceedings 'Microbial Aspects of Dental Caries'. Ed. Stiles, 275-290.

57. Dreizen, S. and Brown, L.R. 1976. Xerostomia and dental caries. Proceedings 'Microbial Aspects of Dental Caries'. Ed. Stiles, 263-273.

58. Bibby, B.G. 1976. Influence of diet on the bacterial composition of plaques. Proceedings 'Microbial Aspects of Dental Caries'. Ed. Stiles, 477-490.

59. Carlsson, J. and Egelberg, J. 1965. Effect of diet on early plaque formation in man. Odont. Revy. 16:112-125.

60. Carlsson, J. and Suncstrom, B. 1968. Variations in composition of early dental plaque following ingestion of sucrose and glucose. Odont. Revy. 19:161-169.

61. Ellwood, D.C. 1976. Chemostat studies of oral bacteria. Proceedings 'Microbial Aspects of Dental Caries'. Ed. Stiles, 785-798.

62. Gilmour, M.N., Green, G.C., Zahn, L.M., Sparmann, C.D. and Pearlman, J. 1976. The C1 - C4 monocarboylic and lactic acids in dental plaques before and after exposure to sucrose 'in vivo'. Proceedings 'Microbial Aspects of Dental Caries'. Ed. Stiles, 539-556.

63. Dellebarre, C.W., Franken, H.C.M., Camp, P.J.M. and van der Hoeven, J.S. 1977. Determination of organic acids in dental plaque by isotachophoresis. J. Dent. Res. 56 Special Issue A, 121.

64. Kleinberg, I., Kanapka, J.A. and Craw, D. 1976. Proceedings, 'Microbial Aspects of Dental Caries'. Ed. Stiles, 433-464.

65. Minah, G.E. and Loesche, W.J. 1976. Development of methods to analyse sucrose metabolism by small dental plaque suspensions. Proceedings 'Microbial Aspects of Dental Caries'. Ed. Stiles, 491-520.

66. Ziegler, C.B., Ziegler, E. and Witzenhausen, R. 1975. Nachweis der stoffwechselaktivitat von microorganismen durch vital-fluorochromierung mit 3'-6' Diacetyl fluorescein. Zbl. Bakt. Hyg. 1 Abt. Orig. A. 330:252-264.

67. Stewart, G.T. 1968. Dogma Disputed: Limitations of the Germ Theory. Lancet 1:1077-1081.

68. Gyllenberg, H., Eklund, E., Carberg, G., Autilla, M. and Vartiovaara, V. 1963. Contamination and deterioration of market mild V_1. Application of taxometrics in order to evaluate relationship between microbiological characteristics and keeping quality of market milk. Acta Agr. Scand. 13:177-194.

69. Sneath, PHA. and Sokal, P.R. 1973. Numerical Taxonomy. Freeman and Company, San Francisco.

70. Harder, W., Kuenen, J.G. and Matin, A. 1977. Microbial Selection in Continuous Culture. J. App. Bact. 43:1-24.

Discussion of microbial analyses related to caries susceptibility

H.V. Jordan

Forsyth Dental Center, 140 The Fenway, Boston, Massachusetts 02115

It is generally agreed that available caries predictive tests are limited because they do not sufficiently account for the complex etiology of dental caries[1,2,3,4]. These tests have been over-simplified at 2 different levels. The primary level involves the well-known triad of host, diet and microflora. The secondary level involves the numerous factors that combine to make up each of these 3 main components. This is the level that concerns us in the present discussion - specifically the mixed bacterial flora that may interact in the course of caries development. In his discussion of this problem, Dr. Bowden has pointed out some possibilities for recording populations of other microorganisms in addition to the usual assays of lactobacilli and Streptococcus mutans. These additional types would be selected on the basis of their suspected involvement in various phases of the plaque ecology. Included would be other acidogenic organisms as well as organisms like the Actinomyces that have been reported to show an association with caries in epidemiological surveys. Another possibility would be organisms such as lactate-utilizing Veillonella that might show a negative correlation and thus be indicative of a non-cariogenic condition. This approach could help to extend the utility of existing tests; however, it eventually comes into conflict with the standard admonishment that a caries predictive test must be cheap, simple to perform, and easy to evaluate if it is to find widespread use in dental practice[5,6,7]. With presently available media and techniques, these surveys would require the services of a trained microbiologist using special equipment and thus, may not be applicable to general use. However, they could be employed in special research situations. For general use, there is a great need for the development of additional simplified techniques such as the dip-slide method for recording salivary lactobacillus populations described by Larmas[7].

It has been suggested that assays of lactobacilli and Strep. mutans in combination could serve as improved indices of caries activity. A study by Swenson, et al[8] utilized plaque samples taken from sound approximal surfaces of first molars to show a correlation between Strep. mutans and subsequent caries development. The correlation was improved when data on lactobacilli were included. These authors have discussed the increased sensitivity attained when multiple diagnostic tests are combined as well as the increased specificity that results when the combination of tests is employed at frequent intervals. Klock and Krasse[9] recorded salivary populations of lactobacilli and Strep. mutans in schoolchildren in order to identify subjects who might require special preventive care. A positive correlation was noted between Strep. mutans and incipient smooth surface carious lesions. In contrast, lactobacillus populations were correlated with open carious lesions. Since these studies and others[10,11,12] indicate a strong involvement of *Strep. mutans* in the initiation of the carious lesion it is suggested that the *Strep. mutans* assay is a logical starting point for an improved test for caries prediction.

These studies also provide a contrast in the manner of sample collection that should be considered in future work because it bears on the desired goals of a predictive test. A plaque sample from a specific tooth surface should be related to the caries risk on that surface. However, it is not necessarily indicative of conditions elsewhere in the mouth. Ideally, a comprehensive sampling of all caries susceptible surfaces would provide the best microbiological profile to be related to caries development on the different surfaces, but this may not be practical. On the other hand, salivary samples are easier to obtain, disperse and quantitate,which could be an advantage in large epidemiological studies or in dental office use. However, saliva tests lack the inherent precision of plaque samples, particularly as applied to specific tooth surfaces. Possibly they can provide a general picture of the micro-biology of the whole mouth that is useful in certain situations. Further studies on the relationship between salivary concentrations of *Strep. mutans* and lactobacilli, and the populations of these organisms in plaque could be very helpful in this respect[13].

Dr. Bowden has pointed out the inconsistency in recording organisms like the streptococci as individual species while the lactobacilli are lumped together at the genus level. This is an important point to be made and is a good example of one of the many discrepancies in our knowledge of the different types of oral bacteria. Considerable information is available about the oral streptococci with regards to the species present[14,15] as well as colonization patterns and comparative pathogenicity of different species[16]. Comparable information about the lactobacilli is less complete although oral species have been identified[17] and some information has become available on their distribution patterns in comparison to the streptococci[18]. Despite early attempts to show an association between specific types of lactobacilli and dental caries[19,20] we still have only scattered reports on the cariogenicity of some species in gnotobiotic rats[21,22,23]. The problem is further compounded by the lack of methods for easy differentiation of the many species of oral lactobacilli.

Dr. Bowden has proposed that there could be an "eclipse" phase when a cariogenic organism enters the decalcified lesion and can no longer be detected in samples. It is possible that once the lesion has developed, the microbial ecology at that site will undergo certain changes and the pre-lesion proportions of organisms will be significantly altered. A phenomenon related to this is suggested by the work of Brown and associates[24] in studies on caries development in xerostomic patients subsequent to radiation therapy. Plaque populations of *Strep. mutans* increased dramatically before and during the appearance of post-irradiation caries. Following caries development, the plaque concentrations of *Strep. mutans* declined steadily. This observation illustrates the difficulty in relating caries to precise numbers of *Strep. mutans* in a mouth with carious lesions in different stages of development.

Dr. Bowden's paper illustrates in part the conflict that arises in any discussion of caries predictive tests. Most workers agree that what is needed is a simple test that accurately reflects present and/or future caries status of the individual. Preferably the test would be administered either by auxillary dental personnel or else with minimal supervision of a dentist[5,7]. Hidden in this statement of purpose, however, is a dilemma that is not easily resolved. The two horns of the dilemma consist of 1) the multifactorial etiology of dental caries per se, and 2) the prevailing attitudes about the relative importance of dental caries as a medical problem. Unfortunately, a complex and chronic disease such as dental caries does not lend itself readily to the development of a reliable single-parameter diagnostic test. At the same time, dental caries is seen as a relatively mild condition in comparison to other more life-threatening situations. Consequently, its prediction, diagnosis and surveillance by laboratory test have not been given a high priority. Snyder[5] has listed the characteristics of an ideal laboratory office test. Perhaps it is time to make some decisions about how much less than "ideal" a test could be and still be useful in different clinical situations. It may be necessary to determine reasonable levels of sensitivity and specificity that provide an acceptable compromise between predictability and utility. Thus, future research efforts will have to consider both horns of the dilemma of caries predictive tests as they are presently envisioned. Theoretically, the first part of the problem that deals with integration of the components in a multifactorial disease should be amenable to some kind of resolution. After that the hardest part may be to convince the public and the profession that dental caries is a problem that is worthy of the time and expense involved in the routine use of a reliable and accurate predictive test.

Some of the important determinants that influence the course of infectious diseases have been discussed by Stewart[25]. Included are susceptibility, genetic constitution, behavior, and social and economic considerations. He points out that an important aspect of behavior is the community's attitude about particular diseases. In some cases in the past, this attitude has been seen as a fatalistic acceptance of diseases that were, in fact, preventable. He concludes that the continuing prevalence of diseases such as schistosomiasis, sleeping sickness, malaria, trachoma, and many others in underdeveloped countries is probably due at least as much to local attitudes as to any other single factor. It would not be inaccurate to describe dental caries as a disease that is fatalistically accepted by a large segment of the population in the developed countries.

LITERATURE CITED

1. Socransky, S.S. 1968. Caries-susceptibility tests. Ann. N.Y. Acad. Sci. 153:137-146.

2. Bowen, W.H. 1969. Caries activity tests. Inter. Den. J. 19:267-272.

3. Stople, J.R. 1970. Chemical and bacteriological tests for determining susceptibility to and activity of dental caries: A review. J. of Pub. Health Den. 30:141-155.

4. Ellen, R.P. 1976. Microbiological assays for dental caries and periodontal disease susceptibility. Oral Sci. Rev. 8:3-23.

5. Snyder, M.L. 1951. Laboratory methods in the clinical evaluation of caries activity. J. Am Den. Ass. 42:400-413.

6. Kroncke, A. and Naujoks, R. 1956. Dental caries susceptibility tests and their significance in dental practice. Inter. Den. J. 6:174-188.

7. Larmas, M. 1975. A new dip-slide method for the counting of salivary lactobacilli. Proc. Finn. Dent. Soc. 71:31-35.

8. Swenson, J.I., Liljemark, W.F. and Schuman, L.M. 1976. A longitudinal epidemiologic evaluation of the association between the detection of plaque streptococci and development of dental caries in children. Proceedings "Microbial Aspects of Dental Caries" Eds. Stiles, Loesche, and O'Brien. Sp. Supp. Microbiology Abstracts. 211-222.

9. Klock, B. and Krasse, B. 1977. Microbial and salivary conditions in 9 to 12 year-old children. Scand. J. Dent. Res. 85:56-63.

10. Ikeda, T., Sandham, H.J. and Bradley, Jr., E.L. 1973. Changes in Streptococcus mutans and lactobacilli in plaque in relation to the initiation of dental caries in negro children. Archs. oral Biol. 18:555-566.

11. van Houte, J. 1976. Oral bacterial colonization: mechanisms and implications. Proceedings "Microbial Aspects of Dental Caries" Ed. Stiles, 3-32.

12. Brown, L.R., Dreizen, S., Handler, S. and Johnston, D.A. 1974. Effect of radiation-induced xerostomia on human oral microflora. J. Dent. Res. 54:740-750.

13. van Houte, J. and Green, D.B. 1974. Relationship between the concentration of bacteria in saliva and the colonization of teeth in humans. Infect. and Immun. 9:624-630.

14. Carlsson, J. 1968. A numerical taxonomic study of human oral streptococci. Odont. Revy. 19:137-160.

15. Colman, C. and Williams, R.E.O. 1972. Taxonomy of some human viridans streptococci. In "Streptococci and Streptococcal Diseases". Eds. L.W. Wannamaker and J.M. Matsen. Acad. Press. N.Y. 281-299.

16. Gibbons, R.J. 1972. Ecology and cariogenic potential of oral streptococci. In "Streptococci and Streptococcal Diseases ". Eds. L.W. Wannamaker and J.M. Matsen. Acad. Press. N.Y. 371-385.

17. Rogosa, M., Wiseman, R.F., Mitchell, J.A., Disraely, M.N. and assisted by Beaman, A.J. 1953. Species differentiation of oral lactobacilli from man including descriptions of Lactobacillus salivarius nov. spec. and Lactobacillus cellobiosus nov. spec. J. Bact.65:681-699.

18. van Houte, J., Gibbons, R,J, and Pulkkinen, A.J. 1972. Ecology of human oral lactobacilli. Infect. and Immun. 6:723-729.

19. Clapper, W.E. and Heatherman, M.E. 1949. Strain differences in oral lactobacilli and the relation to dental caries. J. Bact. 58:261-268.

20. Baird-Parker, A.C., Bisset, K.A. and Pike, E.B. 1957. The distribution of Lactobacillus species in Northern and Southern Italian communities. Bri. Dent. J. 105:137.

21. Fitzgerald, R.J., Jordan, H.V. and Archard, H.O. 1966. Dental caries in gnotobiotic rats infected with a variety of Lactobacillus acidophilus. Arch. oral Biol. 11:473-476.

22. Rosen, S., Lenney, W.S. and O'Malley, J.E. 1968. Dental caries in gnotobiotic rats inoculated with Lactobacillus casei. J. Dent. Res. 47:358-363.

23. Hammond, B.F. 1971. Massive dental caries in gnotobiotic rats infected with a variety of Lactobacillus casei. I.A.D.R. Abst. #350.

24. Brown, L.R., Dreizen, S., and Handler, S. 1976. Effects of selected caries preventive regimens on microbial changes following irradiation-induced xerostomia in cancer patients. Proceedings "Microbial Aspects of Dental Caries". Ed. Stiles, 275-290.

25. Stewart, G.T. 1968. Limitations of the germ theory. Lancet. 1:1077-1081.

Discussion of microbial analyses related to caries susceptibility

F.E. Shovlin, Z. Sheykholeslam, J.E. Skribner

Dental School, College of Medicine & Dentistry, 100 Bergen Street, Newark, New Jersey 07103

First we would like to recognize the preciseness demonstrated by Dr. Bowden and his colleagues in covering the microbiology of dental caries thoroughly and effectively. There is little room for objection to what has been said. Their presentation emphasizes the many difficulties inherent in the study of the relationship of bacteria to dental caries and the enigma that continues as a result of these difficulties.

The area alluded to by Dr. Bowden that hopefully will be amplified in this paper relates to the organisms that have already been demonstrated as showing a positive correlation to caries, i.e., Streptococcus mutans Actinomyces israelii and the Lactobacillus species. Although the correlations show only group significance, it is preferable that these organisms should form the baseline for future investigations rather than undertaking studies of a new spectrum of microorganisms,which in addition to being unwieldy, might not provide new information.

The method we propose as a caries indicator will logically justify the study of Lactobacillus casei for caries prediction. However, similar arguments and like procedures might be equally applicable for the utilization of Streptococcus mutans or Actinomyces israelii as the test organism. In any event, probably all three organisms should be studied using the fluorescent antibody techniques which we favor, in place of the cultural procedures used in previous studies.

The rationale for the selection of L. casei as a caries indicator is as follows:

Many authors have reported a group relationship between the genus Lactobacillus and dental caries[1,2,3].

The above studies were deficient in the sampling procedures used and in the omission of species identification.

Selective culture methods are available for isolation[4] of L. casei.

Fluorescent antibody techniques may provide a rapid and an effective means for identification[5].

L. casei has been reported as the most frequent strain of Lactobacillus associated with carious lesions[6,7,8].

L. casei is the only human strain of Lactobacillus demonstrated to be significantly cariogenic in laboratory animals[9,10,11].

The test system proposed would have three stages, isolation of organisms, their identification, and correlation of findings.

Isolation of organisms: Patients selected on the basis of availability would be divided into three groups according to their dental status. The areas for bacterial sampling would be selected on the basis of susceptibility to caries as described by Newbrun[12]. The test samples would be dispersed in yeast extract solution and cultured on appropriate media. Some of the remaining cell suspension would be centrifuged, to provide cells for species identification using fluorescent antibody techniques,(Kawamura[13]). Colonies developing on the culture plates would be tentatively identified by slide agglutination, and those giving different reactions sub-cultured for biochemical testing.

Identification of organisms: The isolated organisms would be identified utilizing the indirect fluorescent antibody technique. Based on a) the serologic classification of *Lactobacillus* described by Sharpe[14]; b) the serologic typing and cross-reactivity studies reported by Knox and Wicken[15] and Shimohashi, *et al*[16], and c) experiments conducted in our laboratory[8]. These procedures for the identification of the strains of *L. casei* are highly effective and relatively simple.

The indirect method of FA staining would be appropriate in that it could reduce the necessity of preparing labelled anti-serums for each serological group. The accuracy of testing may be increased by the separation of prepared anti-serums into classes by column chromatography. The labelled anti-rabbit anti-serums then would be specific only for the antibody class with activity. Isolated organisms would be tested with absorbed anti-serums representative of the seven antigen groups defined by Sharpe[14], and the results recorded accordingly.

Collection of data: Samples collected in the clinic would be coded and recorded by persons not involved in laboratory identification procedures. Data would be collected separately and collated only after all data is available for each examination period (every 6 months for at least two years). The data could be evaluated utilizing a standardized computer procedure and the significance of the study accurately evaluated.

The suggested isolation procedures are standard and only slight manipulations would be required to make them effective. This is also true of the methods for data accumulation and evaluation. However, the species identification procedures may warrant refinement since cross-reactivity with dubious results is always a possibility when serologic techniques are used for bacterial identification. Most strains of lactobacilli can be divided into seven serologic groups as described by Sharpe[14]. The antigenic determinants for six groups have been summarized by Knox and Wicken[15], and are shown in Table I.

Table I

Group Antigens of Lactobacilli (Knox and Wicken, Identification of Cariogenic Bacteria by FA Technique - 1976)

Group	Antigen	Location	Determinant*
A	Glycerol teichoic acid	Wall membrane	-Glc
B	Polysaccharide	Wall	-Rha
C	Polysaccharide	Wall	-Glc
D	Ribitol Teichoic acid	Wall	-Glc
E	Glycerol teichoic acid	Wall	?
F	Glycerol teichoic acid	Membrane	-Gal

*Glc, D-glucosyl; Rha, L-rhamnosyl; Gal, D-galactosyl.

Based upon the information presently available and on further studies to be completed, the indirect fluorescent antibody method should be highly effective in the accurate identification of serologic group B relative to group C organisms, and in the identification of groups B and C relative to the remaining serologic groups. The selective isolation procedures available for the study of lactobacilli should prevent interference in identification by other gram positive organisms which may contain related teichoic acid antigens or other cross-reacting antigens.

So far the status of L. casei as the cause or as an opportunist associated with the dental lesion has not been discussed. Use of L. casei as an indicator of caries is more dependent upon its association with the lesion than on its function. We have previously reported a ninety-five percent correlation between L. casei and the dentinal lesion[17]. This was supported by studies by McNamara and Friedman[7], and Edwardsson[6] who reported L. casei as the most common isolate from the dentinal lesion. In addition, L. casei, serologic group C organisms, were identified in situ by us[17] in eleven of fifteen lesions using fluorescent antibody techniques which have since been extended to 27 out of 39 lesions.

The involvement of the dentin is indicative of an advanced lesion that may be too extreme for use as a caries predictor. However, the high frequency of the association of L. casei with the lesion may indicate that it is present in the initial lesion at low concentrations and that more sensitive testing methods than those used in previous studies are required for its identification.

The development of an accurate caries susceptibility test should receive high priority. For the practioner, it would serve as a reliable guide for clinical caries preventive procedures; for the researcher, it would provide an accurate measure for clinical testing of caries inhibitory agents; and for the patient, it would provide significant progress toward eradication of caries. Based upon information presently available, a concerted thrust in this direction may prove highly beneficial to the dental professional for which the minimum to be gained is a better understanding of the carious process.

LITERATURE CITED

1. Marshall-Day, C.D. 1949. Oral bacteriological studies in Puerto Rican children. J. Dent. Res. 28:648-653.

2. Slack, G.L. and Martin, W.J. 1956. Salivary lactobacillus counts and Snyder's caries susceptibility test and their relationship to dental caries incidence during a period of 12 months. Brit. D.J. 101:111-115.

3. Snyder, M.L., Porter, D.R., Claycomb, C.K., Sims, W. and Macho, F.R. 1963. Evaluation of laboratory tests for the estimation of caries activity. Correlation with specific surfaces. Archs.oral Biol. 8:541-547.

4. Rogosa, M., Mitchell, J.S., and Wiseman, R.F. 1951. A selective medium for the growth and study of lactobacilli. J. Bact. 62:132-137.

5. Shovlin, F.E. and Gillis, R.E. 1969. Biochemical and antigenic studies of lactobacilli isolated from deep dentinal caries. I. Biochemical Aspects. J. Dent. Res. 48:356-360.

6. Edwardsson, S. 1947. Bacteriological studies on deep areas of carious dentine. Odont. Revy. 25:Suppl. 32:1-143.

7. McNamara, T.F. and Friedman, B.K. 1976. The comparative microflora of plaque from intact enamel surfaces and carious lesions. J. Dent. Res. 55:Spec. issue B Prog. and Abs. Feb.

8. Shovlin, F.E. and Sheykoleslam, Z. Identification of L. casei with the indirect FA technique. Unpublished data.

9. Rosen, S., Lenney, W.S. and O'Malley, J.E. 1968. Dental caries in gnotobiotic rats inoculated with Lactobacillus casei. J. Dent. Res. 47:358-363.

10. Hammond, B.F. 1971. Massive dental caries in gnotobiotic rats infected with a variety of Lactobacillus casei. J. Dent. Res. Proc. and Abs. 49th General meeting, Chicago.

11. Shovlin, F.E. 1970. Initiation and inhibition of rat caries by lactobacilli. J. Dent. Res. Proc. and Abs. 48th General meeting, New York.

12. Newbrun, E. 1975. Cariology: 3rd edition. University of California, San Francisco, 38-39.

13. Kawamura, A. 1969. ed. "Fluorescent antibody techniques and their applications." U. of Tokyo Press, Tokyo, 23-75.

14. Sharpe, M.E. 1962. Dairy Sci. Abst. 24:109.

15. Knox, K.W. and Wicken, A.J. 1976. Grouping and cross-reacting antigens of oral lactic acid bacteria. Spec. issue A. "Identification of cariogenic bacteria by fluorescent antibody and other techniques". J. Dent. Res. 55 Special Issue A, 116-122.

16. Shimohashi, H., Kamiyama, K., and Arai, H. 1973. Studies on group antigens of Lactobacillus casei. Japan J. Microbial 17:205-210.

17. Shovlin, F.E. 1972. Identification of L. casei in deep dentinal caries using fluorescent antiserum. J. Dent. Res. Proc. and Abs. 50th General Meeting, Las Vegas.

Considerations about microbial interactions in relation to modification of the microflora of dental plaque

Frans H.M. Mikx and M. Svanberg

Institute Preventive & Community Dentistry, Nijmegen, The Netherlands
Dept. of Cariology, Dental School, University of Gothenburg Sweden

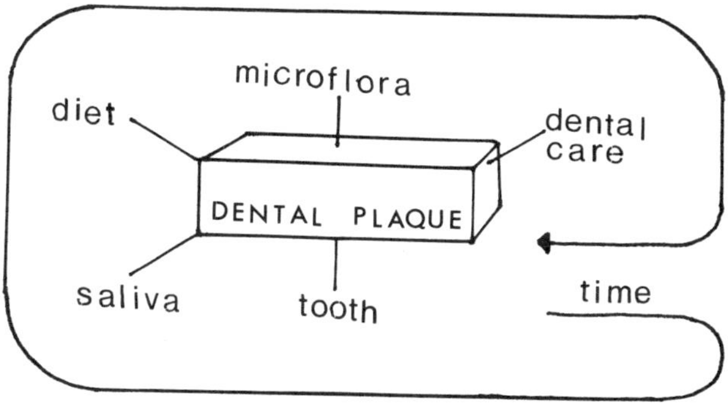

Fig. 1: Elements in the ecosystem of dental plaque.

The dental plaque is considered to be an ecosystem. The elements influencing this ecosystem are: microflora, tooth, saliva, diet, and dental care (oral hygiene routines, restorative dental procedures and anti-microbial treatment). These elements have the property of building blocks, but are also influencing each other. The dental plaque has four dimensions: height, width, depth and time, the latter is shown as an all surrounding circle. (Fig. 1).

The different elements involved in dental plaque will be discussed in so far they support considerations about modification of the microflora into a less cariogenic or even protective microbial layer on the teeth.

Plaque composition and acid production

Most information about plaque micro-organisms is related to streptococci and in particular to *S. mutans*. There is evidence that this organism is related to dental decay (1,2,3,4). However, it is also evident, that other micro-organisms of the complex microflora are involved in the demineralisation process (5,6,59).

A carious lesion develops as the result of acid attack on the enamel. Many organisms in dental plaque are capable of producing acid from carbohydrates (10). Therefore, one might not expect to find a simple relationship of a specific bacterium to caries. For example, it is found that a carious lesion can occur in relation to a high level of *S. mutans* or *Actinomyces israelii* (59), or to a combination of moderate levels of *S. mutans* and lactobacilli, or to low levels of *Veillonella* (6). Gnotobiotic studies have shown that *Veillonella* is able to modify the caries attack by S. mutans or S. sanguis (50). Also other lactate fermenting organisms like Neisseria might alter the acid attack on the enamel (49), indicating the importance of the composition of the microflora for the demineralisation process.

The information about the ecology of dental plaque shows a variation in plaque composition between different sites, each of the sites representing a separate ecological niche (7,54). Therefore, difficulties arise in obtaining a consistent opinion concerning the composition of a non-cariogenic flora, or regarding the way the flora should be modified to be less cariogenic.

Microflora in steady state

Different investigations have shown a general similarity and stability of supra-gingival plaque at the genus level, thus, suggesting the existence of an interspecific association of bacteria on the teeth (8,41). The approximal plaque samples in the longitudinal study of Bowden and co-workers (6), show this stability for the genera Actinomyces, Streptococcus, and Veillonella. Within the genus Streptococcus the largest variations were observed. In some instances the level of S. mutans increased when caries was detected.

These observations are in accord with the characteristics of a climax community (9), in which the inter-actions between microbial and non-microbial components of the ecosystem have reached a form of stabilization. At this stage the species composition of the microflora is maintained in a reasonably constant state. Nevertheless, the climax may be modified as the ecosystem undergoes drastic exogenous forces, like change in diet or disturbance by oral cleansing. Also, the environment might become irreversibly altered, e.g. when a carious lesion is formed. In such circumstances the microbial community gets out of balance and shifts to a different steady state.

Another characteristic of a climax community is that all niches are occupied, so that alien organisms will not be able to establish themselves. The absence of a potential member of a climax community suggests that its possible niche is filled by a more fit organism. However, disturbances of the ecosystem might lead to new unfilled niches or newly available places and subsequent colonization by other species (9).

Colonization by S. mutans

Concerning the factors involved in the formation of dental plaque, much emphasis is put on the adherence processes of bacteria to enamel and the involvment of saliva and carbohydrates in this process (30,31,32). In this paper special attention shall be given to growth as a factor in colonization of S. mutans and the antagonistic effect of the local microflora Several investigations have shown that S. mutans is not recovered from the early erupted teeth, but is found at a later age (23,25,34). Although, there is not general agreement among the different investigations. (Table 1). The question arises whether S. mutans is a primary colonizer or a secondary invader, Newly erupted teeth will not only be readily covered by a pellicle of salivary components (33), but also by bacteria other than S. mutans especially S. sanguis (34). This can be understood by the fact that S. sanguis is predominant in saliva and is much better adhering to the teeth than S. mutans (30). It is likely that tne establishment of S. mutans is a result of succession or of other changes in the ecosystem, like pH-drop (35,36) creating the niche of S. mutans in an existing microflora.

The study of Ruangsri and Ørstavik (37) shows the importance of ecological factors other than attachment to the tooth surface for the establishment of a labelled S. mutans strain. Pellicle free, pellicle coated and plaque coated incisor surfaces were challanged with a heavy suspension in buffer (10^9 CFU/ml) of a streptomycin resistant S. mutans

Table 1.

Isolation frequency of S. mutans in Dental Plaque of different Tooth Sites and Different Age Groups

References	(24)	(23)	(23)	(23)	(26)	(26)	(27)	(28)	(7)	(29)
Age group in years	0.5	0.5	1	5	5	5-8	7-9	13	13	17-22
Bucco/lingual	22*	0	18	30	20	-	3	66	-	30
Occlusal	-	-	0	17	17	50	39	-	-	72
Approximal	-	-	-	44	23	60	0	-	66	70
All subjects	22	0	18	46	-	-	100	-	100	92
Number of subjects	(40)	(14)	(11)	(57)	(104)	(25)	(12)	(128)	(10)	(92)

*Percentage of samples positive for S. mutans.

strain. The recovery of the implanted strain was greatest when the labelled cells were applied directly on newly cleaned tooth surfaces. However, the total counts of the implanted S. mutans strain decreased in time and after 7 days no differences were observed in the recovery of the labelled strain between the three treatment groups, Table 2. These results show the ability of S. mutans to participate in the formation of dental plaque on cleaned and pellicle coated surfaces as well as its capacity to colonize an already existing microbial layer.

The adherence to the enamel and subsequent outgrowth of bacterial cells is depicted by Rosan et al (38,39). Histological sections of dental plaque

Table 2.

Recovery of S. mutans After Implantation on Pellicle-Free, Pellicle-coated and Plaque-coated Tooth Surfaces[a)]

SUBJECT	PELLICLE-FREE			PELLICLE-COATED			PLAQUE COATED		
	24h	3d	7d	24h	3d	7d	24h	3d	7d
I	127[b)]	3	0.4	7	1.3	0.4	11	1.5	0.4
II	52	2	0.005	4	0.9	0.1	8	2	0.3
III	17	0.5	0.02	0.4	0.03	0.005	0.6	0.1	0.05

a) Summarized from Ruangsri and Ørstavid (37)

b) Mean total count of labelled S. mutans (x 10^3)

show pyramid-shaped microcolonies. The authors stress the importance in plaque formation of growth by initially adhering cells rather than by apposition of extraneous bacteria. One picture in the same publication shows an inverted pyramid shape suggesting the ingrowth of a bacterium into dental plaque. Similar observations of ingrowth of filamentous rods are made by Listgarten (40), and Mikx et al (50) have shown the invasion of a Veillonella microcolony by S. mutans.

In artificial fissures a same phenomenon of invasion has been observed (18). Artificial fissures colonized in vitro with a labelled S. mutans strain and placed in the oral cavity were invaded by an indigenous S. mutans strain. The cell numbers of the invading S. mutans strain increased with time (Fig. 2).

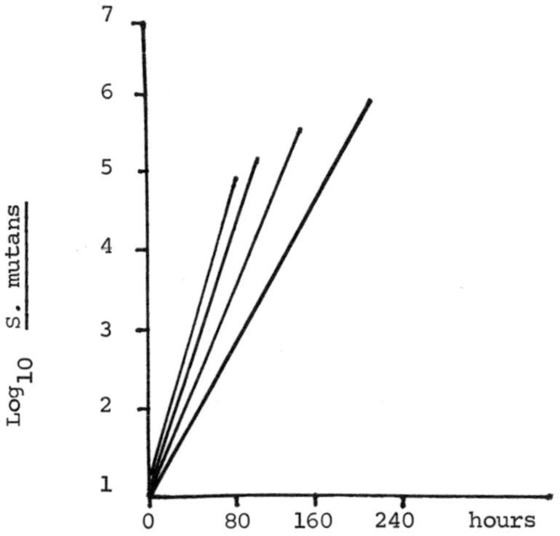

Fig. 2.

These studies offer the possibility that colonization rate could be estimated as the net result of growth and shedding of cells. Samples taken on the first days of implantation make possible a speculative calculation of the mean generation time (MGT) of S. mutans in fissures. Neglecting the shedding of cells during this period, a value of maximal 6-14 hours MGT is found. For supra-gingival plaque Socransky (41) calculated an MGT of 3-4 hours. These observations confirm the notion that different growth conditions exist between supra-gingival and fissure plaque.

In general these results indicate that S. mutans can colonize the tooth surface both because of initial attachment, and also by invading an existing microflora. It might very well be that in both instances the production of extracellular polysaccharide (EPS) by S. mutans plays a role. The EPS might strengthen the initial feeble absorption of the cells to the tooth surfaces or the EPS might provide an area in between the primary attached bacteria that becomes available for penetration by ingrowing cells of their dextranase activity (42,43,44). This might be an explanation for the selective effect of sucrose on the outgrowth of S.mutans.

Microbial antagonism in dental plaque

Microbial antagonisms have been observed by several investigators in implantation experiments of S. mutans in humans and animals (11,12,13,14). In rats the previous establishment of an Actinomyces viscosus strain together with a strain of S. sanguis inhibited the establishment of a S. mutans strain, that was inoculated in a high dose (15). A repetition of this experiment, including strains with bacteriocin activity, showed the same results.

However, the bacteriocin producer got well established suggesting a role of bacteriocin production in the competition with other plaque micro-organisms (see also van der Hoeven, this symposium).

The Actinomyces strain used in these experiments was isolated from rats fed a glucose diet. This diet favored a dental plaque microflora consisting mainly of A. viscosus (51). Similar selection and inhibition effects might have influenced the non-establishment of S. mutans in conventional rats fed a glucose diet by van Houte et al (52).

The effect of aging on the colonization of S. mutans in rats can also be an expression of differences in the plaque microflora (59). Comparable differences are observed between children and adults in the resistance of the throat microflora against group A streptococci (62). Further investigation of these antagonisms might reveal possibilities for reinforcing the resistance of a microflora against unwanted components.

Another experimental approach to the study of microbial inter-actions in dental plaque is the use of artificial fissures (16,17,18). Such fissures were generally colonized by 10^7 CFU within 1 day. In persons with high salivary S. mutans concentrations, this organism readily colonized the fissures in numbers increasing with time, representing about 6% of total CFU after 21 days. When the fissures were inserted during a regimen, that reduced the salivary S. mutans concentrations, this organism did not colonize the fissures. Even 28 days after the cessation of the regimen no S. mutans were detected in the fissure in spite of the fact that the salivary S. mutans concentrations had increased to levels that produced colonization of sterile artificial fissures. This experiment indicates the importance of the pioneer microflora in the fissure for subsequent S. mutans colonization. Another example can be offered.

It is possible that the existence of a microflora antagonistic for S. mutans in the approximal dental plaque of the 7-9 year old children investigated by Ikeda and co-workers (22) might have been responsible for their rare recovery of this organism from a site where it is normally prevalent.

However, at the end of this longitudinal investigation the approximal areas were found to be colonized by S. mutans. A calculation of the isolation frequency of S. mutans during the study reveals a steady increase from 0% at the start of the experiment to 25% after 3 months, 50% after 6 months, and 67% after 12 months, (Table 3).

Table 3.

Isolation Frequency and Prevalence of S. mutans in Approximal Areas of 7-9 Year Old Children[a)]

Months	0	3	6	12
Isolation frequency of S. mutans	0[b)]	25	50	67
Prevalence of S. mutans	0[c)]	1.7	7.4	11

a) derived from Ikeda et al (22)
b) percentage of samples positive for S. mutans
c) percent S. mutans of total streptococci

A remarkable change within this relative short period. It seems likely that disturbance of the approximal plaque because of sampling procedures modified the resistance of the local microflora, thus, enabling the spread of S. mutans from adjacent areas.

Lactoperoxidase system in saliva

An environmental influence on the outgrowth and composition of dental plaque might be the lactoperoxidase system(LPO) in saliva. Hoogendoorn(46) has shown that the LPO-system inhibits the glycolysis by oral bacteria. It has also been claimed to reduce plaque formation and prevent initial caries lesions (47).

The limiting factor in the LPO-system is H_2O_2. The H_2O_2 produced by S. mutans in the presence of lactoperoxidase and SCN^- is enough to stop the acid production of S. mutans in vitro. S. sanguis itself is far less susceptible to the LPO-system than the other plaque forming organisms (48). Therefore, this system might be important for the early outgrowth of S. sanguis in a pioneer population and also for the inter-action between neighbouring micro-organisms in developing dental plaque.

Clinical effects

It is realized that under some circumstances a microflora will develop on certain areas of the teeth that is acidogenic enough to produce caries lesions. In other situations a microflora might be present with a low cariogenic potential. Disturbance of these microflora can induce a change in the composition and cariogenicity of the dental plaque.

In other instances the microflora of plaque allows a mineral deposition on the teeth in the form of calculus. Calculus is commonly found on smooth surfaces, but may also occur in occlusal fissures. Theilade et al (53) found crystallites in dental fissure plaque even when they were challenged by frequent sucrose addition. No demineralisation was observed in these fissures, indicating that they were colonized by a rather resistant non-cariogenic microflora.

Recent research is mainly oriented towards the microflora of decalcifying plaque. It might, however, be of great importance to know the composition of mineralizing plaque as has been studied by Howell et al (55). Further information about such microfloras is needed to recognize non-cariogenic plaque and to indicate, in which way a cariogenic plaque has to be modified.

So far oral-microbiology is not able to predict whether a certain microflora will induce a lesion or not, neither can it indicate, in which way the microflora should be modified to be non-cariogenic.

Practical implications

S. mutans is used as an indicator organism for the cariogenic potential of dental plaque. There are methods to reduce the levels of S. mutans on tooth surfaces. Thus, Loesche (56) got a reduction of this organism in approximal plaque with topical application of an acidulated NaF gel (APF). Treatment with chlorhexidine was effective in reducing the S. mutans population both in plaque (60) and in saliva (61).

Treatment with Vancomycin was effective in reducing the S. mutans levels in occlusal surfaces (64), and gave a caries reduction in fissures especially in newly erupted teeth (65). Reducing the salivary S. mutans concentrations by a dietary and APF-regimen has been shown to prevent the establishment of S. mutans in artificial fissures, if administered at the time the fissures are inserted (17). The same regimen had, however, no effect upon the proportions S. mutans colonizing the fissures, when started two weeks after the insertion, i.e. when the fissures were already colonized.

This is of direct significance for dental practice, since it envisages the possibility of preventing the establishment of S. mutans in certain retentive areas introduced in the oral cavity (like fissures in newly erupted teeth and margins of fillings and crowns), if the efforts are adequately timed.

There is evidence, that intra-oral spread of S. mutans occurs mainly locally, i.e. to adjacent and antagonist tooth surfaces (57,19). Edman et al (57) used dental floss to establish S. mutans in approximal areas, and suggested the possibility, that improper use of dental floss might help to spread S. mutans. The dental explorer has shown to be an effective tool to spread S. mutans from an infected site to a non-infected artificial fissure (58,21).

A situation that exemplifies the need for a better integration of dentistry and oral microbiology is a case of unilateral caries associated with an unilateral S. mutans infection (20), in a 28-year old woman. The caries side had 37 filled and 11 decayed tooth surfaces, but no sub-gingival calculus, which was prevalent on the caries free side. Each year fillings were placed on the caries side and calculus removed from the caries-free side, but this therapy has been apparently insufficient in reducing or eliminating the pathogenic micro-organisms. Although the ordinary symptomatic treatment was not able to stop repeated relapses, it is possible that application of knowledge about the dental plaque ecosystem would have been more successful.

LITERATURE CITED

1. Loesche, W.J., Rowan, J, Straffon, L.H. and Loos, P.J. 1975. Inf. and Immunity 11:1252-1260.

2. De Stoppelaar, J.D., van Houte, J. and Backer Dirks,O. 1969. Caries Research 3:190-199.

3. Shklair, J.L., Keene, H.J. and Cullen, P. 1974. Archs. oral Biol. 19:199-202.

4. Gibbons, R., and van Houte, J. 1975. Annual Rev. of Med. 26:121-136.

5. Harrison, R.W. 1948. J.A.D.A. 37:391-403.

6. Bowden, G.H., Hardie, J.M., Mckee, A.S., Marsh, P.D., Fillery, E.D., and Slack, G.L. 1976. Proc. Microbial Aspects of Dental Caries. Sp. Supp. Microbiology Abstracts 1:223-241.

7. Bowden, G.H., Hardie, J.M., and Slack, G.L. 1975. Caries Res. 9:253-277

8. Hardie, J.M. and Bowden, G.H. 1974. The Normal Microbial Flora of Man, Soc. Appl. Bact. Symp. Series No. 3:47-83, Academic Press, London and New York.

9. Alexander, M. 1971. Microbial Ecology, John Wiley and Sons Inc., New York, Sydney, London, Toronto.

10. Sandham, H.J. and Phillips, H.I. 1976. Proc. Microbial Aspects of Dental Caries, Sp. Spp. Microbiology Abstracts 2:557-562.

11. Keyes, P.H. and Fitzgerald, R.J. 1962. Archs. oral Biol. 7:267-278.

12. Krasse, B., Edwardsson, S., Svensson, I. and Trell, C. 1967. Archs. oral Biol. 12:231-236.

13. Jordan, H.V., Englander, H.R., Engler, W.O. and Kulczyk, S. 1972. J. Dent. Res. 51:515-518.

14. Jordan, H.V. 1976. J. Dent. Res. 55 Spec. No. C 10-17.

15. Mikx, F.H.M., van der Hoeven, J.S., Plasschaert, A.J.M. and König, K.G. 1975. Caries Res. 9:1-20.

16. Löe, H., Karring, T., and Theilade, E. 1973. Caries Res. 7:120-129.

17. Svanberg, M. and Loesche, W.J. 1977. Archs. oral Biol. accepted for publication.

18. Svanberg, M. and Loesche, W.J. Implantation of S. mutans in humans. (in manuscript).

19. Svanberg, M. and Loesche, W.J. Intra-oral spread of S. mutans in humans. (in manuscript).

20. Svanberg, M. and Krasse, B. 1977. J.A.D.A. in press.

21. Loesche, W.J. and Svanberg, M. 1977. J. Dent. Res. 56 Sp. B 56.

22. Ikeda, T., Sandham, H.J., and Bradley, E.L. Jr. 1973. Archs. oral Biol. 18:555-566.

23. Catalanotto, F.A., Shklair, I.L. and Keene, H.J. 1975. J.A.D.A. 91:606-609.

24. Berkowitz, R.J., Jordan, H.V. and White, G. 1975. Archs. oral Biol. 20:171-174.

25. Carlsson, J., Grahnen, H., and Jonsson, G. 1975. Caries Res. 9:333-339.

26. Qureshi, J.V., Goldner, M., Riche, W.H. le, and Hargreaves, J.A. 1977. Caries Res. 11:141-152.

27. Ikeda, T. and Sandham, H.J. 1971. Archs. oral Biol. 16:1237-1240.

28. De Stoppelaar, J.D., van Houte, J. and Backer Dirks, O. 1969. Caries Res. 3:190-199.

29. Shklair, I.L., Keene, H.J. and Cullen, P. 1974. Archs. oral Biol. 19:199-202.

30. Gibbons, R.J. and van Houte, J. 1973. Annual Rev. Microbial 29:19-44.

31. Rölla, G. 1976. Proc. Microbial Aspects of Dental Caries. Sp. Supp. Microbiology Abstracts 2:309-324.

32. Kilian, M. and Rölla, G. 1976. Inf. and Immunity 14:1022-1027.

33. Sönju, T. and Rölla, G. 1973. Caries Res. 7:30-38.

34. Carlsson, J., Grahnen, H., Jonsson, G., and Wikner, S. 1970. Archs. oral Biol. 15:1143-1148.

35. Mikx, F.H.M. 1971. J. Dent. Res. 51:857-858.

36. Bibby, B.G. 1976. Proc. Microbial Aspects of Dental Caries Sp. Supp. Microbiology Abstracts 2:477-490.

37. Ruangsri, P., and Ørstavik, D. 1977. Caries Res. 11:204-210.

38. Rosan, B., Lai, C.H. and Listgarten, M.A. 1976. J. Dent. Res. 55A:124-141.

39. Lai, C.H., Listgarten, M.A. and Rosan, B. 1975. Inf. and Immunity 11:200-210.

40. Listgarten, M.A., Mayo, H.E. and Tremblay, R. 1975. J. Periodontal 46:10-26.

41. Sockransky, S.S., Manganiello, A.D., Propas, S., Oram, V., and van Houte, J. 1977. J. Periodontal Res. 12:90-106.

42. Dewar, M.D. and Walker, G.J. 1975. Caries Res. 9:21-35.

43. Staat, R.H. and Schachtele, C.F. 1974. Inf. and Immunity 9:467-469.

44. Guggenhein, B. and Burckhardt, J. 1974. J. Helv. Odont. Acta 18:101-103.

45. van Houte, J. 1976. Porc. Microbial Aspects of Dental Caries, Sp. Supp. i:3-32.

46. Hoogendoorn, H. 1974. Thesis, Delft. Mouton, The Hague.

47. Huyoson, A., Koch, G., Thilander, H. and Hoogendoorn, H. 1974. Odont. Revy. 25:69-80.

48. Scholtes, W. and Hoogendoorn, H. 1977. ORCA Abstr. 24.

49. Hoshino, E., Yamada, T., and Araya, S. 1976. Archs. oral Biol. 21:677-683.

50. Mikx. F.H.M., van der Hoeven, J.S., König, K.G., Plasschaert, A.J.M. and Guggenheim, B. 1972. Caries Res. 6:211-223.

51. van der Hoeven, J.S. 1974. Caries Res. 8:193-210.

52. van Houte, J. and Upeslacis, V.N. 1976. J. Dent. Res. 55:216-222.

53. Theilade, J., Fejerskov, O., and Karring, T. 1977. ORCA Abstr. 16.

54. Theilade, E., Larson, R.H. and Karring, T. 1973. Caries Res. 7:130-138.

55. Howell, A.,Rizzo, A. and Paul, F. 1965. Archs. oral Biol. 10:307-313.

56. Loesche, W.J., Murray, R.J. and Mellberg, J.R. 1973. Caries Res. 7:283-296.

57. Edman, D.C., Keene, H.J., Shklair, I.L. and Hoerman, K.C. 1975. Archs. oral Biol. 20:145-148.

58. Loesche, W.J., Walenga, A., and Loos, F. 1973. Archs. oral Biol. 18:571-575.

59. van Palenstein Helderman, W.H., Sampaio Camargo, P., and de Stoppelaar, J.D. 1977. (Abstr) Caries Res. 11:119.

60. Emilson,C.G., Krasse, B., and Westergren, G. 1976. Scan. J. dent. Res. 84:56-62.

61. Emilson, C.G., and Fornell, J. 1976. Scan. J. dent. Res. 84:308-319.

62. van Houte, J., Upeslacis, N. and Edelstein, S. 1977. Inf. and Immun. 16:203-212,

63. Sanders, C.C., Nelson, G.E. and Sanders, W.E. Jr. 1977. Inf. and Immun 16:599-603.

64. Jordan, H.V. and De Paola, P.F. 1977. Archs. oral Biol. 22:195-201.

65. De Paola, P.F., Kordan, H.V., and Soparkar, P.M. 1977. Archs. oral Biol. 22:187-191.

Discussion of microbial interactions and modification of the microflora

J.S. van der Hoeven and A.H. Rogers

Dept. of Preventive and Community Dentistry, University of Nijmegen, The Netherlands
Dept. of Oral Biology, University of Adelaide, Adelaide, South Australia

In recent years various aspects of the establishment of Streptococcus mutans in the mouth have been investigated. The presence of hard surfaces as a necessary requirement for the establishment of S. mutans in the mouth was demonstrated (1,2). This corresponded with the recognition later on of selective adherence as an ecological determinant (3). Indeed, the preferential attachment of S. mutans to tooth surfaces is in accordance with its habitat in dental plaque.

The diet was also shown to influence the oral flora (4). Sucrose was found to facilitate the establishment of S. mutans. Glucose favoured Actinomyces viscosus in dental plaque of conventional rats, while extracellular polysaccharide producing streptococci, S. mutans and S. sanguis became predominant if these rats were fed on sucrose diet (5).

The molecular mechanisms of the adherence process of S. mutans to hard tissue have been studied in detail, but not yet completely clarified (6). Despite this knowledge, the outcome of experimental implantation of S. mutans in man or animals is unpredictable and difficult to explain (7,8,9,10), however, that neither initial presence (adherence) of S. mutans nor frequent consumption of sucrose (8,9,15) ensures its final success in becoming established.

In fact, little is known of serotype and strain specific characteristics that could affect the establishment of S. mutans. In addition, host related factors of which the resident microflora is thought to be important have been given little attention.

A widely held view is that the production of bacteriocin accounts for the successful establishment of a bacterium (16). It is well known that the majority of the S. mutans strains isolated from human dental plaque exhibit bacteriocin activity(11,12,13). Like the bacteriocins of other Gram positive species, the S. mutans bacteriocins are also active against unrelated Gram positive bacteria (12). In particular, oral actinomycetes are very sensitive to bacteriocins of S. mutans (van der Hoeven, unpublished data).

Our previous studies (14) have strongly suggested that S. mutans bacteriocins are produced in vivo and are active against sensitive species in the plaque of gnotobiotic rats. Further studies were aimed at demonstrating an ecological role for bacteriocins in dental plaque; in particular, their possible significance in the colonization of S. mutans. These studies were performed in rats harbouring a complex microflora that inhibited colonization of certain S. mutans strains. This so-called "SPF-Ny" microflora was obtained by inoculation of SPF (specific pathogen free) rats with Actinomyces viscosus Ny 1 and Streptococcus sanguis Ny 101. Subsequent inoculation of the rats with S. mutans OMZ 176 failed to show establishment of the strain, but it was readily established in normal SPF rats (15). In our last study various S. mutans strains, differing in bacteriocin activity, were tested for their ability to colonize the SPF-Ny system.

To this end S. mutans strains were inoculated in SPF Osborne Mendel rats that had been inoculated before with A. viscosus Ny 1 and S. sanguis Ny 101.

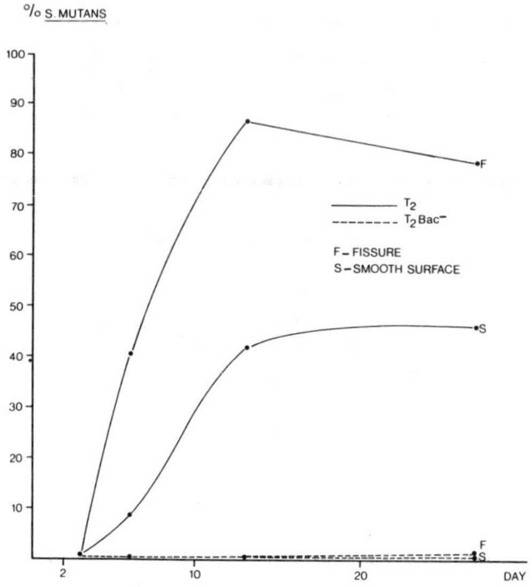

Figure 1. Kinetics of the establishment of S. mutans T2 and its non-bacteriocinogenic mutant T2 bac⁻ in smooth surface and fissure plaque of SPF-Ny rats. The S. mutans strains were inoculated 1 day after A. Viscosus Ny 1 and S. sanguis Ny 101. Plaque was sampled 3, 6, 13, and 28 days after inoculation of S. mutans. S. mutans was expressed as median percentage of the total flora.

The establishment of the bacteriocinogenic S. mutans T2 or its mutagen-induced non-bacteriocinogenic mutant T2 bac⁻ is shown in Figure 1. Strain T2, but not T2 bac⁻ was found to establish on smooth surfaces and in fissures, supporting the hypothesis that bacteriocin was involved. A stable proportion of S. mutans was attained at approximately 14 days after inoculation. In this experiment the S. mutans strains were inoculated one day after Ny 1 and Ny 101. Subsequent experiments were aimed to study the establishment of S. mutans in relation to the state of the resident microflora of the rats. Figure 2 shows the proportion of S. mutans in the total flora, at increasing intervals between the inoculations of Ny 1 plus Ny 101 and S. mutans, that is an increasing stability of the SPF Ny ecosystem. The more stable the SPF-Ny ecosystem became, the lower the eventual proportion of S. mutans. Data are given for two bacteriocinogenic S. mutans strains (T2 and SW31), and for OMZ 176, a strain without any detectable level of bacteriocin production. It is noted that OMZ 176 only became established, in a very low proportion, if it was inoculated one day after Ny 1 and Ny 101.

The establishment of the strains was recorded 28 days after inoculation when a stable situation can be expected (Figure 1). The ability of the SPF-Ny microflora to prevent establishment of S.mutans may be due to the

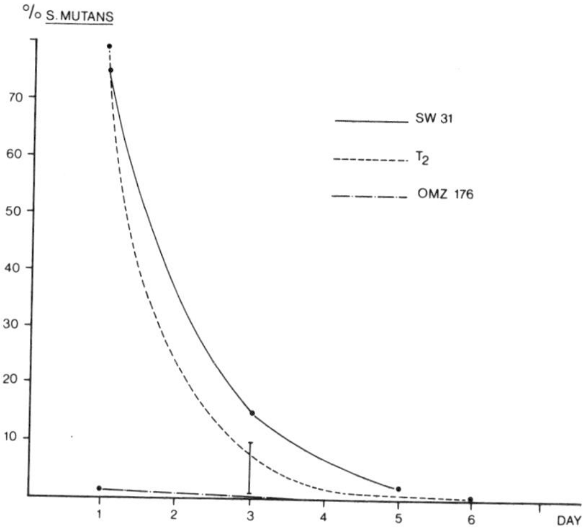

Figure 2. Implantation of S. mutans strains in the developing SPF-Ny ecosystem. Median percentage S. mutans of the total flora at increasing time interval (days) between inoculations of A. viscosus Ny 1 and S. sanguis Ny 101, and the introduction of S. mutans.

producing S. mutans strains may be able to disturb the equilibrium and thereby become established.
fact that it represents a climax community (16). An invading micro-organism would find possible niches occupied by well-integrated members of such a community, and would thus be unable to colonize. It seems logical to assume that the SPF-Ny ecosystem shortly after the inoculation of Ny 1 and Ny 101 does not represent a climax community because microbial equilibrium has not yet been attained.

The results of the implantation of S. mutans at various times during the transient state (Figure 2) support such a view. However, bacteriocin

This is illustrated in Table 1 which gives the data on the implantation of S. mutans strains in the SPF-Ny rats. The strains were inoculated 5 days after Ny 1 and Ny 101 and the table reports their proportions after a further 28 days. The in vitro inhibitory activities against the main components of the SPF-Ny microflora are also recorded. These components were A. Viscosus Ny 1, S. sanguis Ny 101 and SPF biotypes 1 to 4 with decreasing proportions in that order. (No data are available for bacteriocin activity against SPF biotypes 1 and 2, since attempts to grow these strains either as an overlay, or when directly sprayed on plates, have so far been unsuccessful). The data show that bac^+ strains generally colonized in a higher proportion than strains without a detectable level of bacteriocin activity.

Factors other than bacteriocinogeny must be involved in strains with poor or no detectable bacteriocin activity, established quite well. Bacteriocin production in vitro is known to be influenced by the composition of the medium (17), and indeed, these 2 strains have been shown to be bacteriocinogenic, albeit weakly, on a different medium (11,18). The failure of C 67-1 to establish is more difficult to explain since it has been shown to produce bacteriocin in vivo in gnotobiotic rats (14).

Table 1.

Implantation in SPF-Ny Rats of S. mutans Strains with Different Bacteriocin Activities

+ S. mutans Strain	Serotype	Bacteriocin Activity Against: A. viscosus Ny 1	S. sanguis Ny 101	SPF bio-types $1^x 2^x 3$ 4	Establishment of S. mutans % of total flora 28 days after inoculation
T8	c	+	+	+ +	15
T2[xx]	c	+	+	+ +	1
SW31	c	+	+	+ +	4
C67-1	c	+	+	- +	0.1
SM6	c	+	+	- +	5
OIHI	d	+	+	+ +	7
IB	c	±	+	- -	18
FA1	b	-	+	- -	0.01
OMZ175	f	-	-	+ +	0.01
LM7	e	-	-	- +	3
B13	d	-	-	- -	0.01
OMZ65	d/g	-	-	- -	3
KIR	d/g	-	-	- -	0.1
OMZ176	d	-	-	- -	0.01
E49	a	-	-	- -	0.01
T2 Bac⁻	c	-	-	- -	0.01
SW31 Bac⁻	c	-	-	- -	0.05

+ S. mutans inoculated 5 days after A. viscosus Ny 1 and S. sanguis Ny 101
x No data available for SPF biotypes 1&2 xxT2 inoculated 6 da. after Ny1&Ny101

The experiments described here show the existence of an ecosystem that resisted colonization by S. mutans under conditions in which sucrose was amply available. It is of interest to investigate whether such an ecosystem could be developed in man and whether a stable ecosystem, without S. mutans could exist when sucrose was not restricted. The result would be a less cariogenic plaque.

LITERATURE CITED

1. Carlsson, J., Soderholm, G., and Almfeldt, I. 1969. Archs. oral Biol. 14:243-249.

2. Carlsson, J., Grahnen, H., Honson, G., and Wikner, S. 1970. Archs oral Biol. 15:1143-1148.

3. Gibbons, R.J. and van Houte, J. 1973. J. Periodontol. 44:347-360.

4. Bibby, B.G., Proceedings "Microbial Aspects of Dental Caries", Eds. Stiles, Loesche and O'Brien, Sp. Supp. Microbiology Abst. 477-490.

5. van der Hoeven, J.S. 1974. Caries Res. 8:193-210.

6. Rolla, G. Proceedings "Microbial Aspects of Dental Caries", Ed. Stiles 309-324.

7. Krasse, B. 1966. Archs. oral Biol. 11:429-436.

8. Krasse, B., Edwardsson, S., Svensson, I., and Trell, L . 1967. Archs. oral Biol. 12:231-236.

9. Jordan, H.V., Englander, H.R., Engler, W.O., and Kulczyk, S. 1972. J. Dent. Res. 51:515-518.

10. Edman, D.C., Keene, H.J., Shklair, I.L. and Hoerman, K.C. 1975. Archs. oral Biol. 20:145-148.

11. Hamada, S. and OOshima, T. 1975. Archs. oral Biol. 20:641-648.

12. Rogers, A.H. 1976. Archs. oral Biol. 21:99-104.

13. Weerkamp, A., Vogels, G.D. and Skotnicki, N. 1977. Caries Res. 11:245-256.

14. Rogers, A.H., van der Hoeven, J.S. and Mikx, F.H.M. Archs. oral Biol. in press.

15. Mikx, F.H.M., van der Hoeven, J.S., Plasschaert, A.J.M. and Konig, K.G. 1976. Caries Res. 9:1-20.

16. Alexander, M. 1971. "Microbial Ecology", John Wiley, New York.

17. Rogers, A.H. 1972. Appl. Microbiol. 24:294-295.

18. Rogers, A.H. 1976. Archs. oral Biol. 21:243-249.

Discussion of microbial interactions and modification of the microflora

R.A. Kolstad

Baylor College of Dentistry, 3802 Gaston Avenue, Dallas, Texas 75246

In their contribution to the prediction of caries, Mikx and Svanberg (this conference) emphasize the need to be able to recognize and characterize cariogenic, as opposed to non-cariogenic plaque. They point out that microbial inter-actions within the two categories of plaque may differ and suggest that identification of these differences could lead to modification of the plaque flora with resultant decreased caries activity.

One common member, Streptococcus mutans, is continually present in the cariogenic microflora, but not all microbes so named are equally cariogenic. This is not surprising in view of the biotypes, serotypes, and hosts involved. The only consistency about this species is the continuing argument about its unity and diversity.

Although a composite picture revealing the role of individual strains of S. mutans in the development of caries is lacking, independent studies concerning different aspects of the broad topic have been conducted. Strong transmission of strains of S. mutans between mothers and children has been documented by Jordan (1976), who monitored the passage with bacteriocin tagging. Because caries experience is likewise familial, the possibility exists that the strains of S. mutans detected in the caries active group are especially cariogenic.

If the frequency of caries is related to variations among bacterial flora, one reason may be the bacteriocin-promoted colonization advantage of some strains of S. mutans. In order for S. mutans to demineralize enamel, it must first colonize the hard surface to be attacked. Van der Hoeven and Rogers (this conference) demonstrate positive correlation between microbial inhibition by strains of S. mutans and the ability to colonize. In these experiments with rats infected with S. mutans and Actinomyces viscosus, colonization ability varies over a wide range. Especially impressive is the decrease of colonization by bacteriocin-negative mutants. This dramatic shift clearly establishes that bacteriocins produced by oral streptococci have significance beyond the petri plate. Retrospective studies with individual strains of S. mutans recovered from plaque associated with caries will be required to demonstrate a relationship between bacteriocins and caries. High versus low caries expectation could, then, be monitored with oral bacteriocins. Such information would be most useful if it were coupled into a program of flora modification targeted for families in which high caries activity is predicted. Modification should be considered for those persons particularly susceptible to caries, namely children and young adults and persons epidemiologically active, especially pregnant women and parents of very young children.

To speed such developments I would like to suggest that the collection of pertinent data be entered into the NIDR microbiological data bank, managed by Dr. Krichevsky in Bethesda. It is particularly valuable to exploit central data processing and analysis for projects involving several independent workers. Interest in the inhibitory patterns and mechanisms of S. mutans is rapidly expanding. Differences among strains with respect to host range and intensity have been investigated by Delisle et al (1977), Macrina et al (1977), Morhart and Fitzgerald (1977). and Nakamura et al (1977), other workers are cited by van der Hoeven and Rogers (this conference) Although it would be foolish to act as if caries revolved exclusively about S. mutans, the time may be ripe to evaluate the basic and clinical data already at hand to determine relationships among bacteriocin activity, colonization and cariogenicity of S. mutans. The NIDR microbiology data bank and software is designed for this kind of project.

Apart from strain variation in the ability to colonize, time plays a role. Mikx and Svanberg discussed experiments with hard surface implants in an environment of suppressed S. mutans growth. As the time of suppression increased, the ability of S. mutans to colonize diminished. Apparently, the colonization of particular sites blocks subsequent colonization by the same or related species. Amplification of this shift may be promoted if initial colonization involves microbes with strong antagonistic defenses.

That antagonism is not monopolized by S. mutans has been demonstrated by Mikx et al (1972). The biculture, A. naeslundi/S. sanguis, inhibits the colonization of S. mutans. Consideration of this "two-way street", in which microbes both inhibit and are subject to inhibition, is yet another reason not to jump rapidly to conclusions about oral ecology.

In studies at Baylor the native ability of S. sanguis to inhibit S. mutans in the absence of molecular oxygen is always weak. However, because S. sanguis is not associated with caries in humans and because it enjoys an early dominance in plaque development, this species could be an interesting inhibitor of S. mutans were it provided with the capability to generate the appropriate bacteriocins. We have isolated a number of Lancefield Group D streptococci which strongly inhibit S. mutans. Patterns of sensitivity involving Bratthall groups a through e condense into three clusters (Kolstad, 1977). The most interesting inhibition passes through all three clusters and is resistant to proteases. Presently we are working towards transformation to achieve the desired hybrids.

LITERATURE CITED

1. Delisle, A., Marks, H., and Weaver, D. 1977. J. Dent. Res. 55 (Special Issue) Abst. #266.

2. Jordan, H.V. 1976. J. Dent. Res. 55 Sp. Issue C, 10-14.

3. Kolstad, R.A. 1977. J. Dent. Res. 55 Sp. Issue, Symposium IV.

4. Macrina, F.L., Reider, J.L., and Virgili, S.S. 1977. J. Dent. Res. 55 Sp. Issue, Abst. #538.

5. Mikx, F.H.M., van der Hoeven, J.S., Konig, K.G., Plasschaert, A.J.M., and Guggenheim, B. 1972. Caries Res. 6:211-223.

6. Morhart, R.E. and Fitzgerald, R.J. 1977. J. Dent. Res. 55 Sp. Issue, Abst. #542.

7. Nakamura, T., Suginaka, Y., Obata, T., and Takazoe, I. 1977. J. Dent. Res. 55 Sp. Issue, Abst. #541.

Discussion of microbial interaction and modification of the microflora

Jason M. Tanzer

Department of Oral Diagnosis, School of Dental Medicine, University of Connecticut, Farmington, Connecticut 06032

Utility of Bacteriological Monitoring in Secondary Prevention and Management of Caries

While *Streptococcus mutans* is surely not the sole significant cariogenic microorganism, there is much evidence that it is possibly the prime cariogenic microorganism in man and in experimental animals, both on the smooth surfaces of teeth and in their fissures (1-6). Consequently, the logical focus of studies of the ecology of the tooth surface as it relates to coronal caries has been this microorganism.

Very little is known about bacterial antagonisms in caries-associated plaque. Much has been hypothesized. One of the most striking and regularly observed ecological relationships revealed during cross sectional and longitudinal studies of the tooth flora is a seemingly inverse relationship of the percentages of *S. mutans* and *Streptococcus sanguis* on the tooth coronal surface (4,5). In distinction to *S. mutans* there is very little evidence of a potent direct cariogenic role of *S. sanguis*, either from human or experimental animal studies (7,8).

As we retrospectively examine the bacteriological and pathological records of a rather large number of caries active patients in whose management we began to participate in 1970, we are struck by the strong correlation of the percentages of *S. mutans* on early carious surfaces (white spots). We are even more impressed by the remarkable submergence of *S. mutans* and concommitant emergence of *S. sanguis* at those same surfaces when followed longitudinally in patients advised about and educated to the avoidance of high frequency sucrose consumption. In fact, we have come to believe that the longitudinal monitoring of *S. mutans* and *S. sanguis* at tooth surfaces give conveniently obtained hard data as to patient compliance with dietary counseling. Thus, our monitoring of patients has not been used to predict those who are at risk of developing caries, but rather to predict the outcome of treatment, the prognosis and therefore the selection of approaches to the management of the dental caries patient. We feel it is probably the easiest and most reliable way to evaluate the probable cariogenicity of a plaque at specific, longitudinally monitored tooth loci.

This brief paper proposes to discuss some of the mechanisms which may bear upon this and other clinical caries-relevant ecological relationships on the tooth surface and to suggest at least one chemotherapeutic approach to shifting the plaque flora to favor survival of less cariogenic microorganisms than *S. mutans*.

Figure 1 represents a variety of types of hypothesized and established ecological relationships upon the balance between cariogenic and noncariogenic plaque flora. This paper will be restricted to discussion of bacteriological and antimicrobial agents. Discussions of salivary, gross anatomical

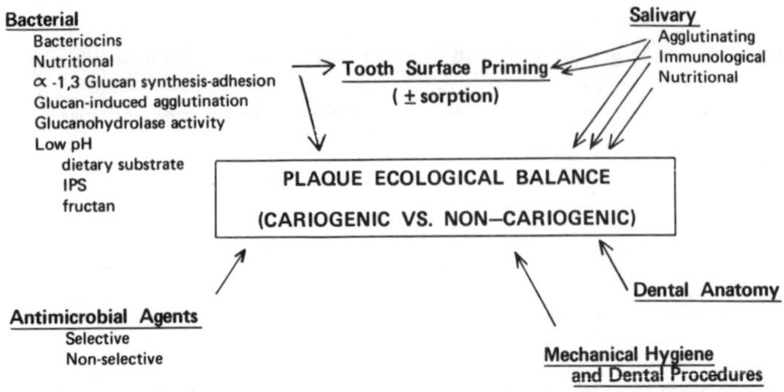

Figure 1. Relationships between cariogenic and noncariogenic plaque flora

and dental mechanical influences will be found in the papers of others in these proceedings.

Some Mechanisms of Interest

Bacteriocin production as a selective pressure

Responsive to my charge not to recapitulate areas discussed by the disquisitors in this segment of our meeting, I will not add to the nice discussion of the possible role of bacteriocins (9,10). It should be noted, however, that the factuality of bacteriocin significance is now passing the conjectural (hypothetical) stage and is being subjected to test.

Nutritional selective pressures

There have been several suggestions of the importance of nutritional selective pressures resulting directly from the bacterial metabolism of some microorganism types upon the metabolism and thus survival of other bacterial types (7,8). However, there have been no direct in vivo tests of the import of these hypothetical nutritional pressures. Nutritional selective pressures resulting from the diet of the host will be discussed below.

Priming of the tooth surface as a selective pressure

It is quite likely that the prime colonization of a "clean" enamel surface by a microorganism and its proliferation there as a clone may alter the surface and exclude or foster colonization by other microorganisms (11). This may be a result of the inherently dense colonization of the surface by the first colonizer with a resultant lack of "Lebensraum" for others, as well as the compulsion of growth in an oralward direction, as described both in vivo and in vitro (12-14).

In addition current studies by Tinanoff and Tanzer (15) of pure culture plaque growth in vitro on clean intact enamel surfaces suggest that pellicle, long thought to be involved in either ecological establishment or prohibition of establishment (11), may substantially originate from bacterial biosynthetic processes, independent of the presence of salivary substances. The real role of such bacterially produced pellicular substances, and indeed of salivary produced ones, in flora establishment and interactions appears uncertain.

Low pH as a selective pressure

It has been proposed by several workers that the potent acidogenicity of S. mutans from both exogenous and endogenous carbohydrates not only serves as the probable prime force in driving dimineralization of the tooth but as an important modifier of the flora on the tooth surface (16). It is reasoned that in the face of rapid acid production by a carbohydrate-replete cariogenic flora that non-aciduric microorganisms could fail to survive in the ecology of the tooth surface while aciduric ones would survive and be favored. Conceivably the well known increase of lactobacillus numbers in saliva of caries active patients may at least in part reflect this phenomenon. However, the only data of which we are aware directly pertaining to the ecological force of acidogenicity in the plaque are those revealed by our laboratory's studies of IPS synthesis-defective mutants of S. mutans Bratthall serotype c. These mutants substantially lose their pathogenicity on smooth tooth surfaces of rats, and to a lesser extent, in tooth fissures also. However, they do not detectably fail to colonize animals when compared to their normal IPS-producing progenitor wild type (wt) or to emerge and survive within the plaque ecology. It would seem likely that if the IPS synthesis trait, and its resultant longterm production of acid and low plaque pH in the absence of exogenous carbohydrate, were important in selecting against the survival of less aciduric organisms than S. mutans, the IPS synthesis-defective mutants of S. mutans sould have become less numerous than the wt. But they didn't (17). In addition, wt cells of Bratthall serotype d form little IPS (3,18) yet they are perfectly capable of colonizing an animal with an established tooth flora, ascending in the flora, and indeed dominating it (3). Hence, we presently can see no evidence that acidogenesis from the IPS of S. mutans has a potent effect on the ecology although it clearly does have a potent effect on the virulence of serotype c cells which do produce IPS (17).

Fructan synthesis and fructanase activity as a selective pressure.

It has also been suggested that fructans synthesized by S. mutans (or other cells such as S. salivarius) may be important exogenous substrates in the absence of dietary exogenous carbohydrates. It is thought that fructans (levans or inulins) may be degraded by inducible fructanases of S. mutans (or perhaps other plaque cells), thereby generating free fructose as substrate for prolonged acid production (16,19-22). From this point, the argument as to the ecological selection pressure potentially resulting from prolonged acid production in the plaque from fructan substrate is analogous to that from IPS of S. mutans. However, there is one exception; only those cells forming and degrading IPS can benefit from its energy yield while any cell capable of catabolizing fructose may possibly be favored by the ability to consume extracellular fructans. Present work with fructanase-defective mutants of S. mutans (Tanzer and Freedman, unpublished data) may help clarify the ecological and pathological significance of fructans.

-1,3-linked glucan synthesis and accumulative adhesion as a selective pressure

Much has been studied about the synthesis of extracellular and cell-associated glucans of S. mutans (17). It now appears clear that the formation of cell-associated glucans of the -1,3 rich class is not only germane to virulence but apparently is required for successful emergence of S. mutans in the plaque flora of rats (3) and hamsters (23). Mutans defective in this trait fail to compete (3,23).

Glucan-induced agglutination as a selective pressure

It has been suggested that exogenous glucan-induced agglutination (dextran-induced agglutination) of S. mutans is functionally equivalent to the glucan-mediated adhesion of S. mutans to heterologous surfaces. Such agglutination has been hypothesized thus as important to cohesion of S. mutans within its plaque "growth" (11,23). It is now clear, however, that the glucan-induced agglutination phenomenon is genetically, functionally, and biochemically distinct from the glucan-associated aspect of the adhesion phenomenon (3,23, 25-30). Mutants defective in adhesion but normal with respect to agglutination have been described. They fail to form plaque on the teeth (3,23,25) as pointed out above. In addition, mutants of the same strain of *S. mutans* which are defective in agglutination but normal in adhesion have now been studied. In rat caries models they are either as virulent or more virulent than their wt progenitor, forming plaque and competing well in the plaque flora (26,27). These data thus suggest that the glucan-induced agglutination trait fosters clearance of non-adherent *S. mutans* from the oral cavity, much as antibodies fostering agglutination of bacterial antigens foster their clearance from infected loci.

Glucanohydrolase activity as a selective pressure

Several plaque microorganisms form glucanohydrolases (glucanases) (31-34). The glucanhydrolases of *S. mutans* appear specific for --1,6 linkages most common among extracellular water-soluble glucans of *S. mutans*. Indeed, a role of such glucanases in modification of *S. mutans* glucans and cross linking of its cell surface-associated glucans has been proposed (35,36). It has been suggested that resultant branched -1,3-rich glucans foster adhesive and accumulative plaque formation of the teeth (37). However, mutants of *S. mutans* defective in -1,6 glucanohydrolase production form adhesive colonizations on solid surfaces in pure culture *in vitro* just as well as their wt progenitors (38). Hence, this glucanase production trait of *S. mutans* may not directly yield ecological advantage. However, it is notable that such glucanase-defective mutants are decidedly less virulent than their wt's and while they persist in the plaque flora after successfully infecting experimental animals, they fail to emerge as dominant members of the plaque flora (38). It could well be that the glucanohydrolase trait functions to degrade -1,6 glucans of other plaque microorganisms, thereby allowing invasion of the life space of non-*S. mutans* clones, perhaps most especially those *S. sanguis* which synthesizes -1,6 glucans. Because the glucanase of *S. mutans* is an endohydrolase it is unlikely that the resultant oligosaccharide fragments produced by its action can serve as substrate for its growth and acidogenesis (34,36,39).

Common denominator of sucrose as an ecological selective pressure

It should not escape notice that virtually all of these functions of *S. mutans* are either sucrose-related or sucrose-dependent. Indeed this appears correlated with the association of aggressive caries activity with high frequency consumption of sucrose (40). It has certainly become clear that humans or animals may become infected and sustain infection by *S. mutans* when they consume either little, infrequent or no sucrose (41,42). However, the consumption of sucrose may call forth all of the above-discussed phenomena (and probably others) to give *S. mutans* the ecological advantage fostering its ascendency in the plaque flora, and its eventual elicitation of tooth demineralization by virtue of its rapid acidogenesis against the tooth's surface.

Possible chemotherapeutic selection of the plaque flora

Because one cannot be wildly optomistic about controlling sucrose consumption of caries active patients or of those at risk for caries development, one must consider plaque ecological modification by other means. One of the more intriguing possibilities is illustrated by the differential potency of inorganic iodine as an antiseptic against plaque microorganisms. It has been observed that one can select iodine concentrations which are bactericidal to plaques of *S. sanguis*, *Actinomyces naeslundii* or *A. viscosus*, plaque-forming microorganisms of relatively little demonstrated pathogenicity on the crowns of teeth (43). Indeed, some workers have demonstrated the ability to suppress *S. mutans* at selected colonized tooth sites by inorganic iodine scrubs (44). Other data (45) suggest that a variety of chlorhexidine analogs could be used to differentially suppress the most cariogenic of the plaque-forming oral microflora. It is our feeling that such selective antimicrobial agent-mediated suppression of the most cariogenic elements of the oral flora and allowance of survival of the least cariogenic elements may provide a potent approach to caries prevention and management and is a fertile area for research.

LITERATURE CITED

1. Fitzgerald, R.J. and P.H. Keyes. 1960. Demonstration of the etiologic role of streptococci in experimental caries in the hamster. J. Amer. Dent. Res. 61:9-19.

2. Shklair, I.L. 1973. Streptococcus mutans and the epidemiology of dental caries. In: Streptococcus mutans and Dental Caries. R.J. Fitzgerald (ed). U.S.D.H.E.W. Pub. No. (NIH) 75-286:7-13.

3. Tanzer, J.M., M.L. Freedman, R.J. Fitzgerald and R.H. Larson. 1974. Diminished virulence of glucan synthesis-defective mutants of Streptococcus mutans. Infec. Immun. 10:197-203.

4. deStoppelaar, J.D., J. van Houte and O. Backer Dirks. 1969. The relationship between extracellular polysaccharide-producing streptococci and smooth surface caries in 13-year-old children. Caries. Res. 3:190-200.

5. Loesche, W.J., J. Rowan, L.H. Straffon and P.J. Loos. 1975. Association of Streptococcus mutans with human dental decay. Invec. Immun. 11:1252-1260.

6. Swenson, J.I., W.F. Liljemark and L.M. Schuman. 1976. A longitudinal epidemiologic evaluation of the association between the detection of plaque streptococci and development of dental caries in children. In: Microbial Aspects of Dental Caries. Vol. I (H.M. Stiles, W.J. Loesche, and T.C. O'Brien, eds). I.R.L. p. 211-222.

7. Fitzgerald, R.J. (ed). 1973. Streptococcus mutans and Dental Caries. U.S.D.H.E.W. Pub. No. (NIH) 75-286. pp. 1-51.

8. Stiles, H.M., W.J. Loesche and T.C. O'Brien (eds). 1976. Microbial Aspects of Dental Caries, Vol. 3, pp. 878. I.R.L.

9. Mikx, F.H.M. and M. Svanberg. 1977. Considerations about microbial interactions in relation to modification of the microflora of dental plaque. These proceedings p.

10. van der Hoeven, J.S. and A.H. Rogers. 1977. The establishment of Streptococcus mutans in rats in relation to bacteriocinogeny and stability of the resident flora. These proceedings p.

11. Gibbons, R.J. and J.H. van Houte. 1975. Bacterial adherence in oral microbial ecology. Ann. Rev. Microbiol. 29:19-44.

12. Tanzer, J.M. and M.C. Johnston. 1976. Gradients for growth within intact Streptococcus mutans plaque in vitro demonstrated by radioautography. Arch. Oral Biol. 21:555-559.

13. Newman, H.N. and D.F.G. Poole. 1974. Structural and ecological aspects of dental plaque. Soc. Appl. Bact. Symp. Ser. 3:111-134.

14. Lai, C., M.A. Listgarten and B. Rosan. 1975. Immunoelectron microscopic identification and localization of Streptococcus sanguis with peroxidase labeled antibody: Localization of Streptococcus sanguis in intact plaque. Infec. Immun. 11:200-210.

15. Tinanoff, N. and J.M. Tanzer. Parameters involved in the sorption of S. mutans to enamel. J. Dent. Res. (IADR. Abst.) 1978.

16. Tanzer, J.M. 1973. Sucrose metabolism of Streptococcus mutans. In: Streptococcus mutans and Dental Caries. R.J. Fitzgerald (ed). U.S.D.H.E.W. Pub. No. (NIH) 75-286 p. 25-32.

17. Tanzer, J.M., M.L. Freedman, F.N. Woodiel, R.L. Eifert and L.A. Rinehimer. 1976. Association of Streptococcus mutans virulence with synthesis of intracellular polysaccharide. In: Microbial Aspects of Dental Caries. Vol. III. (H.M. Stiles, W.J. Loesche, and T.C. O'Brien, eds). IRL p. 597-616.

18. Freedman, M.L. and A.L. Coykendall. 1975. Variation in internal polysaccharide synthesis among Streptococcus mutans strains. Infec. Immun. 12:475-479.

19. daCosta, T. and R.J. Gibbons. 1968. Hydrolysis of levan by human plaque streptococci. Arch. Oral Biol. 13:609-617.

20. Manly, R.S. and D.T. Richardson. 1968. Metabolism of levan by oral samples. J. Dent. Res. 47:1080-1086.

21. van Houte, J.H. and H.M. Jansen. 1968. Levan degradation by streptococci isolated from human dental plaque. Arch. Oral Biol. 13-827-830.

22. Parker, R.B. and H.R. Creamer. 1971. Contribution of plaque polysaccharides to growth of cariogenic microorganisms. Arch. Oral Biol. 16:855-862.

23. Fitzgerald, R.J., D.B. Fitzgerald and J.M. Tanzer. Loss of virulence of glucan synthesis-defective mutants of S. mutans in hamsters. In preparation.

24. Gibbons, R.J. and R.J. Fitzgerald. 1969. Dextran-induced agglutination of Streptococcus mutans and its role in the formation of microbial dental plaques. J. Bacteriol. 98:341-346.

25. Freedman, M.L. and J.M. Tanzer. 1974. The dissociation of plaque formation from glucan-induced agglutination in mutants of Streptococcus mutans. Infec. Immun. 10:189-196.

26. Tanzer, J.M., M.L. Freedman and R.J. Fitzgerald. Role of glucan-induced agglutination in virulence of Streptococcus mutans. J. Dent. Res. (IADR. Abst. 1978).

27. Freedman, M.L. and J.M. Tanzer. Mutants of S. mutans defective in glucan-induced agglutination but capable of adhesive growth on solid surfaces. In preparation.

28. Mukasa, H. and H.D. Slade. 1973. Mechanism of adherence of Streptococcus mutans to smooth surfaces. Infec. Immun. 8:555-562.

29. McCabe, M.M. and E.E. Smith. 1975. Relationship between cell-bound dextransucrase and the agglutination of Streptococcus mutans. Infec. Immun. 12:512-520.

30. Nalbandian, J., M.L. Freedman, J.M. Tanzer and S.M. Lovelace. 1974. Ultrastructure of mutants of Streptococcus mutans with reference to agglutination, adhesion, and extracellular polysaccharide. Infec. Immun. 10:1170-1179.

31. Staat, R.H., T. Gawrowski and C.F. Schachtele. 1973. Detection and preliminary studies on dextranase-producing microorganisms from human dental plaque. Infec. Immun. 8:1009-1016.

32. Staat, R.H. and C. Schachtele. 1975. Characterization of a dextranase produced by an oral strain of Actinomyces israelii. Infec. Immun. 12:556-563.

33. daCosta, T., L. Bier and F. Gaida. 1974. Dextran hydrolysis by a Fusobacterium strain isolated from human dental plaque. Arch. Oral Biol. 19:341-342.

34. Dewar, M.D. and G.J. Walker. 1975. Metabolism of the polysaccharides of human dental plaque. I. Dextranase activity of streptococci and the extracellular polysaccharide synthesized from sucrose. Caries Res. 9:21-35.

35. Ebisu, S., A. Misaki, K. Kato, S. Kotani. 1974. The structure of water-insoluble glucans of cariogenic Streptococcus mutans, formed in the absence of or presence of dextranase. Carbohydrate Res. 38:374-381.

36. Guggenheim, B. and J. Burckhardt. 1974. Isolation and properties of a dextranase from Streptococcus mutans OMZ-176. Helv. Odont. Acta 18:101-113.

37. Guggenheim, B. 1970. Enzymatic hydrolysis and structure of water-insoluble glucan produced by glucosyl transferases from a strain of Streptococcus mutans. Helv. Odont. Acta 14 (Suppl V): 89-108.

38. Tanzer, J.M., M.L. Freedman, L.A. Rinehimer, R. Eifert, S. Griffith and F. Woodiel. 1977. Loss of virulence of glucanohydrolase-defective mutants of S. mutans. J.D.R. 56 (Special Issue A), A132.

39. Staat, R.H. and C.F. Schachtele. 1974. Evaluation of dextranase production by a cariogenic bacterium Streptococcus mutans. Infec. Immun. 9:467-469.

40. Mandel, I. 1970. Effects of dietary modifications on caries in humans. J. Dent. Res. 49 (Suppl): 1201-1211.

41. van Houte, J.H., V.N. Upeslacis, H.V. Jordan, Z. Skobe and D.B. Green. 1976. Role of sucrose in colonization of Streptococcus mutans in conventional Sprague-Dawley rats. J. Dent. Res. 55:202-215.

42. van Houte, J.H. and S. Duchin. 197 . Streptococcus mutans in the mouths of children with congenital sucrose deficiency. Arch. Oral Biol.

43. Tanzer, J.M., A.M. Slee, B. Kamay and E.R. Scheer. 1977. In vitro evaluation of three iodine-containing compounds as antiplaque agents. Antimicrob. Agts. Chemother. 12:107-113.

44. Gibbons, R.J., P.F. dePaola, D.M. Spinell and Z. Skobe. 1974. Interdental localization of Streptococcus mutans as related to dental caries experience. Infec. Immun. 9:481-488.

45. Tanzer, J.M., A.M. Slee and B. Kamay. 1977. Structural requirements of guanide, biguanide, and bisbiguanide agents for antiplaque activity. Antimicrob. Agts. Chemother. (in press. Dec. 1977).

Some disease-predictive biochemical activities of plaque microbes

M.L. Freedman

University of Connecticut Health Center, Farmington, Connecticut 06032

The biochemical activities of plaque are certainly as multifarious as those of other assemblages of cells, pro- or eukaryotic. However, plaque microbes conduct many anabolic and catabolic processes which are wholly non-distinctive and which may be common to systems as diverse as the gut flora and muscle. Examples of such processes include elements of glycolysis and the biosynthesis of macromolecular precursors such as amino acids, purines, etc. Thus, while there are certainly differences in enzymes of like function, in their structure, control, and regulation, at the present time there seem to be relatively few plaque-distinctive, caries-associated processes compared to the total biochemical potential of this tooth-surface ecosystem. While the "common"reactions provide energy and proliferative potential for plaque, without which tooth decay would cease, a few biochemical activities hypothesized to be directly linked to disease in an equally small number of bacterial species have garnered the most research effort. The study in vitro of the correct process in the wrong bacterium, or the converse, is both distressing and possible inasmuch as studies of pure cultures cannot take into account the synergism and antagonism, the syntropy and symbiosis among plaque microbes. Despite these caveats, organic acids produced by many growth-associated, degradative biochemical activities and two synthetic processes, intracellular and extracellular glucan production, stronly favor disease causation by promoting the adhesive retention of cells with abilities to produce acids for a prolonged time.

Acid production.

The production of organic acids by plaque catabolism (1-3) of exogenous dietary carbohydrates, intracellular storage polymers such as glycogen (IPS) (5,7), and extracellular fructans such as levan or inulin (8-12) has long been regarded as the mechanism by which the tooth is demineralized (4) leading to the formation of the carious lesion. Many oral microbes including streptococci, lactobacilli and actinomyces species are acidogenic (13) and produce a broad assortment of acids: formic, acetic, propionic, butyric, and in the case of lactic, both D- and L+ isomers (14-16).

Plaques not associated with caries are both low in S. mutans (3,17-21), and produce predominantly volatile acids (3,13,15) with pK values higher than that of lactic acid. Bacteria isolated from the oral cavity of tube-nourished individuals likewise have reduced fermentative capacity (76,77). It has also been reported that starving plaque and glucose-limited chemostat cultures of S. mutans produce more volatile acids (3,15,16,22) than do the same systems responding to an abruptly elevated level of fermentable carbohydrate. There is, therefore, an apparent shift to lactic acid production in virulent plaques (3) and in a number of plaque strains isolated and studied in pure culture (13,22,23). S. mutans best reflects and most probably causes this fermentative shift (13). It has been reported that S. mutans, in fact, synthesizes quantitatively more acid from exogenous (78) as well as endogenous carbohydrates (26), and by virtue of being aciduric does so at lower environmental pH values (79). Veillonella species which are capable of metabolizing lactic acid have been detected in inverse quantitative relationship to S. mutans (21) as, of course, have other species, notable S. sanguis.

Acid production as a predictive tool

From a mechanistic standpoint acid production should be useful as a biochemical activity predictive of disease. Starved, cariogenic plaques might be expected to shift to production of qualitatively and quantitatively less volatile acids and more lactic acid when presented with excess exogenous fermentable carbohydrate. Conversely, plaques neither virulent nor associated with disease should show smaller shifts. There exists evidence that such changes occur in vitro and can be quantified in small plaque samples (13,3) using isotopically labelled substrates and gas chromatography.

Also, broths supplemented with sucrose and bacitracin or mannitol and arginine and containing a pH indicator, coupled with colony enumeration on agar plates, have been used to establish the presence of S. mutans and S. sanguis in plaque and saliva, their proportions of the total cultivable flora, and their ratio (80). Despite false positives, this acid-production-linked predictive test shows promise for detecting S. mutans establishment and perhaps ascension (82).

Intracellular polysaccharide (IPS)

IPS, an iodophilic α-(1$\rightarrow$4) - linked homopolymer of glucose with a high degree of α-(1$\rightarrow$6) branching (24) can compose a significant fraction of the dry weight of plaque bacteria (5,25,26). It has been detected in several oral microbes, S. mitis (30), S. salivarius (26,28), S. mutans (5,25,33), and L. casei (7,27) as well as in plaque diphtheroids, fusobacteria, and Bacteroides (29,31). Although not studied in all strains, two enzymes, ADP-glucose synthase which requires ATP and glucose-1-phosphate and ADP-glucose transferase which requres ADP-glucose and an acceptor glucan appear involved in IPS synthesis at least in S. mitis (32) and S. salivarius (26), and probably in S. mutans as well (25). It has been reported (i) that bacteria harboring glycogen-like intracellular granules are recoverable from plaque samples associated with carious lesions (29), (ii) that the possession of such granules is a trait more stable in caries-active plaque bacteria than in bacteria associated with caries-inactive plaque (31,3), (iii) that positionally the most abundant granule-formers lie deepest in the plaque (36), and (iv) that the presence of IPS in plaque bacteria correlates with a carbohydrate-rich diet as does disease (13,34,35). Recent studies using macromolecular synthesis inhibitors have indicated that abundant IPS sequestration correlated most strongly with unbalanced RNA synthesis (25). Prolonged periods of internally- or externally-controlled balanced growth, in which all cell parameters increase with time at the same rate governed by the cell's synthetic capabilities and availability of nutrients, may not exist in vivo to any appreciable extent given the feast-or-famine mode of plaque nutrition. Thus, IPS synthesis should be favored as capable cells vacillate between states of unbalanced (RNA) synthesis.

S. mutans, which has been positively associated with caries, synthesizes less IPS and degrades it more slowly than S. salivarius strains (26). Metabolism of stored IPS by S. mutans leads to (long-term) acid production and energy for inducible enzyme formation (38). However, it has been shown in vitro that not all S. mutans serogenetic groups synthesize or degrade equal amounts of IPS (5), and that many microbes which synthesize IPS are not prime candidates as caries pathogens. Although, studies have shown that there is little turnover of IPS until mobilized for catabolism, perhaps in response to the return of a favorable pH, or a low level of metabolic intermediate (5,23), or the absence of other fermentable carbohydrates, there is some IPS breakdown during growth even in the presence of exogenous carbohydrates (26). Thus, the net results of plaque microbes' abilities to synthesize and degrade IPS is (i) the prolonged maintenance of low pH, (ii) the establishment of an acid-tolerant flora, (iii) a source of energy for continued syntheses and perhaps proliferation, and (iv) the production of demineralizing acids for extended periods of time.

Studies with IPS synthesis-defective mutants isolated from serogenetic groups I-c strains known to synthesize IPS (38) and to be virulent in a rodent caries system have shown that the mutants became established in the mixed flora of specific-pathogen-free rats, but produced significantly less sulcal and smooth surface decay than their IPS synthesis-proficient progenitors (39). The loss of sulcal virulence was greater when animals had restricted, seven-hour access to food, a ploy designed to stress the IPS trait. Therefore, IPS is an apparent biochemical determinant of virulence, but apparently not a determinant of establishment or persistance in the plaque. This seems true only in those S. mutans that synthesize and degrade IPS but not in members of serogenetic group III-d which synthesized and degraded little IPS to acid (9). Thus, this bio-chemical activity may positively correlate with the existence of or potential for disease causation by plaques containing S. mutans groups other than III-d.

Utility of IPS as a predictive agent.

If IPS is the between-meal-snack of virulent plaque, then the presence of plaque rich in IPS-synthesizing bacteria is probably a reasonable caries (risk) indicator, bearing in mind that (i) plaque samples vary in microbial composition between surfaces and even within areas of the same surface (3), (ii) not all virulent S. mutans are fecund IPS synthesizers, (iii) the trait might be more crucial to smooth-surface decay in an individual eating fermentable carbohydrates especially glucose- or sucrose-containing foods incessantly, and more crucial to sulcal decay in an intermittent dietary regimen, (iv) many organisms not implicated as prime caries pathogens synthesize and presumably degrade IPS, and (v) the presence of IPS granules in a micrograph of mixed plaque bacteria does not mean that these bacteria are viable and capable of metabolizing their IPS presumably to demineralizing acid.

For IPS to serve as an indicator, very-well-starved plaque should probably be examined microscopically, or for iodophilic properties, or for glucose content following neutralization of acid hydrolysates, or by methylation analysis to disclose 2, 3-di-methyl and 2,3,6-tri-methyl glucose, or for endogenous acidogenicity. A comparison should be made with contiguous, adjacent plaque exposed to a glucose pulse and an acidic buffer chase --- the glucose does not serve as a precursor of extra-cellular glucans, and the acidic buffer chase prevents prompt metabolism of the intra-cellular polysaccharides. Clearly a correlation should ultimately be made between the existence of known pathogens or current disease at the site sampled, inasmuch as it has been shown that S. mutans strongly correlates with the presence of a caries-active flora, and is frequently an IPS former. Studies of this type, but using plaque samples removed from caries-active and inactive children and exposed to isotopically labelled sucrose for the simultaneous quantitation and qualitation of intra-cellular (and extra-cellular) polysaccharides and metabolic acids have recently been reported (3).

Extra-cellular glucan synthesis.

α-(1→3) linkage-rich, water-insoluble and α-(1→6)-rich water-soluble polymers synthesized from the glucose half of sucrose by one or more constitutive glucosyl transferase enzymes (43,44,48-50) appear to be of crucial importance in stabilizing the initial reversible association of bacteria (46,47), especially, but not exclusively S. mutans to the primed tooth surface (67). These polymers provide an adhesive structure that tends to retain newly divided cells thereby augmenting plaque mass (50,51). They serve as diffusion barriers which may keep metabolic products, especially acids, in the tooth area longer and which may also (81) reduce the magnitude of concentration transients, thus providing a degree of nutritional constancy in the plaque. Glucans perhaps serve also as an attractive surface to which circulating microbes with appropriate receptors can bind (40,45,52-54) and with time proliferate, so fostering plaque heterogeneity.

Recently many papers have described the isolation and characterization of glucosyl transferase enzymes (55-59) predominantly from S. mutans and the physical structures of the enzymes' products (43,44,48-50). The synthesis of glucans seems separable from their association with apparently proteinaceous (40) cell-surface receptors (45) which are distinct from the synthetic enzymes(40). Also entering into the picture, are endohydrolytic glucanohydrolases, termed dextranases, from S. mutans (41), which appear to provide acceptor molecules for continued glucan synthesis (68) and possibly a degree of post-synthetic structural alteration of the glucans (42).

It has been found that an antagonism, possibly mediated by dextranase, exists between Actinomyces viscosus (63), a frequent inhabitant of non-caries associated plaque, perhaps other oral microbes as well (60-62), and S. mutans. Thus, territoriality of specific genera and species and cariogenicity of their associated plaques may have some basis in the elaboration of glucanases and sensitive glucans. It should be noted that the α-(1→3)-rich glucan seems resistant to the glucanases of S. mutans (41), and perhaps also to the hydrolases of other bacteria associated with an α-(1→3)-linkage-rich plaque.

Again, through the use of mutants, it has been possible to establish a regionality for the ability to form an adherent plaque (64). Mutants which form an abundance of α-(1→6)-rich, water-soluble glucan do not form adherent smooth-surface plaque nor do they cause severe disease at sites which rely on active glucan-mediated retention(65). Virulence in sulci is less affected; the results hold for both specific-pathogen-free and gnotobiotic animals. Recent methylation analyses of the glucans produced by the wild type and mutants of S. mutans strain 6715-13 show specific loss of the α-(1→3) component (66). Thus, smooth-surface virulence would seem to be vitally dependent upon classes of α-(1→3)-linkage-rich, water-insoluble glucans, while sulcal caries appears far less demanding and can be fostered by mechanical entrapment.

Extra-cellular glucans and glucanases as predictive agents.

In view of the established importance of glucans, especially α-(1→3) linked, to plaque formation and virulence, quantitation of these polymers in plaque should be a useful predictive tool. The procedures for such analyses are well established, require relatively small amounts of material, and can adequately distinguish these glucan polymers from intra-cellular polysaccharides and fructans. A large α-(1→3)-linkage quantity might well correlate positively with a virulent plaque, assuming plaque structural glucans are predominantly those of S. mutans and that glucan synthesis in vivo is quantitatively and qualitatively parallel to the processes already studied in vitro. Again, the ploy of sampling plaque before and after glucan-precursor exposure should expose the plaque's capacity to synthesis α-(1→3)-rich glucans and conceivably indicate adhesive and pathogenic capabilities. Methylation analysis lends itself to this type of study with a high ratio of 2,4,6,=to-2,3,4-tri-methy. glucose indicating α-(1→3)-rich plaque.

The converse approach, an assay of α-(1→3)- or α-(1→6)-rich glucan hydrolase activity in plaque using appropriate chromogen-tagged substrates, or quantitation by methylation analysis following dialysis to remove hydrolyzed fragments of polymers, might indicate the presence of a less virulent, more S. mutans- antagonist plaque.

There are reports with extensive bibliographies of such studies using pooled plaque from children and adults and various preparative regimens, but no correlation with the extent of disease (69,70). α-(1→3)-rich material was detected with variable frequency and might well reflect a low average biased by considerable amounts of non-caries-associated tooth deposits.

CONCLUSION

There is a distressing anachronism in the use of biochemical activities of plaque and its microbes as predictive measures. This is: the traits commonly considered and discussed above are caries-associated, most frequently found in S. mutans, and, thus, do not presage disease but rather, depending upon quantity, are pathognomonic of disease. Thus, virulent caries-associated plaque is IPS-former and probably α-(1→3)-linkage-rich, and produces abundant lactic acid. A very short distance away can exist a flora not disease-associated containing many of the same microbial species, probably in different ratios, and diminished biochemical activities of the types specified. Assay of these biochemical activities in caries-associated plaque is too late, while study in plaque not associated with disease may suggest at that time and site no cause for concern. While bacteriocins(71), plasmids (72), phage (73), teichoic acid moieties(74.75). etc. may prove to be useful disease-predictive traits in the future, distinctive biochemical activities of plaque as it makes the transition from non-virulent to virulent still need to be identified.

LITERATURE CITED

1. Bowen, W. and Eastoe, J. 1967. Caries Res. 1:130-136.

2. Charlton, G., Fitzgerald, R., and Keyes, P. 1971. Archs. oral Biol. 16:649-654.

3. Minah, G. and Loesche, W. 1977. Infect. Immun. 17:43-54.

4. Miller, W. 1898. Die Mikroorganismen der Mundhöle. Georg Thieme Liepzig.

5. Freedman, M. and Coykendall, A. 1975. Infect. Immun. 12:475-479.

6. van Houte, J., Winkler, K., and Jansen, H. 1969. Archs. oral Biol. 14:45-61.

7. Hammond, B. 1971. Archs. oral Biol. 16:323-338.

8. Rosell, K, and Birkhed, D. 1974. Acta Chem. Scand. B28:589.

9. Carlsson, J. 1970. Caries Res. 4:97-113.

10. DaCosta, T. and Gibbons, R. 1968. Archs. oral Biol. 13:609-617.

11. van Houte, J. and Jansen, H. 1968. Archs. oral Biol. 13:827-830.

12. Parker, R. and Creamer, H. 1971. Archs. oral Biol. 16:855-862.

13. Minah, G. and Loesche, W. 1977. Infect. Immun. 17:55-61.

14. Gilmour, M. et al. 1976. in"Microbial Aspects of Dental Caries." Eds. Stiles, Lo sche, and O'Brien. IRL. p. 539-556.

15. Geddes, D. 1975. Caries Res. 9:98-109.

16. Gilmour, M. and Poole, A. 1967. Caries Res. 1:247-260.

17. Ikeda, T., Sandham, H. and Bradley, E. 1973. Archs. oral Biol. 18:555-566.

18. Englander, H. and Jordan, H. 1972. J. Dent. Res. 51:1505.

19. deStoppelaar, J., van Houte, J. and Baker, O. 1970. Caries Res. 4:114-123.

20. Loesche, W., Hockett, R., and Syed, S. 1972. Archs. oral Biol. 17:1311-1325.

21. Loesche, W. and Syed. S. 1973. Caries Res. 7:201-216.

22. Cooney, C., Keung, J. and Sinskey, A. 1976. in "Microbial Aspects of Dental Caries." Eds. Stiles, Loesche, and O'Brien, IRL p.799-807.

23. Yamada, T. and Carlsson, J. 1975. J. Bacteriol. 124:55-61.

24. Meyer, K. 1942. "Natural and Synthetic High Polymers." Interscience Publishers. p. 419.

25. Mattingly, S., Daneo-Moore, L, and Shockman, G. 1977. Infect. Immun. 16:967-973.

26. Hamilton, I. 1976. in "Microbial Aspects of Dental Caries." Eds. Stiles, Loesche, and O'Brien. IRL. p. 683-701.

27. Kobayashi, Y. and Takei, M. 1972. Jap. J. Microbiol. 16:70-72.

28. van Houte, J. and Jansen, H. 1968. Caries Res. 2:47-56.

29. Gibbons, R. and Socransky, S. 1962. Archs. oral Biol. 7:73-80.

30. Berman, K., Gibbons, R. and Nalbandian, J. 1967. Archs. oral Biol. 12:1133-1138.

31. Berman, K. and Gibbons, R. 1966. Archs. oral Biol. 11:533-542.

32. Builder, J. and Walker, G. 1970. Carbohyd. Res. 14:35-51.

33. van Houte, J., DeMoor, C. and Jansen, H. 1970. Archs. oral Biol. 15:263-266.

34. van Houte, J. 1964. Archs. oral Biol. 9:91-93.

35. Loesche, W. and Henry. C. 1967. Archs. oral Biol. 12:189-194.

36. Saxton, C. 1975. Caries Res. 9:418-437.

37. Gibbons, R. 1964. J. Bacteriol. 87:1512-1520.

38. Freedman, M., Tanzer, J. and Eifert, R. 1976. in "Microbial Aspects of Dental Caries." Eds. Stiles, Loesche, and O'Brien. IRL. p. 583-596.

39. Tanzer, J., Freedman et al, M. 1976. in " Microbial Aspects of Dental Caries." Eds. Stiles, Loesche, and O'Brien. IRL. p. 597-616.

40. Kelstrup, J and Funder-Nielsen, T. 1974. J. Gen. Microbiol. 81:485-489.

41. Guggenheim, B. and Burckhardt, J. 1974. Helv. Odont. Acta. 18:101-113.

42. Ebisu, S. et al. 1974. Carbohyd. Res. 38:374-381.

43. Baird, J., Longyear, V. and Ellwood, D. 1973. Microbiol. 8:143-150.

44. Ceska, M. et al. 1972. Acta Chim. Scand. 26:2223-2230.

45. McCabe, M. and Smith, E. 1976. in "Immunologic Aspects of Dental Caries." Bowen, Genco, and O'Brien eds. IRL. p.111-119.

46. Gibbons, R. and van Houte, J. 1973. J. Periodontol. 347-360.

47. Gibbons, R. and van Houte, J. 1975. Ann. Rev. Microbiol. 29:19-44.

48. Guggenheim, B. and Schroeder, H. 1967. Helv. Odont. Acta. 11:131-152.

49. Nisizawa, t. et al. 1976. Archs. oral Biol. 21:207-213.

50. Gibbons, R. and Nygarrd, M. 1968. Archs. oral Biol. 13:1249-1262.

51. Gibbons, R. and Banghart, S. 1967. Archs. oral Biol. 12:11-24.

52. Gibbons, R. and Fitzgerald, R. 1969. J. Bacteriol. 98:341-346.

53. Germaine, G. and Schachtele, C. 1976. Infect. Immun. 13:365-372.

54. Borgeah, G. and McBride, B. 1976. Infect. Immun. 13:1228-1234.

55. Guggenheim, B. and Newbrun, E. 1969. Hlev. Odont. Acta. 13:84-97.

56. Carlsson, J. and Elander, D. 1973. Caries Res. 7:89-101.

57. Chludzinski, A., Germaine, G. and Schachtele, C. 1974. J. Bacteriol. 118:1-7.

58. Ciardi, J., Hageage, G. and Wittenberger, C. 1976. J. Dent. Res. 55:C87-C96.

59. McCabe, M. and Smith, E. 1977. 16:760-765.

60. DaCosta,t., Bier,L. and Gaida, F. 1974. Archs. oral Biol. 19:341-342.

61. Staat, R. and Schachtele, C. 1976. J. Dent. Res. 55:1103-1110.

62. Staat, R., Gawrowski, T. and Schachtele, C. 1973. Infect. Immun. 8:1009-1016.

63. Staat, R. and Schachtele, C. 1975. Infect. Immun. 12:556-563.

64. Freedman, M. and Tanzer, J. 1974. Infect. Immun. 10:189-196.

65. Tanzer, J., Freedman, M., Fitzgerald, R. and Larson, R. 1974. Infect. Immun. 10:197-203.

66. Freedman, M. and Birkhed, D. Unpublished Observations.

67. Schachtele, C, et al. 1976. in "Microbial Aspects of Dental Caries." Eds. Stiles, Loesche, and O'Brien. IRL. p. 401-412.

68. Chludzinski, A., Germaine, G. and Schachtele, C. 1976. J. Dent. Res. 55:C75-C86.

69. Birkhed, D. and Rosell. 1975. Odont. Revy. 26:281-290.

70. Hotz, P., Guggenheim, B. and Schmid, R. 1972. Caries Res. 6:103-121.

71. Delisle, A. 1976. Infect. Immun. 13:619-626.

72. Higuchi, M., Araya, S. and Higuchi, M. 1976. J. Dent. Res. 55:266-271.

73. Greer, S. et al. 1971. J. Dent. Res. 50:1594-1604.

74. Bleiweis, A., Hurst, S. and Craig, R. in "Immunologic Aspects of Dental Caries." Eds. Bowen, Genco, and O'Brien. p. 45-49.

75. Shockman, G. et al. 1976. in "Microbial Aspects of Dental Caries." Eds. Stiles, Loesche, and O'Brien, IRL. p. 631-647.

76. Littleton, N. et al. 1967. Arch. oral Biol. 12:601-609.

77. Littleton, N., Carter, C. and Kelley, R. 1967. J. Amer. Dent. Assn. 74:119-123.

78. Onose, H. and Sandham, H. 1976. Archs. oral Biol. 21.291-296.

79. Sandham, H. and Phillips, H. 1976. in "Microbial Aspects of Dental Caries." Eds. Bowen, Genco and O'Brien. IRL. p. 557-562.

80. Loesche, W. and Bhat, M. 1976. in "Microbial Aspects of Dental Caries." Eds. Bowen, Genco, and O'Brien. IRL. p. 291-301.

81. Hojo, S., Higuchi, M. and Araya, S. 1976. J. Dent. Res. 55:169.

82. Ellen, R. 1976. Oral Sci. Rev. 8:3-23.

Discussion of some disease-predictive biochemical activities of plaque microbes

W.M. Edgar

Department of Oral Physiology, University of Newcastle on Tyne, Newcastle, England

Dr. Freedman's thoughtful and well-documented communication deals with 3 important biochemical activities of potential value in caries prognostication. It is a measure of the distances dental scientists have travelled along the road to hoped-for success that we are in a position to consider so fully these factors, yet as Dr. Freedman points out, two fundamental problems remain: first, tests of biochemical activities associated with caries are hitherto of diagnostic rather than predictive value; and secondly, sensitive indicators of the cariogenicity of plaque remain to be identified.

The history of lactobacillus counts and Snyder tests tells us that we cannot expect to learn about causal relationships from correlations between caries prevalence and biochemical or microbiological studies, but can only check on predictions by following them up longitudinally with observations of disease incidence (1,2). The conduct of such experiments in normal human populations is complex, expensive and slow, and may engender more fundamental problems - for instance, does sampling change the environment,or ecology of the sites studies? Equally, it might be argued that the time-scales of changes in plaque biochemistry and caries are so different that a single biochemical measurement, however well controlled the sampling, cannot give more than a crude indication of the probability of subsequent caries.

As caries is considered as being a multi-factorial etiology, biochemical studies related to caries prevalence (comparing caries active and inactive subjects, or sites) might in theory at least be expected to have greatest predictive value if the measurement(s) reflect a combination of caries-related factors. From the older literature, the Karshan (3) and Fosdick (4) tests on saliva represent tests of this kind. Another such measurement, more in line with modern thinking, is that of plaque pH - often regarded as a prime parameter of cariogenicity, and which is the resultant of at least five contributory factors (microbial acidogenicity, base production, plaque buffering, access to saliva, dietary history). Analysis of any of these contributory factors, each a function of a number of processes, is likely to be inadequate to predict the pH behaviour of plaque <u>in situ</u> unless the factor is of overriding importance, a situation which on present knowledge does not appear to hold.

However, while plaque pH has been shown in a number of studies (5-8) to be to a degree related to caries prevalence, other biochemical factors in plaque are likely to inter-act to reduce the closeness of this association. Calcium and phosphate concentrations in the plaque environment are usually considered to be of importance in governing the rate of withdrawal of mineral from the underlying enamel, and are associated inversely with caries (9,10,11) although a secondary relationship with plaque pH may complicate this relationship (10). Similar considerations apply to plaque fluoride concentrations, which are negatively associated with caries (12), but also with plaque quantities (13,14) and acidogenicity (14). Refinement of the mathematical analysis of the effects of these inter-related factors, perhaps using multiple regression techniques, might possibly lead to a derived parameter with superior powers of discrimination between cariogenic and non-cariogenic plaques.

Nevertheless, plaques with similar rates of acid production, intra- and extra-cellular polysaccharide synthesis, and concentrations of calcium, phosphate and fluoride, may yet differ in cariogenicity owing to differences in other factors in the biochemistry of the plaque, in the nature of the tooth surface colonised, or in the salivary environment. An ideal biochemical test of the aggressiveness of plaque would measure directly the loss of mineral from the enamel. A test described by Coolidge (15) measured the change in phosphate concentration of plaque in situ after exposure to glucose; a rise in phosphate (observed in a caries-prone 12-year-old, but not in a caries-free site in a 45-year-old subject) was held to represent phosphate withdrawn from the tooth, as access of saliva to the plaque was prevented. Experiments on similar lines (16) have given some confirmation of the effect, although interpretation of these latter experiments is complicated by the fact that salivary access was permitted - of course, salivary factors should, notwithstanding, be admitted into consideration of cariogenicity as will, no doubt, be described later by Dr. Mandel.

It is conceivable that a number of biochemical indicators of plaque cariogenicity could be linked through the properties of a single predominant microorganism. The studies of Minah and Loesche (17,18) described by Dr. Freedman highlight the place of Streptococcus mutans in such a role. The relatively high proportion of S. mutans (40% of C.F.U.) in caries-associated plaque compared with plaque from adjacent caries-free sites is accompanied by increased rates of lactate production and IPS, and extra-cellular polysaccharide synthesis when the plaques were incubated in vitro with low levels (0.06%) of sucrose. These three biochemical activities can be considered alongside the differences in plaque pH between carious and non-carious subjects or sites referred to earlier; study of their role in controlling the initial pH, and pH minimum after sucrose exposure in situ merits attention, in view of other evidence that plaque pH tends to reflect salivary pH and buffering power (6,7,8), or the supply of urea from the saliva or gingival fluid (19).

Search for a sensitive indicator of predictive value may yet succeed. Dr. Freedman brings to our attention a range of microbial traits which require further study. To these we might add the examination of activities within the broader range of chemical inter-actions with the enamel, in plaque as a whole, preferably in situ. Whether or not such studies will prove of value beyond the narrow confines of a controlled laboratory experiment, they may repay the effort in terms of our recognition of the factors controlling the cariogenicity of plaque.

LITERATURE CITED

1. Davies, G.N., King, R.M. and Collins, A.A. 1959. Archs. oral Biol. 1:62.

2. Gardner, M.K. and Snyder, M.L. 1960. J. Dent. Res. 39:320.

3. Karshan, M. 1939. J. Dent. Res. 18:395.

4. Fosdick, L.S., Hansen, H.L. and Epple, C. 1937. J. Amer. Dent. Assn. 24:1275.

5. Stephan, R.M. 1944. J. Dent. Res. 23:257.

6. Englander, H.R., Carter, W.J. and Fosdick, L.S. 1956. J. Dent. Res. 35:792.

7. Kleinberg, I. and Jenkins, G.N. 1964. Archs. oral Biol. 9:493.

8. Edgar, W.M. 1976. Caries Res. 10:241.

9. Dawes, C. and Jenkins, G.N. 1962. Archs oral Biol. 7:161.

10. Kleinberg, I., Chatterjee, R., Kaminsky, F.S., Cross, G.H., Goldenberg, D.J. and Kaufman, H.W. 1971. J. Periodontol. 42:497.

11. Ashley,F.P. 1975. Caries Res. 9:351.

12. Agus, H.M., Schamschula, R.G., Barmes, D.E. and Brunzel, M. 1976. Community Dent. Oral Epidemiol. 4:210.

13. Hardwick, J.L. 1970. In: McHugh, W.D. (ed) Dental Plaque. Livengstone Edinburgh, p. 171.

14. Jenkins, G.N. and Edgar, W.M. 1977. Caries Res.11.(Suppl I)226.

15. Coolidge, T.B. 1947. J. Dent. Res. 26:43.

16. Ferguson, D.B. and Thomas, P.D. 1974. J. Dent. Res. 53:1071 and personal communication.

17. Minah, G.E. and Loesche, W.J. 1977. Infect. Immunity 17:43.

18. Minah, G.E. and Loesche, W.J. 1977. Infect. Immunity 17:55.

19. Kleinberg, I. 1967. Archs. oral Biol. 12:1475.

Salivary factors in caries prediction

Irwin D. Mandel

School of Dental and Oral Surgery, Columbia University, 630 West 168th Street, New York, New York 10032

New analytic techniques, advances in equipment and the ready availability from commercial sources of a large variety of reagents have stimulated a considerable amount of research on the normal composition of saliva, especially the salivary proteins. Several recent reviews summarize the current state of knowledge[1-4]. Salivary secretions are rather modest in protein concentration, but are rich in diversity and include high molecular weight glycoproteins (alias mucin), low molecular weight glycoproteins, phospho-proteins, proline-rich basic proteins, proline-rich anionic proteins, histidine-rich proteins, tyrosine-rich proteins (no poor proteins in saliva), immunoglobulins, lactoferrin, amylase, lysozyme, lactoperoxidase, albumin and serum proteins in low concentration, and a number of other proteins as well as a variety of peptides. The large range of biologic activities resulting from this diversity is only beginning to be appreciated[5,6]. These proteins (and peptides), aided by the cations, anions and organic non-electrolytes in saliva, afford the host considerable protection against dental caries[2,5].

The widely accepted view is that saliva provides protection against cariogenic challenge via four general mechanisms: (1) bacterial clearance (reduced adherence to tooth surfaces) by mechanico-anatomic means and by immunologic and non-immunologic mediated aggregation, (2) direct antibacterial activity, (3) buffering neutralizing or modifying acid production or acid transport in the plaque, (4) counteracting demineralization (or encouraging remineralization) through cations (calcium, magnesium), anions (phosphate, fluoride), and other anti-solubility factors (specific proteins). For pertinent references, see reviews by Mandel[5.6], van Houte[7], and Kleinberg <u>et al</u>[8,9].

<u>Bacterial Clearance (reduced adherence)</u>

It is only in the past few years that there has been a full appreciation of the importance of bacterial clearance (the interference with bacterial adherence to tooth and mucous membrane surfaces), as the basic protective mechanism in the oral cavity[10]. The comparability of salivary flow and oral muscle action to: (a) tearing and blinking, (b) blowing, expectorating and mucociliary movement and (c) peristaltic action has always been apparent. The comparability of oral immunologic and non-immunologic aggregating mechanisms to similar activities on a variety of mucous membrane surfaces is, however, only lately becoming apparent[11]. Bacterial adherence to teeth (and inhibition of same) represents a unique human situation and, for analogous activity one has to go to marine biology[12]; from the bacteria's point of view, however, a flowing stream analogy is apt.

When one relates bacterial clearance to caries activity, it is difficult to picture anatomic mechanisms (lip, tongue, oral-facial muscle movement) as major factors. Patients with marked impairment (stroke, cerebral palsy, etc.) would, of course, be at greater risk, but within the normal situation, anatomic variations would not be an important determinant. Salivary flow, however, would have more pertinence. This is most readily apparent in patients with severe xerostomia, especially the extreme situation that accompanies irradiation. This area has recently been reviewed by Dreizen and Brown[13] and offers strong testimony as to the protective quality of saliva.

When one moves beyond this extreme situation to studies involving the correlation between flow rate and caries attack rate, no consistent relationship can be shown. The most comprehensive study was conducted by Shannon and Terry[14], who measured parotid fluid flow rate without exogenous stimulation in 3,786 healthy, young adult males. In the lowest caries group, zero through ten DMF surfaces, there was a significantly higher flow rate (0.041 ml/min) than in all the other subjects (0.037 ml/min).

Although the difference was significant statistically, the degree of overlap of the flow rates between the groups limits the biologic significance of the finding. The caries status of an individual could not be predicted from the flow rate measurement. Similar findings have been reported even when completely caries-resistant individuals have been compared to highly susceptible subjects[15]. Only when flow rate is noticeably reduced by pathologic or pharmacologic agents is the effect on caries consistent. Flow rate measurements should be recommended to objectively establish a major impairment in flow. Such measurements are easily made by standard procedures

Since flow rate per se does not appear to account for resistance, other aspects of the clearance mechanism need to be considered. Within tissues, bacteria are usually cleared by phagocytosis, aided by the products of the complement activation cascade (both regular and alternate pathways). Such a clearance mechanism can operate in the crevicular area, but because of a paucity of functional phagocytes and lack of complement, not in most of the oral cavity. The only portion of the teeth that could benefit from phagocyotic activity would be the area immediately adjacent to the gingival margins. The oral cavity, however, is open on both ends and hence, appropriately clumped or aggregated bacteria, with a diminished capacity for adherence to mucous membrane or tooth surfaces, would be expectorated, or more usually, swallowed.

We all possess a rather tortuous, but effective sewage system and the high concentration of bacteria in feces attests to its efficacy. Bacterial aggregation can result from both immunologic[7] and non-immunologic mechanisms[5].

Immunologic Aspects of Bacterial Clearance

A workshop and the resulting publications reviewed the rapidly growing literature on the role of secretory IgA as an inhibitor of bacterial adherence to tooth surfaces[16]. Animal immunization studies provide the most direct evidence that "Salivary antibody to cariogenic streptococci inhibits implantation of these organisms in dental plaque and may be protective against dental caries"[17]. The evidence in humans is, as yet, neither direct nor clear[18]. Several groups reported elevated levels of SIgA in caries free, as opposed to caries active, subjects; others, the reverse (see reference 18 and 19 for review). In all of these studies total SIgA (concentration or secretion rate) was measured, not specific antibody. The current availability of appropriate antigens and the development of sensitive techniques (ELISA)[20] make it possible to engage in quantitative antibody measurements. The recent demonstration by Crawford et al[21], that the minor salivary glands contribute a major share of the salivary SIgA suggest that secretions from these glands should be assayed as well.

Secretory IgA antibody titer measurements against specific antigens such as the serotype "C" cell wall antigen of S. mutans or a specific S. mutans glucosyltransferase would appear to be a desirable measurement to predict host resistance against caries. Commercially available plastic tubes with a given amount of specific antigens could be treated with an appropriate amount of parotid or submaxillary saliva and in turn treated with an enzyme linked anti-human secretory IgA (also commerically available). The antibody could be readily quantitated via an appropriate chromogenic reaction.

Non-Immunological Aspects of Bacterial Clearance

Work in several laboratories suggests that, in addition to tailor-made, precisely fitting antibodies, ready-made salivary macromolecules may also react with appropriate receptors on the surface of bacteria, cause agglutination, and reduce the proclivity of these organisms to join pellicle proteins on the tooth surface -- in short, to noticeably modify adherence and colonization. Since many of the same salivary proteins are present in the pellicle as well as in the fluid environment of the pellicle, adherence and agglutination or aggregation are potentially co-operative or competitive processes, depending upon circumstances.

An excellent recent review by Gibbons and Van Houte[22] pointed out the variety of reactions that occur among bacteria because of the special properties of the cell walls of different bacteria and the intriguing interactions that result from the chemical affinity of specific groups on host proteins for receptors on the bacterial cell walls. The permutations and combinations that might arise from the couplings and polygamous liaisons that could develop stagger the imagination. Thanks to several groups of investigators[22,32], however, some order is emerging. The findings to date support the contention that aggregating factors in saliva may include a "general type that cross reacts with a number of different cells as well as a specific type reacting with particular cell surface configurations[24]. The degree to which the specificity is a function of the host molecule or the bacteria or both remains to be established.

The only bacterial aggregating factors that have been examined chemically are an apparent high molecular weight (or aggregated) glycoprotein in parotid saliva[26] and high molecular weight glycoproteins in whole saliva [23,24,33], resembling "mucins". One would expect considerable individual variation in agglutination activity, since these mucins give evidence of considerable heterogeneity. They possess blood group activity, which is one of the reasons for the variation in composition, and hence, could be one of the pathways of expression of a genetic relationship to caries activity[34].

Regulation of Bacterial Clearance

Consideration of blood group activity and heterogeneity suggests that we have reached a second stage in the description of oral bacterial clearance, namely, regulation of the process.

Extrapolating from the observations in non-oral as well as oral studies, it is possible to suggest a number of determinants of the rate of clearance of potentially cariogenic organisms: (1) Ericson,[35] summarizing the findings of his group on the role of salivary agglutinins in plaque formation, suggested that at a low concentration of the factor only a limited number of sites on the bacterial cell surface are blocked, allowing for formation of multilayers of aggregates of organisms on the tooth surface with rapid plaque formation. At high concentrations of the salivary factor, sites on the bacterial surface become saturated and binding of the bacteria to the tooth surface occurs in monolayers and plaque formation proceeds at a slower rate.

The implication of this observation is that the relative concentration of the potential agglutinin in the saliva vs. the plaque or pellicle would be a major rate determinant. In time this could become a valid indication of caries activity. More information on specific agglutinins would be a necessary requisite. (2) Evidence is rapidly accumulating that terminal sugars are responsible for the specificity of mammalian lectins (see Ashwell and Morell[36] for review). If, indeed, the integrity of terminal sugars on the potential agglutinin is essential for interaction with the specific bacterial receptor site, then the effective concentration of enzymes mammalian or bacterial sources capable of hydrolyzing these sugars would be an important determinant of rate of clearance. The effective concentration of the enzymes would, in turn, be a function of their rate of liberation into the oral cavity and the presence of inhibitors of this activity.

Since the bacterial enzymes are quite abundant in the oral cavity, the determinant of rate may be the inhibition of the enzymes. Several studies indicate that such inhibition is present and measurable. Fukui *et al*[37] demonstrated inhibition of oral bacterial neuraminidase by SIgA; bacterial neuraminidases from non-oral sources were affected to a much less degree. Theoretically, SIgA could partially or completely inhibit all of the bacterial hydrolases, just as it appears to have the potential to inhibit at least some glucosyltransferases[38,39]. Quantitation of specific enzymes such as neuraminadase, fucosidase, galactosidase, etc. as well as SIgA antibody titers to these enzymes is worth considering. Non-immunological inhibitors of bacterial and possible mammalian enzymes also exist in the oral cavity[40,41] hence, it might be more appropriate to measure interference with enzyme activity rather than antibody titer.

Measurements of Aggregation

Until such time as specific agglutinins are characterized, measurement of aggregation by salivary secretions against specific organisms should be a worthwhile procedure. Some aspects of the inter-relations of aggregating agents and bacteria can be studied in *in vitro* systems in which either rate or degree of aggregation is quantitated, usually by spectrophotometric analyses. The usual procedures and their limitations were reviewed by Harris and Mitchell in 1973[42]. Quantitative spectrophometric measurements are currently in use by Iancono *et al*[43], and Ericson *et al*[44], a Coulter counter method by Kashket and colleagues[24,33]. It should be possible to utilize these techniques, especially the one described by Ericson *et al*[44] for quantitative comparison of aggregating ability of subjects against a variety or organisms or combinations of organisms. As pointed out by Harris and Mitchell[42], however, the changes in turbidity measure are the result of settling of large aggregates containing at least 150 cocci and, consequently, not a measure of the initial phase of aggregation. Harris and Mitchell[42] suggested light-scattering techniques.

A light-scattering technique par excellence is produced when a helium-neon laser beam is scattered from bacteria in suspension. Such a system is being currently developed by Ryan and colleagues at Stevens Institute in Hoboken, N.J.[45]

Direct Anti-Bacterial Activity, Non-Immunologic Aspects

Saliva shares with other exocrine glands and phagocytic cells a common defense system against bacteria - lysozyme, lactoferrin, and lactoperoxidase[5,46-48]. Phagocytic cells, of course, possess a much more extensive weaponry because of the unavailability of mechanical clearance mechanisms in most tissues. It is possible that there are more than just the 3L counterparts in saliva. For instance, the large number of cationic proteins of parotid and submaxillary saliva[1,2,49] might include some with antibacterial properties similar to those in the phagocytic cell. This area deserves attention. It is being focused on lysozyme, lactoferrin and lactoperoxidase at this time.

The work to date on lysozyme activity in the oral cavity would support the view that lysozyme concentration may not be a major determinant of caries activity. Gibbons, de Stoppelar, and Harder[50] found that none of the thirteen groups of oral organisms they tested were susceptible to lysozyme at concentrations of more than ten times that usually found in saliva. Mandel and Zengo[15] could find no significant difference in parotid or submaxillary lysozyme concentration or secretion rate when caries resistant and caries susceptible subjects were compared.

It would be premature, however, to infer from these few studies that lysozyme is without effect on oral organisms. The negative findings may be a reflection of the test systems used for examination of lysozyme activity[51]. Considerable impetus has been given to lysozyme investigations in the oral cavity by the elegant experiments of Pollack *et al*[52]. They demonstrated that lysozyme binding to *S. mutans* was receptor site specific, but that it was *not* due to muramidase activity per se. Binding was followed by aggregation and, under appropriate conditions (such as addition to sodium chloride), lysis. Even without actual lysis, however, the binding of lysozyme to bacteria results in loss of viability[52]. These observations strongly suggest the importance of continued examination of lysozyme in caries prediction.

Earlier studies on lysozyme levels in saliva employed a turbidometric method. The popular current method is the lysoplate assay of Osserman and Lawlor[53]. This method, too, has many problems[54]. The strong binding of lysozyme to anionic proteins, such as the high molecular weight glycoprotein of salivary gland mucous cells, creates additional difficulty. Improvements in lysozyme quantitation and use of measurements against specific oral organisms should be encouraged.

Lactoferrin

Lactoferrin (Lf) has been shown to possess bacteriostatic properties for a variety of aerobic and facultative organisms (see reference 5 for review). The bacteriostatic properties have been attributed to the ability of the unsaturated protein to bind two iron atoms per molecule. This ability of a host protein to withhold iron from invading bacteria has been termed "nutritional immunity" and is receiving increasing interest. It is an important protective mechanism against aerobic and facultative bacteria, since they require ferric iron for their metabolism. It has also been postulated that Lf can enhance the antibacterial activity of lysozyme by chelating iron and copper, both metals reducing the efficacy of lysozyme[55].

Information on the specifics of the Lf inhibition of bacteria has recently been provided by Bishop *et al*[56] who demonstrated *in vitro* growth inhibition of coliform bacteria by bovine APO-Lf and the reversal of this inhibition by citrate. This study demonstrated the importance of the competitive aspects of iron capture in the immediate environment of iron dependent bacteria. The plaque must be a highly competitive prospecting environment where iron mining by bacteria becomes the host equivalent of gold mining.

The potential importance of iron and Lf to caries was shown by Cole *et al*[57]. They found that in their *in vitro* system human colostrum Lf (and presumably salivary as well) was *bacteriocidal* for *S. mutans*. They pointed out that "the elimination of the bacteriocidal effect of Lf following saturation with iron strongly indicates that this effect can be attributed to the iron binding capacity of the molecule". The effect could be blocked by SIgA with anti *S. mutans* activity, suggesting that Lf acts via specific cell wall receptors.

Lactoferrin is elevated and easily measurable in parotitis by a rocket electrophoresis method[58]. In normal subjects a more sensitive technique is necessary. The ELISA procedure[20] offers promise as does a solid phase radioimmunoassay currently being employed to measure the small amount of plasma Lf in diseases involving white blood cells[59].

Lactoperoxidase

Lactoperoxidase activity and its antibacterial role in exocrine secretions and phagocytic cells has been receiving increased attention in recent years (see references 5 and 46 for review). In the phagocytic cell, major emphasis is being placed on oxidative killing of bacteria, generation of highly reactive oxygen "products", such as superoxide, singlet oxygen and hyproxyl radicals (see reference 60 for review). The role of myeloperoxidase in these reactions is a major area of research.

Although lactoperoxidase is very similar to myeloperoxidase (although antigenically distinct), they are part of systems operating in a different milieu and have to be studied independently. Most of the recent work in saliva has been conducted by Hoogedoorn and summarized in a recent paper[61]. His data indicate that the inter-action of the salivary enzyme with the thiocyanate ion and hydrogen peroxide results in the formation of the hypothiocyanate ion which reacts with RSH groups in hexokinase. The subsequent reduction in glycolysis can be shown to result in an inhibition of S. mutans growth in vitro and in reduced accumulation of plaque in vivo[62,63] (when lactoperoxidase is introduced in a suitable formulation).

Some recent work by Gothefors and Marklund[64] showed that the amounts of lactoperoxidase and thiocyanate in the saliva of human infants was sufficient to inhibit bacterial growth in vitro systems. Interest in lactoperoxidase in saliva has been stimulated by the work of Makinen et al[65], which indicates that xylitol consumption increases salivary lactoperoxidase activity four to ten times. It has been speculated that part of the marked caries reduction that accompanies xylitol substitution for sucrose arises via the lactoperoxidase system.

There are several methods in use for examination of lactoperoxidase activity[61,64,65], essentially variations on the standard procedures for peroxidase measurement. The best procedure for examination for potential value in caries prediction testing has to be established.

Antacid and Antisolubility Factors

The current status of research in this area was reviewed by Mandel and Kleinberg[9]. A number of components contribute to the ability of saliva to neutralize the acid procuded in the plaque or introduced directly in the diet. These include the buffer systems (carbonic acid-bicarbonate, phosphate, proteins) ammonia, urea and recently described pH rise factor[9]. This salivary peptide can rapidly clear glucose from plaque, increase base formation, and elevate the level of pH in plaque. Most of the studies relating calcium, phosphate, magnesium, ammonia and urea to caries activity have been at best, equivocal[2]. Some of the early studies on buffer capacity seemed to indicate an inverse relationship)see reference 2 for review), and should be repeated . Perhaps the role of saliva as an antacid and antisolubility entity should be looked at in a somewhat different way than in the past - perhaps more as a regulatory agency[6]. In this frame of reference, pH regulators, such as sialin[9] and proteins that interact with calcium[66-68] may have a major impact on critical processes within the plaque and at the tooth-plaque (pellicle) interface. Hay and Grøn[66] clearly demonstrated that specific salivary proteins (designated as tyrosine and proline rich), by interacting with calcium, could prevent precipitation and phase transformation of basic calcium phosphate to hydroxyapatite. They suggested that such a stabilization would act to maintain super-saturation of calcium phosphate in plaque and act to reduce the rate of demineralization.

Inter-action with calcium can also affect aggregation, since calcium bridging and calcium neutralization of the electro-negative surface of most bacteria is an important aspect of aggregation. Crystal formation and dissolution should also be considered as part of the regulatory mechanism in plaque.

With the delineation of specific proteins that have potential regulatory functions, a reasonable first step in establishing their association with caries would be a quantitative comparison in parotid and submaxillary saliva of caries resistant and susceptible subjects. Initially, this might be pursued as part of a comparison of acrylamide gels examined densitometrically after electrophoresis or iso-electric focusing. In time, the comparison should be on the basis of quantitative immunochemistry with appropriate antisera. A similar strategy should be employed in determining whether there are any quantitative differences in "sialin"[9]. Comparisons in saliva can first be conducted on an activity basis and then by quantitative immunochemistry when appropriate antisera are available.

Theoretically, at least, and with some experimental support[69,70] salivary proteins could affect demineralization via the pellicle and a role in controlling rate of diffusion into and out of the enamel surface. Specific components in the pellicle might also modify the permselective properties at the enamel interface. Examination of pellicle for specific proteins could prove a fruitful area of research and serve as a basis for the next generation of caries activity testing.

It is abundantly clear that saliva is closely related to caries; but it is a relative once removed. The immediate family is tooth pellicle and plaque. Perhaps the next generation of caries predictors will focus on salivary components in pellicle or plaque, not on saliva per se.

SUMMARY

Past studies on salivary parameters with potential for predicting caries activity have not resulted in any positive recommendations. The only salivary characteristics that may be valuable are salivary flow rate in cases of marked impairment (less than .2 ml/min/gland) and buffer capacity.

The present generation of studies offer promise in a number of areas: 1) quantitation of salivary aggregation of specific bacteria, since salivary aggregation can be an effective clearance mechanism; 2) measurements of carbohydrases and inhibitors of carbohydrases as indicators of clearance regulation; 3) secretory IgA antibody levels against specific bacterial antigens and enzymes (i.e. sero-type "C" S. mutans cell wall antigens and glucosyltransferase) on the basis of inhibition of adherence to tooth surfaces; 4) direct anti-bacterial activity via lysozyme, lactoferrin and lactoperoxidase. This may be the promise of the courtship period; whether the expectations are met remains to be seen.

Recent work suggests that specific salivary peptides may become incorporated into pellicle and plaque and: 1) affect rate of acid production, (Sialin, an arginine peptide) and 2) regulate calcium and phosphate concentration, (Statherin a tyrosine rich anionic peptide). On a theoretical basis quantitation of these peptides might be valuable measures of host resistance.

LITERATURE CITED

1. Levine, M. J. and Ellison, S.A. 1973. Immuno-Electrophoretic and Chemical Analyses of Human Parotid Saliva. Archs. oral Biol. 18:839.

2. Mandel, I.D. 1974. Relation of Saliva and Plaque to Caries. J. Dent. Res. 53:246.

3. Arneberg, P. 1974. Secretroy Proteins from Primate Glands. Thesis. University of Oslo.

4. Mandel, I.D. Human Submaxillary, Sublingual and Parotid Glycoproteins and Enamel Pellical in the Glycoproteins. eds. Horowitz, M. and Pigman, W. Academic Press. In press.

5. Mandel, I.D. 1976. Nonimmunologic Aspects of Caries Resistance. J. Dent. Res. 55:C22.

6. Mandel, I.D. 1977. Salivary Products in Plaque and Saliva in Relation to Caries. "Microb. Aspects of Dent. Caries" eds. Stiles, Loesche, and O'Brien, Sp. Supp. Microb. Abstracts 859.

7. Van Houte, J. 1977. Oral Bacterial Colonization: Mechanisms and Implications. Sp. Supp. Microbiol. eds. Stiles, Abstracts 3.

8. Kleinberg, I. 1970. Biochemistry of the Dental Plaque p. 43-90. In: Staple, P.H. (ed.) Advances in Oral Biology, Vol. 4, Academic Press, New York.

9. Kleinberg, I., Kanapka, J.A. and Craw, D. 1977. Effects of Saliva and Salivary Factors on the metabolism of the mixed Oral Flora. Sp. Supp. Microbiol. Eds. Stiles, Abstract 433.

10. Van Houte, J., Gibbons, R.J. and Pulkkinan, A.J. 1971. Adherence as an Ecological Determinant for Streptococci in the Human Mouth. Archs. oral Biol., 16:1131.

11. Savage, D.C. 1977. Microbiol Colonization of Epithelial Surfaces in the Intestinal Tract: A Review. Sp. Supp. Microbiol. Ed. Stiles. Abstract 33.

12. Mitchell, R. 1977. Mechanism of Attachment of Microorganisms to Surfaces. Sp. Supp. Microbiol. Ed. Stiles, Abstract 47.

13. Dreizen, S. and Brown, L.R. 1977. Xerostomia and Dental Caries Sp. Supp. Microbiol. Ed. Stiles, Abstract 263.

14. Shannon, I.L. and Terry, J.M. 1965. A Higher Parotid Flow Rate in Subjects with Resistance to Caries. J. Dent. Med. 20:128.

15. Mandel, I.D. and Zengo, A.N. 1973. Genetic and Chemical Aspects in Caries Resistance in Comparative Immunology of the Oral Cavity. Washington, D.C. U.S. Gov't Printing Office.

16. O'Brien, T. 1976. Rationale for Continued Investigations on a Vaccine as an Approach to Dental Caries Prevention. Sp. Supp. Immunol. Eds. Bowen, Genco and O'Brien. Abst. 3.

17. Evans, R.T. Emmings, F.G. and Genco, R.J. 1975. Salivary Antibody Inhibition of S. Mutans. Infect. and Immun. 12:293.

18. Bowen, W. 1976. Relevance of Caries Vaccine Investigations in Rodents, Primates and Humans. Sp. Suppl. Immunol. Abst. 1:11.

19. Everhart, D.L. et al 1977. Dental Caries and Salivary IgA in Children. Caries Res. 11:211.

20. Evans, R.T. et al 1971. Measurement of Antibody to Purified Carbohydrates of S. mutans with RLISHA. Sp. Supp. Microbiol. Abst. 375.

21. Crawford, J.M., Taubman, M.A. and Smith, D.J. 1975. Minor Salivary Glands as a Major Source of Secretory IgA in Human Oral Cavity. Science 190:1206.

22. Gibbons, R.J. and van Houte, J. 1975. Bacterial Adherence in Microbial Ecology. Ann. Rev. Microbiology, 29:19.

23. Hay, D.I., Gibbons, R.J. and Spinell, D.M. 1971. Characteristics of Some High Molecular Weight Constituents with Bacterial Aggregating Activity. Caries Res., 5:111.

24. Kashket, A. and Donaldson, C.G. 1972. Saliva Induced Aggregation of Oral Streptococci. J. Bact. 112:1127.

25. Chatterjee, R.and Kleinberg,I.1974Formation of Salivary Aggregates. Proc. I.A.D.R. Supp. J. Dent. Res. Abst. #180.

26. Ericson, T., Carlen, A. and Dagerskun, E. 1977. Salivary Aggregating Factors. Sp. Supp. Microbiol. Ed. Stiles, Abst. 151.

27. Kashket, S. and Hankin, S.R. 1977. Interaction of Streptococcal Aggregating Factors with Thio and Disulphide Reactive Compounds. Archs. oral Biol. 22:49.

28. Ericson,T., Pruitt, K. and Bratthall, D. 1973. On the Specificity of Bacterial Aggregation. J. Dent. Res. 52:205.

29. Ericson, T., Sandham, J.& Magnusson,I.1975. A Sedimentation Method for Study of Adsorption of Microorganisms onto Apatite Surfaces. Caries Res. 9:325.

30. Magnuson, I. and Ericson, T. 1970. Effect of Salivary Agglutinins on Reactions Between Hydroxapatite Serotype C Strain of S. mutans. Caries Res. 10:277.

31. Magnusson, I., Ericson, T., and Pruitt, K. Effect of Salivary Agglutinins on Bacterial Colonization of Tooth Surfaces (Submitted for Publication).

32. Orstavik, D., Kraus, F.W. and Henshaw, I.C. 1974. In vitro Attachment of Streptococci to the Tooth Surface. Infect. and Immun. 9:794.

33. Williams, R.C. and Gibbons, R.J. 1975. Inhibition of Streptococcal Attachment to Receptors on Human Buccal Epithelial Cells. Infect. and Immun. 11:711.

35. Ericson, T. 1972. A Possible Role for Salivary Lectins in the Early Stages of Plaque Formation. Eur. Org. Caries Res. Meeting, London.

36. Ashwell, G. and Morell, A.G. 1977. Membrane Glycoproteins and Recognition Phenomena. TIBS, Page 76, April.

37. Fukui, Y. et al 1973. Inhibition of Enzymes by Human Salivary IgA, Infect. and Immun. 8:375.

38. Klein, J.P. et al 1977. Inhibition of Glucosyltransferase by Human Salivary IgA. Infect. and Immun. 15:329.

39. Challacombe, S.J., Lehner, T., and Guggenheim, B. 1972. Serum and Salivary Antibodies to Glucosyltransferases in Dental Caries in Man. Nature, 238:219.

40. Sakamoto, W. et al. 1976. B-Glucuronidase Inhibitor Activity in Human Activity in Human Saliva. Archs. oral Biol. 21:761.

41. Gillard, B.K. 1976. Cystic Fibrosis: Enzymatic Detection of a Ciliostatic Factor. Pediat. Res. 10:907.

42. Harris, R.H. and Mitchell, R. 1973. Role of Polymers in Microbial Aggregation. Ann. Rev. Microbiol. 27:27.

43. Iacono, V.J. et al. 1975. Spectrophometric Assay for Quantitation of Bacterial Antibody. J. Dent. Res. 54, Sp. Issue A, Abst. L394.

44. Ericson, T. et al. 1975. The Reaction of Salivary Substances with Bacteria. J. Oral Path. 4:307.

45. Ryan, V. et al. Aggregation Rate Study of Streptococcus Mutans FA-1 Using Laser Homodyne Spectorscopy. Submitted for Publication.

46. Bowen, W. 1974. Defense Mechanisms in the Mouth and their Possible Role in Prevention of Dental Caries: A Review. J. Oral Path. 3:266.

47. Coleman, S.E., Van de Rign, I. and Bleiweis, A.S. 1971. Lysis of Cariogenic and Non-Cariogenic Oral Streptococci with Lysozyme. J. Dent. Res. 50:939.

48. Iwamoto, Y., Watanabe, T., Tsunemitsu, A., Fukui, K. and Moriyama, T. 1971. Lysis of Streptococci by Lysozyme from Human Parotid Saliva and Sodium Lauryl Sulfate. J. Dent. Res., 50:1688.

49. Bonilla, C. 1971. Comparative Biochemistry and Pharmacology of Salivary Gland Secretions. J. Chromatog. 56:368.

50. Gibbons, R.J., de Stoppelar, J.D. and Harder, L. 1966. Lysozyme Insensitivity of Bacteria Indigenous to the Oral Cavity of Man. J. Dent. Res. 45:877-881.

51. Bleiweis, A.S., Craig, R.A., Coleman, S.E. and Van de Rign, I. 1971. The Streptococcal Cell Wall: Structure, Antigenic Composition and Reactivity with Lysozyme. J. Dent. Res. 50:1118.

52. Pollack, J. et al. 1977. The binding Aggregation and Lytic Properties of Lysozyme. Sp. Supp. Microbiol. Ed. Stiles. Abst. 325.

53. Osserman, E. and Lawlor, D.P 1966. Serum and Urinary Lysozyme in Monocytic and Mono-Myelocytic Leukemia. J. Expt. Med. 124:921.

54. Greenwald, R.A. and Mot, W.W. 1976. Effect of Agarose Variability on the Measurement of Lysozyme Activity. Clin. Chim. Acta. 73:299.

55. Bullen, J., Rogers, H.J. and Leigh, L. 1972. Iron-Binding Proteins in Milk and Resistance to E. Coli Infection in Infants. Br, Med. J. 1:69.

56. Bishop,J. et al. 1976. In Vitro Growth Inhibition of Coliform Bacteria by APO-Lactoferrin. Infect. and Immun. 14:911.

57. Cole, M.F. et al. 1977. Studies with Human Lactoferrin and S. mutans Sp. Suppl. Microbiol. Abst. 359.

58. Tabak, L. et al. Alterations in Lactoferrin in Salivary Gland Disease. J. Dent. Res. In press.

59. Bennett, R.M. and Mohla, C. 1976. A Solid-Phase Radioimmunoassay for Measurement of Lactoferrin in Human Plasma. J. Lab. Clin. Med. 80:156.

60. Roos, D. 1977. Oxidative Killing of Microorganisms by Phagocytic Cells. TIBS, p. 61, March.

61. Hoogendoorn, H. 1977. The Inhibitory Action of the Lactoeroxidase System on S. mutans and Other Organisms. Sp. Suppl. Microbiol. Abst. 353.

62. Hoogendoorn, H, and Moorer, W.R. 1973. Lactoperoxidase in the Prevention of Plaque Accumulation, Gingivitis and Dental Caries: I. Odontol. Revy. 24:355-366.

63. Koch, G., Edlund, K. and Hoogendoorn, H. 1973. Lactoperoxidase in the Prevention of Plaque Accumulation, Gingivitis and Dental Caries: II. Odontol. Revy., 24:367.

64. Gothefors, L. and Marklund, S. 1975. Lactoperoxidase Activity in Human Milk and in Saliva of Newborn Infants. Infect. and Immun., 11:1210.

65. Makinen, K. et al. 1976. Xylitol-Induced Increase in Lactoperoxidase Activity. J. Dent. Res. 55:652.

66. Hay, D. and Grøn, P. 1977. Inhibitors of Calcium and Phosphate Precipitation in Human Whole Saliva. Supp. Microbiol. Eds. Stiles Abst. 143.

67. Mandel, I.D. and Concool, B. 1974. Metal Binding Proteins of Human Parotid and Submaxillary Saliva. I.A.D.R. Abstracts.

68. Mandel, I.D. and Concool, B. 1975. Salivary Protein Interactions with Cations and Anions. I.A.D.R. Abstracts.

69. Tung, M.S. 1976. Characterizations of Permselective Properties of Apatite Membranes. J. Dent. Res. 55:D77.

70. Zahradnik, R.T., Moreno, E.C. and Burke, E.J. 1976. Effect of Salivary Pellicle on Enamel Subsurface Demineralization in vitro. J. Dent. Res. 55:664.

Discussion of salivary factors in caries prediction

C. Dawes

Faculty of Dentistry, University of Manitoba, 780 Bannatyne Avenue, Winnipeg, Manitoba Canada

Dr. Mandel has discussed the different components of saliva which, on a theoretical basis, might be expected to contribute to resistance to caries. Since the acidogenic potential of the salivary microflora has been shown to be poorly correlated with caries susceptibility[1], this leaves, as Dr. Mandel pointed out a severely depressed flow rate as the only salivary factor so far shown to have any predictive value with respect to caries. Two other very recent studies confirm this general conclusion[2,3].

This paper will suggest reasons for the lack of correlation in previous studies between salivary flow rate, or salivary composition and caries incidence.

Estimation of Caries susceptibility

It is generally agreed that initiation of caries in a particular patient requires that the patient consume fermentable carbohydrate relatively frequently, and also that the oral cavity, and more specifically the dental plaque, be colonized by acidogenic microorganisms. Of these two factors the dietary one would seem the more important as there is evidence that the acidogenicity of the plaque microbial flora is related to the amount of fermentable carbohydrate in the diet[4].

In all of the studies so far carried out in which attempts were made to relate salivary composition and caries susceptibility, the latter was estimated by use of the existing def or DMF scores. Although at certain ages incremental changes in DMF scores have been shown to correlate with the initial DMF score. The DMF index is basically a static index of previous caries experience. As such, it cannot be expected to have much predictive value of future caries, particularly if oral hygiene practices or dietary habits change. The DMF index gives no indication of the intensity of the cariogenic challenge to which the patient was exposed. Two patients may have the same DMF index, one who was very susceptible to caries, having been exposed to a low cariogenic challenge, the other who was relatively resistant to caries, having been exposed to a severe cariogenic challenge. Therefore, a clear distinction must be made between the natural caries susceptibility of patients on their usual diets and what I will term inherent caries susceptibility which would relate to the caries development on exposure to a standardized cariogenic challenge. Obviously, if a patient is on a non-cariogenic diet, no caries will develop irrespective of the flow rate or composition of the saliva. Thus, it is desirable that correlations be sought between salivary flow rate or composition, and inherent caries susceptibility.

Determination of salivary flow rate and composition

The composition of human saliva is dependent on glandular source, flow rate, duration of stimulation, time of day of saliva collection, nature of the stimulus, the genetic constitution of the donor and stimulated saliva is subject to serial dependency of sampling[5]. Similarly, the flow rate of saliva is dependent on the glandular source, the size of the gland, the time of day of saliva collection and the nature of the stimulus[5]. Thus, the question arises as to what type of saliva should be studied and under what conditions it should be collected. Previous workers have collected, usually on a single occasion, either unstimulated or chewing gum-stimulated parotid or whole saliva. In the absence of evidence regarding the stability of salivary composition with time, it is questionable whether the composition of saliva collected is related to the composition of saliva present at the time of caries development, possibly many years earlier.

Assuming the validity of the acidogenic theory of the etiology of dental caries, caries is largely initiated or progresses only when the pH of dental plaque is decreased by bacterial acid production during the approximately ½ - 1 hour following consumption of fermentable carbohydrate. Saliva could theoretically exert a caries-protective effect both during the period of plaque pH depression following oral exposure to fermentable carbohydrate or during the longer periods between meals or snacks when plaque pH is about neutral.

If the beneficial effects of saliva operate during the periods between meals, the type of saliva involved would most likely be unstimulated whole saliva. The beneficial effects could conceivably be due either to remineralization of early carious lesions, or to alteration of the plaque flora to make it less acidogenic.

If the beneficial effects of saliva are exerted during the actual period of acid production by the plaque, then the saliva involved would be that stimulated saliva secreted at a flow rate and for a duration in response to the food eaten. Whether flow rate decreased again to unstimulated levels prior to the return of plaque pH to neutrality, might be of some importance. There is little information on the duration of increased flow rates following gustatory stimulation, but that following a glucose or sucrose rinse appears to be relatively small[6]. Any beneficial effects of the saliva would most likely be due to a reduction of plaque acid accumulation to an increase in plaque base formation, or to an alteration in the plaque flora rendering it less acidogenic. With respect to the latter possibility it should be noted that the salivary concentrations of IgA and lactoferrin actually decrease as flow rate increases[7].

Desirable features for needed studies

To determine inherent caries susceptibility it would be desirable to study the increment in caries over a period of time with a standardized cariogenic challenge.

In practical terms, probably only dietary factors could be reasonably standardized and a possible experimental design would be the use of a short term, intense cariogenic challenge such as the multiple sucrose rinse technique[8]. The sucrose concentration or frequency of application could be adjusted to ensure a wide variation between individuals in the degree of early caries development. Since the caries is scored on the buccal surfaces of the teeth it has to be assumed not only that this is representative of fissure and approximal caries, but also that the mechanisms for the beneficial effects of saliva are the same for the different types of caries and are the same during intense cariogenic challenge as during the more usual weak cariogenic challenge

Since the effects of saliva could be working either during the time of pH fall caused by the sucrose rinses or at other times, it would be of interest to collect whole saliva under different conditions.

Firstly, unstimulated saliva should be collected at times when plaque pH is not expected to be depressed and, since any beneficial effects would most likely be mainly due to remineralization of early carious lesions, the inorganic components of interest would be the calcium, phosphate and fluoride concentrations and the pH; and the organic components of interest might be the various aggregating factors, statherin, lysozyme, lactoperoxidase and lactoferrin (3 Ls).

Secondly, whole saliva should be collected both within the few minutes just after a sucrose rinse (when the flow rate will be somewhat higher than the resting or unstimulated flow rate) and also about 30 mins. after the sucrose rinse, when the plaque pH would still be depressed. Since any beneficial effects would probably be due to modification of the Stephan curve, the inorganic components of interest might be the calcium, phosphate, fluoride and bicarbonate concentrations and the pH and pO_2 whilst the organic components of interest might be urea, the 3 Ls, sialin and statherin. Because of the circadian rhythms in salivary flow rate and composition it may be that caries susceptibility varies with time of day and there may be merit in making saliva collections at several different times of day (and night)[5].

In summary, except when salivary flow rate is severely depressed, previous studies of correlations between salivary factors and caries have given inconclusive results. This is perhaps primarily because estimates of caries susceptibility have been quite inadequate, but also because the relevant type of saliva collected under the appropriate conditions has not been studied.

LITERATURE CITED

1. Socransky, S.S. 1968. Caries-susceptibility Tests. Ann. N.Y. Acad. Sci. 153, Art 1, 137-146.

2. Crossner, C.G. and Holm, A.K. 1977. Saliva tests in the prognosis of caries in children. Acta Odont. Scand. 35:135-139.

3. Adorjan, S.A. and Stack, M.V. 1976. Oral sugar clearance in children. Br. dent. J. 141:221-222.

4. Littleton, N.W., McCabe, R.M. and Carter, C.H. 1967. Studies of oral health in persons nourished by stomach tube. II. Acidogenic properties and selected bacterial components of plaque material. Archs. oral Biol. 12:601-609.

5. Dawes, C. 1974. Rythms in salivary flow rate and composition. Internat. J. Chronobiol. 2:253-279.

6. Edgar, W.M. 1976. The role of saliva in the control of pH changes in human dental plaque. Caries Res. 10:241-254.

7. Brandtzaeg, P. 1971. Human secretory immunoglöbulins-VII. Concentrations of parotid IgA and other secretory proteins in relation to the rate of flow and duration of secretory stimulus. Archs. oral Biol. 16:1295-1310.

8. Von der Fehr, R.F., Löe, H. and Theilade, E. 1970. Experimental caries in man. Caries Res. 4:131-148.

Discussion of salivary factors in caries prediction

Ira L. Shannon

University of Texas, 6516 John Freeman Avenue, Houston, Texas 77025

Dr. Mandel has presented an admirable review of recent studies that consider the possible relationship of certain salivary variables to dental caries experience. He is to be commended for his purposeful and appropriate avoidance of the older literature on this subject. We have all waded laboriously through the multitude of reports that have identified calcium, phosphorus, amylase, chloride and any number of additional salivary constituents as key factors in the process of dental caries, and we have all seen these bubbles burst when subjected to well-controlled testing. He has presented results of investigations that might serve as platforms from which more searching probes can be launched, but of course, it is not possible to predict which of these will provide most understanding of the process of dental caries. It was emphasized that there is presently no procedure available by which we can analyze a sample of saliva from a single subject and predict with a high degree of reliability the caries status or caries experience of this individual. He concluded that the only salivary characteristic that might be valuable in predicting caries activity is salivary flow rate and buffer capacity in cases of pronounced glandular impairment. There are, however, further considerations relating to salivary flow rates and caries status that merit attention.

In the past years we were fortunate to be in a position in which groups of 50 healthy male military recruits were available to us each day for study. This provided the opportunity to conduct large scale studies of the biochemical constituents of blood, urine and saliva as they might relate to oral disease. Our primary work suggested that stimulated whole saliva varied excessively among subjects. Therefore, we began to study parotid saliva. We became convinced that we could derive more meaningful data from parotid saliva if we worked with the unstimulated secretion. Ultimately, biochemical studies of resting parotid flow as it related to DMFS were completed on more than 500 participants. It was found that when the 45 minute unstimulated parotid flow rate was compared between groups with six levels of caries experience, ranging from 0-10 DMFS to more than 50 DMFS, there was an apparent inverse relationship.

In a second study of 512 subjects from the same population, it was clear that recruits with the higher flow rates of unstimulated parotid saliva had the healthier mouths, but there was not a perfect stepwise negative correlation throughout the DMFS groups.

A third study of 503 subjects gave a very similar picture. However, in this study population there was a higher rate of flow in the 0-10 DMFS group, but a virtual plateau of flow rate in all of the other DMFS groups. When the mean flow rates for a total of 2,563 subjects sampled throughout all seasons of the year to obviate the seasonal factor were studied, an analysis of variance revealed a difference significant at the 0.025 level between the six DMFS groups. When the data for the groups were subjected to a rank sum test it was found that both the means and variances differed at the 0.05 level. Subsequent t tests pointed out that this difference was due primarily to the higher flow rate for the 0-10 DMFS group. A rank sum test carried out on the other five DMFS groups, excluding the 0-10 group, showed that neither the means nor the variances differed significantly even at the 0.10 level. It was thus clear that the only difference of true significance was that between the 0-10 DMFS groups and the remaining 5 DMFS groups.

These findings exemplify the importance in differentiating between statistical significance, biological importance, or usefulness for purposes of prediction. If one is interested only in predictability of caries, he would not be impressed by these analyses of flow rate. To the serious student of glandular physiology and cariology, it would be unthinkable to drop the study at this point. After all, the studies have demonstrated a significant negative correlation between resting parotid flow and caries experience, and it is abundantly clear that patients with very healthy mouths have significantly higher saliva flow rates than do those with much caries.

One must then direct his attention to how we might be falling short in not being able to demonstrate a difference that is indeed present and highly significant. There are two completely simple variables under study -- the DMFS status and the resting parotid flow rate. Methodology for clinical and roentgenographic examinations is now so well established that we believe that, if an investigator has examined literally thousands of mouths in a careful manner, we can indeed accept the DMFS scores as valid. The remaining points to be considered are:

1. Is there a defect in the sampling procedure that might be adding to the variance in such a way that our differences have to be extremely great for significant conclusions to result? Another way to phrase this question is, "Is the collection procedure satisfactory in providing a fluid that we may hopefully classify as nearly as possible,the resting secretion of the parotid gland? and

2. Is the sampling period appropriate to collect a truly representative sample from each participant?"

With a properly outfitted collection area, with adequately instructed subjects, and with an extended period of experience in the collection of this fluid, there is no pronounced problem in obtaining a fluid from the parotid duct that can realistically be accepted as the resting secretion. Repeated consecutive samplings in groups of individuals authenticate that the collection device can be positioned without significant glandular stimulation. Certainly continuous close supervision and an inviolate set of ground rules are essential, but these are rather obvious considerations. To decide the appropriate length of the sampling period, the flow characteristics of the parotid gland have to be known.

We obtained such information during an experiment that was basically an attempt to determine the time course of secretion of the resting human parotid gland, both in routine laboratory light and in complete darkness. Statistical analysis of rate of drop formation showed that a harvested sample of resting parotid saliva is in a sense a heterogeneous mixture of many very small portions of saliva all of which were secreted in a completely unpredictable time frame. Standardization and reproducibility testing are thus demanded of the investigator who will in the future offer inferences based upon such flow rate changes.

Since there are such well estiblished correlations between flow rate and the xonstituent chemistry of saliva, the need for standardization is even more acute. I would, therefore, offer the suggestion that the critical need in studies having to do with salivary flow, and the biochemistry of saliva is in the realm of developing more satisfactory sampling procedures. While this is true for collections of resting secretions, it is even more applicable to the even more variable type of flow found when exogenous stimulants are employed. Based upon our experience with unstimulated human parotid, saliva and its relation to caries experience, I am firmly convinced that appropriate refinement of the collection procedure, to the point that reproducibility is the rule, will demonstrate that flow rate is a factor in the caries process. It would be logical that this would bring into focus those biochemical constituents of saliva which are altered as a result of changes in flow and would clarify their relationship to caries experience.

While it is unquestionably appropriate to concentrate research effort on promising areas, such as salivary aggregation of bacteria, measurement of carbohydrases and their inhibitors, secretory IgA, lysozyme, lactoferrin, lactoperoxidase and to concentrate effort on those which continue to show promise. I submit that salivary flow rate studies, with associated studies of constituents of saliva as they relate to both flow and caries experience, stand on a base that is just as firm, and that if as much effort were devoted to this area, the probability of contributing new and valuable information to the field of cariology would be high.

MODERATOR'S SUMMARY OF DISCUSSION OF TOPIC IV PRESENTATIONS

In response to doubts that were expressed about trying to relate salivary bacteria to dental caries when it is the plaque bacteria which are actually involved in caries initiation it was pointed out that plaque bacteria end up as part of the salivary bacterial effluent and may, therefore, to a certain extent be related. It was noted that even low numbers of L. casei in plaque may be a good predictor of future cavitation. However, fluorescent anti-body techniques may be necessary to detect them at the early stage before a lesion focuses and its lower pH leads to an increase in the numbers of L. casei with resultant spilling over into the saliva.

The difficulty in dispersing plaque before culturing places obstacles in the way of using the bacterial composition of plaque for caries prediction. It was suggested that an answer to this problem might be found in freezing, sectioning, and staining plaques with fluorescent dyes. Such methods need to be developed. Attention was redirected to the fact that the Snyder's test shows a high correlation coefficient of the order of 0.7 with caries. No answer was provided to the question of why this high correlation existed with mixed bacteria in saliva in the face of a poorer correlation in cultures with the incidence of specific bacterial isolates as S. mutans or lactobacilli.

The significant effect of between-meal eating on the growth of caries bacteria was reiterated. It was explained that such eating will increase, not only the number of periods of direct rapid acid formation and pH depression, but also the storage of intra-cellular polysaccharide in plaque bacteria. Increasing the duration of the period between exposures to carbohydrates may be of considerable importance in reducing the liability to caries.

It was pointed out that volatile acid formation by plaques was not higher in caries-active individuals. It was also noted that while decreases in plaque pH are inversely related to caries, this pH is modified by other factors than acid formation.

Various points were brought out in response to questions about plaque. These included information that the "white spots" that are recognized on smooth surfaces as initial caries also occur at the entrance to fissures; that IGA may affect glucosyl transferase by other than an antibody effect; that while IGA may coat organisms and prevent adherance, gel-like aggregation has not been demonstrated; that Australian work has confirmed that increased buffering capacity of plaque is related to lower caries, and that plaque fluid should be studied. A plea was made to keep in mind that mathematically significant correlation coefficients are meaningless if they do not have a logical biological basis.

The discussion of salivary factors dealt with the depression in salivary secretion in darkness, and related this to the reduced salivary flow during sleep. The question of whether parotid secretion was less closely related to caries than sub-maxillary or whole mixed saliva was not resolved.

TOPIC V

TOOTH FACTORS AND CARIES PREDICTION

Moderator:

Paul F. De Paola
Forsyth Dental Center
140 The Fenway
Boston, Massachusetts 02115

Caries prediction by means of tooth morphology and physical characteristics

John P. Brown

Department of Preventive Medicine, Dental School, University of Queensland, Brisbane, Australia

Dental papilla mesenchyme derived from cranial neural crest cells is thought to determine tooth size and shape by inductive and instructive roles in tooth formation. In addition the unique gene sequences in different collagen producing cells may be extremely sensitive to environmental modifications.[1] Herein may lie a source of variability in enamel and dentin matrix elaboration, which is expressed as variations in those tissues in the mature state. Can these differences in morphology and structure be responsible for predictable variations in caries susceptibility between and within teeth?

Morphology

One of the most studied environmental effects on tooth size has been that of fluoride. Ericsson[2] in a recent review concluded that the observed effects on tooth size have not been consistent. There are several reports of more caries resistant teeth being smaller in size[3-6], but Grahnen and Ingervall[7] did not find such a relationship. Hunter[8] found restored primary teeth to be larger than non-carious ones. Larger teeth tend to erupt later. Even though more caries susceptible, they are in the mouth a shorter time and possibly even less resistant than supposed.

Certain racial morphologic characteristics predispose to caries e.g. lingual pits of shovel or barrel shaped incisors, buccal pits without enamel lining in the mongoloid dentition of American Indians and Eskimos[9], and various morphologic traits in different racial groups[10]. Within a population teeth with the greatest number of cusps, and therefore fissures, are most likely to be carious, (Anderson cited by Mayhall[9]). The typical Inuit molar may be more efficient, but is also a more caries prone tooth. Racial differences in caries prevalence are not always observed[11]. Simpler occlusal form, smaller size and more frequent congenital absence of teeth are associated with lower point prevalence of caries in Down's Syndrome[12].

Although variability in caries resistance is to a large extent environmental, the concordance of caries patterns in twins[13-16], and their pattern of inheritance of tooth morphology[17,20] point towards a genetic component expressed through morphology. Shimizu[21] believed this could in turn be expressed as a food retention factor for a given population. Others believe there are genetic implications in observed non-random patterns of caries distribution[22-24].

The genetic and environmental relationships between fissure shape and caries predisposition in animals have been reviewed by Paynter[25] and Konig[26].

Trace element effects, and nutritional effects have also been recorded. In rats, narrower deeper fissures tend to decay more frequently, the greater extent of caries not being directly related to enamel thickness[27].

Attempts to classify the shape of fissures in human teeth[28,30] have not been substantiated by more recent work[31,43]. Narrow and deep fissures are associated, but otherwise distinct morphologic groupings are not justified. The histology of carious attack on fissures is not essentially different to that on other surfaces, although in all but the widest grooves, two initial wall lesions usually develop and later coalesce[34-37].

Bibby[38-39] believed that acquired surface organic material modified the form of early enamel caries and contributed to the increased caries resistance and pigmentation of older teeth. Silverstone[40] has shown that the outer zone of the early lesion is not dependent upon the structure of outer enamel. Surface protein diffusion barriers are, however, common to <u>in vivo</u> and <u>in vitro</u> conditions.

Newman[41] has demonstrated that the approximal caries lesion does not develop until the contact area is established and plaque replaces the acellular vestigal enamel organ beneath it. It is possible that these proteins must be lysed before acid dissolution can begin[42]. Replica studies could not differentiate the surfaces of non-carious and early carious teeth[43], and it is at a relatively late stage that surface penetration is observed[44]. Arguments as to whether prism cores or peripheries are first dissolved have faded as the great variability in enamel surface structure has been described[45], which reflects the range of events surrounding cessation of ameloblastic activity. The ultimate structural association with early carious dissolution is now thought to involve dislocations present in enamel apatite crystals. These linear lattice defects are revealed as etch pits[46].

Tooth surface roughness has racial variations[47], but enamel cracks or lamellae occur at carious sites fortuitously[48]. Although associations of tooth surface roughness with caries predisposition are no longer taken to be causative, much less due to faulty nutrition, they do have a contemporary counterpart. Odontoclasia is a form of caries associated with structural defects, usually in primary teeth, of some Pacific Islanders[49]. These teeth are said to be hypo-mineralised, enamel matrix being normal. A dietary factor is thought to interfere with enamel maturation[50]. Superimposed caries is described as being akin to that described for hypomineralised enamel in rat molars[51]. Fluoride altered the susceptibility of this immature enamel, which preferentially takes up the element. Unerupted human teeth are also hypo-mineralised[52], and as some of this porosity remains at time of eruption, the pre- and post-eruptive maturation is crucial to the caries disposition of teeth. Crabb[53] has described other structural aberrations in unerupted teeth, which might be confused both histologically and clinically with caries. Crabb and Mortimer[54] related rapid progress of lesions to more porous inner enamel, and to areas which lacked prism structure.

The more recent animal[55] and human[56] studies agree that tetracycline incorporation during development, without formation of clinical hypoplasia (abnormal roughness or deficiency of enamel) makes those teeth less caries prone. This is ascribed to unknown structural rather than bacterial factors.

Conflicting reports on whether or not clinically hypoplastic enamel is more or less caries prone depend in part on the level of caries experience in the population[57]. Shaw[58] observed more caries in rats with missing enamel than in normal animals of the same strain. Newman and Poole[45] on the other hand described the ultrastructure of micro-pits in enamel, which were not necessarily demineralised despite the presence of bacteria. These pits appeared different from those associated with Tomes' process of the ameloblast[59]. Porous narrow channels exist at prism junctions in hypoplastic enamel, giving the potential for ions to diffuse more freely[60]. Radiation damage during tooth development causes hypoplasia and predisposes to caries[61] but a causal link through latered enamel structure is not as well established as are radiation effects on salivary glands.

Dental fluorosis is a most positive sign of reduced caries predisposition. The classifications of fluorosis[62] have not been shown to correspond to increasing levels of fluoride uptake or progressive decreases in caries proneness although Forsman[63] demonstrated increased caries in teeth with moderate and severe fluorosis in people consuming 5-10 ppm fluoride in water. The questionable, very mild and mild degrees of fluorosis are often difficult to distinguish from idiopathic opacities. At less than 6 ppm fluoride in water, replica studies do not allow differentiation of fluorosed and normal enamel[64].

Few studies have been made of the nature of idiopathic mottling, and until a true differentiation from fluorosis is made their clinical separation, especially when of slight degree will,be open to question. It could be expected that the highly differentiated ameloblast might respond similarly to various toxic stimuli, with similar results in mature enamel. Dean and Elvove[65] suggested that elements other than fluorine might be responsible for mottling and also for altered caries susceptivility. Such associations have been made in animals[66]. Geographic variations in prevalence of idiopathic opacities and of caries have been made[67], but these are unlikely to reflect trace element variability in the different regions[68]. It was found that compared with low fluoride levels intermediate and optimal water fluoride levels are associated with reduced prevalence of these opacities. In children with similar fluoride intake history, caries predisposition in idiopathically mottled teeth was no different than in teeth without developmental faults[68]. The implication is that in a population, fluorosis and other opacities can be differentiated on the basis of the caries predisposition of those teeth.

In children with a history of low fluoride intake, primary incisors with any developmental defect were less caries prone; first permanent molars with 'fluorosis like' areas were more caries prone than unaffected teeth while those scored for idiopathic opacities were not[68]. This suggests that there is more than one type of idiopathic developmental fault.

Since all hypocalcified enamel tends to accumulate fluoride, enamel biopsy methods cannot be relied on to distinguish fluorosis from other faults. Acid solubility[69], nitrogen content and density[70] differences do not help and histological investigations[71,72] have not so far produced clear differentiation. Although the general histologic appearance of idiopathic opacities often approximates that of mildly fluorosed enamel[73], it is said they can be differentiated from caries under ultra-violet light[74].

Recent unreported observations on idiopathically mottled enamel in acidified gels show that specimens do not behave uniformly. Their caries predisposition varies. Although they take up more fluoride than normal enamel, they do not seem to be more caries resistant.

Conclusions

Inherited morphologic characteristics of the teeth are important caries predictors for some racial groups.

Fissure morphology in human teeth cannot be shown to be related to caries predisposition.

It is yet to be clearly established how the various types of enamel defects differ from one another in caries susceptibility.

The histology, ultrastructure, chemistry or biophysical properties of various enamel defects have not yet been differentiated.

Moderate fluorosis of enamel is a sign of increased caries resistance.

Enamel opacities that are not easily differentiated from fluorosis appear to be at least as caries prone as normal enamel.

Pre- and post-eruptive maturation of outer enamel is crucial in determining its caries predisposition.

Progress in caries prediction in approximal and fissure surfaces requires imporved methods of caries diagnosis.

LITERATURE CITED

1. Slavkin, H.C. 1974. Embryonic tooth formation, Oral Sci. Rev. No. 4 Copenhagen Munksgaard.

2. Ericsson, S.Y. 1977. Cariostatic Mechanisms of fluorides: Clinical observations, Caries Res. 11:(Supp. 1) 2-41.

3. Shiller, W.R., Wolcott, R.B. 1961. Morphologic differences in teeth of caries susceptible and caries immune males (abs), J. Dent. Res. 40:660.

4. Keene, H.J. 1971. Epidemiologic study of tooth size variability in caries free Naval recruits. J. Dent. Res. 50:1331-1345.

5. Schamschula, R.G., Barmes, D.E., Adkins, B.L. 1972. Caries aetiology in Papua New Guinea. Associations of tooth size and dental arch width. Aust. Dent. J. 17:188-195.

6. Stern, S.P., Curzon, M.E.J. 1975. Variations in tooth dimension and geographic caries prevalence. J. Dent. Res. 54:910.

7. Grahnen, h., Ingervall, B. 1963. Tooth width and morphology of the dentition in a group of caries resistant men. Odont. Revy. 14:70,

8. Hunter, W.S. 1967. Tooth size and approximal decay in human teeth. Archs. oral Biol. 12:315.

9. Mayhall, J.T. 1977. The oral health of a Canadian Inuit Community: An anthropological approach. Int. Conf. Oral Biology, J. Dent. Res. in press. Copenhagen,

10. Ludwig, F.J. 1957. The mandibular second premolars: Morphologic variation and inheritance. J. Dent. Res. 36:263.

11. Bagramian, R.A., Russell, A.L. 1971. An Epidemiologic Study of dental caries in race and geographic area. J. Dent. Res. 50:1553-1556.

12. Brown, J.P., Schodel, D. 1976. A review of controlled surveys of dental disease in handicapped persons. J. Dent. Child. 43:313-320.

13. Brucker, W.H. 1944. Influence of heredity and Environment on the caries pictures on monozygotic twins. J. Am. Dent. Assoc. 31:931.

14. Mansbridge, J.N. 1959. Heredity and dental caries. J. Dent. Res. 38:337.

15. Grahnen, H. 1962. Heredity factors in relation to dental caries and congenital missing teeth, p. 194 in "Genetics and Dental Health". McGraw Hill, New York.

16. Bordoni, N. et al 1973. Prevalence of dental caries in twins. J. Dent. Child. 50:440.

17. Lewis, D.W., Grainger, R.M. 1967. Sex-linked inheritance of tooth size. A Family Study. Archs. oral Biol. 12:539.

18. Garn, S.M. 1966. Bilateral asymetry and concordance in cusp number and crown morphology of the mandibular first molar. J. Dent. Res. 45:1820.

19. Garn, S.M., Lewis, A.B., Kerewsky, R.S. 1965. X-linked inheritance of tooth size. J. Dent. Res. 44:439.

20. Garn, S.M. et al 1966. Sexual dimorphism in the buccolingual tooth diameter. J. Dent. Res. 45:1819.

21. Shimizu, T. 1964. On the factor of anatomical form in the epidemiological principles in dental caries attack. Bull. Tokyo Dent. Coll. 5:43-58.

22. Jackson, D., Burch, P.R.J. 1972. Non-random distributions of caries attacks among mesial and distal surfaces of human permanent maxillary incisors. Archs. oral Biol. 17:119-125.

23. Jackson, D., Fairpo, C.G., Burch, P.R.J. 1973. Human lingual pit caries: Distribution between right and left maxillary incisors. Archs. oral Biol. 18:181-187.

24. Jackson, D., Fairpo, C.G., Burch, P.R.J. 1973. Distribution of symetric and asymetric patterns of caries attack in human permanent maxillary incosor teeth: Genetic Implications. Archs. oral Biol. 18:189-195.

25. Paynter, K.J., Grainger, R.M. 1962. Relationship of morphology and size of teeth to caries. Internat. Dent. J. 12:147.

26. Konig, K.G. 1965. "Caries Resistance in Experimental Animals", in caries resistant teeth p. 87-113, Eds. G. Wolstenholme and M. O'Conner, Churchill, London.

27. Brown, J.P. 1970. Rat molar morphology and dental caries. Caries Res. 4:49-55.

28. Bossert, W.A. 1933 The relation between the shape of the occlusal surfaces of molars and the prevalence of decay I. J. Dent. Res. 13:125.

29. Bossert, W.A. 1937. The relation between the shape of the occlusal surfaces of molars and the prevalence of decay II. J. Dent. Res. 16:63.

30. Nagano, T. 1961. Relation between the form of pit and fissure and the primary lesion of caries. Dent. Abs. 6:426.

31. Zuhrt, R., Reussel, G., Vierus, H. 1971. Fissure cross section and caries susceptibility. Dtsch. Stomatol. 21:160-163.

32. Braun, L. 1973. Accuracy of a biometric method for fissure determination. Dtsch. Stomatol 23:24-32.

33. Fejerskov, O., Nelsen, B., Karring, T. 1973. Morphometric analysis of occlusal fissures in human premolars. Scand. J. Dent. Res. 81:505-509.

34. Wachtel, L.W. 1958. Chemical and morphological factors in susceptibility of enamel to acid attack.(Abs) J. Dent. Res. 37:59.

35. Brown, L.R., Wheatcroft, M.G. 1958. Effect of enamel morphology in susceptibility to bacterial attack. (Abs), J. Dent. Res. 37:59.

36. Newbrun, E. et al. 1959. Microradiographic evaluation of occlusal fissures and grooves. J. Am. Dent. Assoc. 58:26.

37. Mortimer, K.U. 1964. Some histological features of fissure caries in enamel. Proceedings O.R.C.A. 2:85-95.

38. Bibby, B.G. 1932. The organic structure of dental enamel as a passive defence against caries. J. Dent. Res. 12:99.

39. Bibby, B.G. 1971. Organic enamel material and caries. Caries Res. 5:305-322.

40. Silverstone, L.M. Structure of carious enamel including the early lesion. In Oral Sci. Rev. No. 3, Eds. Melcher, A.H. and Zarb, G.A. Copenhagen, Munksgaard.

41. Newman, H.N. 1973. Zone demarcation of organic films present on human enamel surfaces in vivo. Br. Dent. J. 134:273-278.

42. Hoffman, S. 1971. Study of enamel surface-bacteria relationships by scanning electron microscopy. J. Dent. Res. 50:1355.

43. Scott, D.B. et al. 1949. Replica studies of changes in tooth surfaces with age. J. Dent. Res. 28:31-47.

44. Lustman, J., Sela, M., Sela, J., Klnansky, M. 1974. White enamel patches - a SEM study of approximal surfaces following removal of plaque. J. Oral Path. 3:123-126.

45. Newman, H.N., Poole, D.F.G. 1974. Observations with scanning and transmission electron microscopy on the structure of human surface enamel. Archs. oral Biol. 19:1135-1143.

46. Jongebloed, J.W. 1976. An ultrastructural study of the caries process. Thesis, University of Groningen.

47. Pedersen, P.O., Scott, D.B. 1951. Replica studies of the surface of teeth from Alaskan eskimo, West Greenland Native, and American White. Acta Odont. Scand. 9:262-292.

48. Scott, D.B., Wyckoff, R.W.G. 1949. Studies of tooth surface structure by optical and electron microscopy. J. Am. Dent. Assoc. 39:275-282.

49. Barmes, D.E. 1967. Dental and nutritional surveys of primitive peoples in the Pacific Islands. Austral. Dent. J. 12:442-454.

50. Baume, L.J., Vulliemoz, J.P. 1972. Variations in the Mineral content of the enamel of Polynesian teeth. Int. Dent. J. 22:193-218.

51. Francis, M.D., Briner, W. 1966. The development and regression of hypo mineralized areas of rat molars. Archs. oral Biol. 11:349.

52. Crabb, H.S.M. 1976. The porous outer enamel of unerupted human premolars. Caries Res. 10:1-7.

53. Crabb, H.S.M. 1964. Observations on the enamel structure of unerupted teeth, with special reference to dental caries. Adv. Fluorine Res. and Dent. Caries Prev. 2:69-76.

54. Crabb. H.S.M., Mortimer, K.U. 1966. Dental caries and Enamel structure. Nature 209:611-612.

55. Harndt, R. 1974. The incidence of caries in the teeth of Syrian hamsters observed after administration of tetracycline during tooth development. Abs. No. 63, O.R.C.A. 21st Congress, London.

56. Brearley, L.J., Porteous, J.R. 1973. Characteristics and caries experience of tetracycline - affected dentitions. J. Dent. Res. 52:508-516.

57. Davies, G.N. 1965. The significance of epidemiological studies in relation to caries resistance. In caries resistant teeth. Eds. G.E. Wolstenholme and M. O'Connor, Churchill, London.

58. Shaw, J.H. 1972. The susceptibility to experimental dental caries of rats from a strain with totally or partially missing enamel. Archs. oral Biol. 17:349-354.

59. Boyde, A. 1970. The surface of the enamel in human hypoplastic teeth. Archs. oral Biol. 15:897-898.

60. Vahl, J., Riede, H. 1968. Mikromorphologishe strukturanomalien des zahnshcmelzes bei mindermineralisation (Schmelzhypoplasie). Dtsch. Zahn Z. 23:289-297.

61. Koppang, H.S. 1975. Dental damage after radiotherapy for maligant lesions in the head and neck region. Nor Tannlaegeforen Tid 85:159-165.

62. Dean, H.T. 1942. The investigation of physiological effects by the epidemiological method. In fluorine and dental health. Am. Assoc. Adv. Sci. In Fluorine and Dental Hlth. Wash. D.C.

63. Forsman, B. 1974. Dental fluorosis and caries in high fluoride districts in Sweden. Comm. Dent. Oral Epidem. 2:132-148.

64. Mannerberg, F. 1968. Appearance of the tooth surface of teeth showing dental fluorosis as observed by shadowed replicas. Odont. Revy. 19:271-291.

65. Dean, H.T., Elvove, E. 1935. Studies on the minimal threshold of the dental sign of chronic endemic fluorosis. Pub. Health Rep. 50:1719-1729.

66. Irving, J.T. 1944. "Fluorine-like" action of various substances on teeth. Nature 154:149-150.

67. Pearce, E., Ludwig, T.G., Darwin, J. 1974. Dental caries Prevalence in seven soil areas of New Zealand. Archs. oral Biol. 19:157-162.

68. Brown, J.P. 1977. The epidemiology of tooth calcification defects and dental caries in Queensland children. PhD Thesis, Univ. of Queensland.

69. Hodson, J.J. 1955. Identification of hypocalcified and demineralised areas in sections of human enamel. Nature (Lond) 175:261-262.

70. Bhussry, B.R. 1958. Chemical and physical studies of enamel from human teeth III. S.G., N_2 Content and histological characteristics of opaque white enamel. J. Dent. Res. 37:1054-1059.

71. Kostlan, J., Plackova, A. 1962. The histological investigation of the development hypomineralized areas of the enamel and their comparison with the carious lesion. Archs. oral Biol. 7:317-326.

72. Plackova, A., Vahl, J. 1967. Mineralization defects in hard dental tissues. Int. Dent. J. 17:709-718.

73. Brown, J.P., Silverstone, L.M. 1976. The histology of idiopathic opacities of human dental enamel. I.A.D.R. British Div. Meeting Manchester.

74. Crabb, H.S.M. 1966. Observations on the histology of the carious attack on enamel and related developmental faults. Adv. in Fluorine Res. 4:225-238.

Discussion of caries prediction by means of tooth morphology and physical characteristics

Leon M. Silverstone

Division of Cariology, University of Iowa, College of Dentistry, Iowa City, Iowa 52242

I agree with Dr. Brown's conclusion that the ability to influence the susceptibility of human teeth to caries by changes in tooth morphology is not proven for fluoride or other trace elements. However, there is little doubt that the caries preventive effect of systemic fluoride differs with respect to different tooth surfaces. Smooth surfaces benefit the greatest, whereas occlusal fissures show least benefit. Whilst this finding is well accepted, it is difficult to find an explanation in the literature. In this respect, the following may be of relevance. With smooth surface caries, an enamel depth of 1,000-1,500 µm must be penetrated in order for the lesion to reach the dentine. Most workers agree that caries is not the result of a simple continuing demineralization, but a dynamic series of events. Thus, during progress of the lesion through the enamel there is ample time for a number of physico-chemical events to occur, influenced by fluoride, which result in a slowing down or arrestment of the lesion (e.g. aquisition of fluoride by surface enamel, influence of fluoride on plaque micro-organisms, remineralization phenomena). In addition, it is well to remember that a lesion penetrating one half to two-thirds through the depth of the enamel is extensive on a histological scale, but is still undetectable both at the clinical level and by bite-wing radiography.

With an occlusal fissure, the base of the fissure is relatively close to the enamel-dentine junction, and sometimes even extending into the dentine. It is well established that the lesion of fissure caries occurs bi-laterally on the walls of the fissure and not at its base. However, the lesions need not penetrate far in order to reach the dentine. On reaching the enamel-dentine junction, spread occurs rapidly in all directions along this junction (i.e. secondary caries of enamel). Therefore, at a time when the carious lesion is small histologically, and certainly not detectable clinically, the disease process has already undermined a relatively large area of sound enamel and has made its presence felt on the pulpo-dentinal unit. It is not surprising, therefore, that fluoride has a relatively small effect in the prevention of occlusal caries in comparison to smooth surface caries.

Although this effect on different tooth surfaces is well defined for populations, it is not so for individuals, as stated in Dr. Brown's paper. Thus, the relative depth of individual fissures on an occlusal surface probably has relatively little effect on caries susceptibility on each site on a single tooth, it being almost an "all-or-none" response.

Whilst on the subject of systemic fluoride and morphology, it is of relevance to examine the state of affairs in fluorotic enamel in the light of recent work. The report by Fejerskov, Silverstone, Melsen and Moller (1975) described the histological features of teeth showing either mild or severe fluorosis. The general morphology and histological structure of fluorotic enamel did not differ from normal enamel, contrary to previous reports, but the tissue showed areas of hypomineralization which, in sever cases, exhibited pore volumes of 25 percent or more. Recent work on testing the susceptibility of severely fluorotic enamel to artificial caries in vitro has produced some interesting results. Areas of fluorotic enamel having up to 25 percent pore volumes were exposed in vitro, together with sound 'normal' enamel, to an artificial caries acidified gel test (Silverstone, 1967). Under identical conditions of attack and exposure, lesions created on the sound enamel were always more extensive than those created on fluorotic enamel, in spite of its initial high porosity)Kidd, Thylstrup, Fejerskov and Silverstone, 1977). These results tend to support the theory proposed recently by Brown and Chow (1977) with respect to the cariostatic effect of fluoride. These authors believe that the dominant effect of fluoride is on the driving forces for diffusion. Their initial experiments support the theory that fluoride reduces the driving force for diffusion of $Ca(OH)_2$ from the lesion, increases that of H_3PO_4 and reduces the diffusion of HCl into a lesion. These effects all favour arrestment of a lesion.

During the past twenty years, the microstructure of enamel was thought to play a significant role in caries susceptibility, and many workers defined specific pathways of caries attack through the enamel. However, more recent work at the ultrastructural level has not supported the concept that structural pathways are the specific tracts for entry and progression of the lesion. For example, features such as cross striations of the prisms and striae of Retzius are seen readily in ground sections of enamel, especially after acid etching or carious involvement. However, to date, no one has unequivocally identified cross striations or striae of Retzius at the ultrastructural level.

Recent work has suggested that small imperfections or dislocations present in the center of enamel crystals could be responsible for the relatively fast penetration of acids along the c-axis of the apatite crystals. In short, these linear lattice defects can determine the demineralization behaviour of the tissue. The joint evidence from high resolution electron microscopy (Selvig, 1970), theoretical calculations (Welch, 1968; Arends et al, 1971) and solubility studies (Jongebloed et al, 1973) all point directly to the existence of dislocations in enamel and apatites. This is an interesting concept, not new in crystallography, but one which might have relevance with respect to dental caries.

Another physical parameter of enamel that has been used extensively by some workers is hardness. Hardness measurements are relatively easy and rapid to carry out of all of the many tests available and this, no doubt, has been responsible for its popularity in the study of both enamel and dentine. The Knoop Hardness Test has been used most widely in dental hard tissues. Enamel is much harder than dentine by a factor of four or five. There appears to be little difference between the compressive failure properties of enamel and dentine in terms of stress, and enamel has much lower strain values. In the case of enamel, which generally has a higher modulus than dentine, the deformation is probably not completely plastic, and some recovery occurs on removal of the indenter. But does hardness of enamel really mean anything in terms of either caries susceptibility or degree of damage? A great deal of work has been carried out by Koulourides (1968) who has employed micro-hardness testing of enamel surfaces prior to softening with dilute acids, after acid exposure and then again after attemps at remineralization. It has been assumed by many of these workers that rehardening of acid-softened enamel is similar to remineralization. Feagin, Koulourides and Pigman (1969) have shown that the increase in surface hardness is accompanied by an uptake of calcium and phosphate by softened enamel. Such studies have gone a long way to demonstrate that the rehardening process is similar to remineralization. However, due to the curvature of the enamel surface , it is difficult to carry out meaningful hardness measurements on the true outer surface. In addition, the heterogeneity of enamel must raise questions as to the relevance of using micro-hardness as a meaningful parameter. The indenter may contact an anatomic variation, or a stria of Retzius on the surface, and there are bound to be differences. The experimental studies of Koulourides and his co-workers have concentrated on the softening and rehardening of the outer 5 µm of enamel. Polarized light studies show that in caries, the outer 30 µm of the enamel is a relatively unaffected surface zone (Silverstone, 1968) which remains at approximately 1 percent mineral loss in spite of the subsurface body of the lesion being extensively demineralized. What does micro-hardness of the outer few microns of enamel mean in terms of the subsurface lesion?

Dr. Brown quoted the work of Bibby (1971) with respect to the acquired surface organic material being able to modify susceptibility of the tissue to caries. There is little doubt that the exogenous organic layers on enamel do modify the attack on enamel both by caries and acid solutions. Previously it was thought that acid solutions and chelators produced specific and different etching patterns on human enamel (Poole and Johnson, 1967). However, it was shown (Silverstone, Saxton, Dogon and Fejerskov, 1975) that a single acid solution could produce the entire range of etching patterns reported previously. Etching patterns of human enamel were classified into three types, Type 1, where there was a preferential dissolution of prism cores, Type 2, dissolution of prism peripheries and Type 3, where the etched pattern showed no apparent relationship to prism morphology. The interesting point being that all three etching patterns occurred on a single tooth surface when employing a single acid solution. Such differences are difficult to explain, but must reflect differences in structure, orientation and chemistry even in adjacent regions at the ultrastructural level.

It is well accepted that the enamel surface can be modified with respect to its chemistry, and this will be dealt with in the following report. However, the surface of sound enamel can also be modified with respect to its micro-morphology by the application of a synthetic calcifying fluid. Test areas of sound enamel were exposed to a synthetic calcifying fluid in vitro, examined at the light and electron microscope levels, and compared with adjacent unexposed control areas (Silverstone, 1971). Transmission electron microscopy (TEM) showed the control regions to have many "wedge-shaped defects" along the enamel surface, measuring up to 10 µm wide and 15 µm deep. Such surface defects, which have been demonstrated by a number of workers, were filled in by organic material of exogenous origin. Examination of test regions by TEM showed two features which differed from control regions. In the first, a layer of mineral composed of fine granules was deposited on the enamel surface after exposure to the calcifying fluid. In the second, the wedge-shaped defects were filled with densely packed crystals which were smaller and more rounded than those of the apatite proper. There was also an increase in the amount of oriented apatite in the surface layers as shown by quantitative imbibition studies.

When erupted teeth were employed in the experiments, surface changes were detected to a depth of approximately 20 µm. However, when unerupted teeth were employed in the experiments, changes were much deeper relative to unexposed control tooth halves, extending 100-200 um into the enamel. This effect was likened to a type of post-eruptive maturation. When test halves of teeth, together with their corresponding unexposed controls, were suspended in acidified gels, the caries-like lesions produced were significantly different. In all cases, lesions created on control tooth halves were significantly larger and more extensively demineralized than those produced on the corresponding test halves of teeth.

One of the important characteristics of caries of human dental enamel is that the greatest degree of demineralization occurs at a subsurface level. Thus, the small enamel lesion remains covered by a surface layer which appears relatively unaffected by the attack. The surface zone has been shown to act as a rate-limiting barrier to the progression of a lesion in vitro (Silverstone, 1968). Although it was assumed prviously that this surface resistance was related to the special intrinsic properties of surface enamel relative to subsurface enamel, it was shown that a surface zone, indistinguishable from the surface zone in caries, could be produced even when the original surface enamel was removed prior to in vitro caries (Silverstone, 1968). The relevance of this zone to remineralization phenomena and caries susceptibility has been discussed elsewhere (Silverstone, 1977). However, it does illustrate that the intrinsic structure and morphology of the tissue is not the sole consideration in determining caries prediction, especially since the disease process is a dynamic one. Thus, factors which promote the remineralization phase of the cycle may be far more important with respect to lesion progression than structural and other factors which affect solely the demineralization phase of the dynamic equilibrium.

Caries prediction for different tooth sites is relatively well defined for populations. On an individual basis, modification of single tooth surfaces can have a significant effect on the susceptibility of such surfaces to carious attack. Other factors described in this paper also have relevance in respect to the initiation and progress of a lesion through the hard tissue. However, these factors are likely to have relatively little bearing on the ability to predict the susceptibility to caries of either a surface, a tooth, or an individual.

LITERATURE CITED

1. Arends, J., Royce, B.S.H., Welch, D.O. and Smoluchowski, R. 1971. Lattice defects and the electrical and transport properties of apatite. Inst. Symp. on the Structural Properties of Hydroxyapatite (Ed. Young). Gaithersburg 1969 (Benjamin, New York,1971).

2. Bibby, B.G. 1971. Organic enamel material and caries. Caries Res. 5:305-322.

3. Brown, W.E. and Chow, L.C. 1977. Mechanism of F^- cariostasis. 55th General Session IADR, Copenhagen, Abst. #444, J. Dent. Res. 56:Spec. Issue 154.

4. Feagin, F., Koulourides, T. and Pigman, W. 1969. Formation of hydroxyapatite under various conditions of remineralization of dental enamel. Archs. oral Biol. 14:1407-1417.

5. Fejerskov, O., Silverstone, L.M., Melsen, B. and Moller, I.J. 1975. The histological featüres of fluorosed human dental enamel. Caries Res. 9:190-210.

6. Kidd, E.A.M., Thylstrup, A., Fejerskov, O. and Silverstone, L.M. 1977. The susceptibility of fluorosed human enamel to artificial caries in vitro. Caries Res. (in press).

7. Jongebloed, W.L., Molenaar, I. and Arends, J. 1973. Orientation dependent etchpit penetration and dissolution of fluorapatite. Caries Res. 7:154-165.

8. Koulourides, T. 1968. Experimental changes of enamel mineral density. IN: Harris, Art and Science of Dental Caries Research. pp.355-378, Academic Press, New York.

9. Poole, D.F.G. and Johnson, N.W. 1967. The effects of different demineralizing agents on human enamel surfaces studied by scanning electron microscopy. Archs. oral Biol. 12:1621-1634.

10. Selvig, K.A. 1970. Periodic lattice images of hydroxyapatite crystals in human bone and dental hard tissues. Calcif. Tiss. Res. 6:227-238.

11. Silverstone, L.M. 1967. The histopathology of enamel lesions produced in vitro and their relation with enamel caries. Ph.D. Thesis University of Bristol, England.

12. Silverstone, L.M. 1968. The surface zone in caries and in caries-like lesions produced in vitro. Brit. dent. J. 125:145-157.

13. Silverstone, L.M. 1972. The effect of topical application of calcifying fluids on human dental enamel in vitro. J. Int. Ass. dent. Child. 2:39-54.

14. Silverstone, L.M. 1976. Remineralization phenomena. IN: Proc. Workshop on Cariostatic Mechanisms of Fluoride. Caries Res. 11:(Suppl) 59-84.

15. Silverstone, L.M., Saxton, C.A., Dogon, I.L. and Fejerskov, O. 1975. Variation in the pattern of acid etching of human enamel examined by scanning electron microscopy. Caries Res. 9:373-387.

16. Welch, D.O. 1968. The physical and biological properties of apatite. IN: Royce et al, Princeton Univ. Conf. 1968. Princeton Paper No. 5 (Princeton Univ. Press, Princeton).

Tooth chemistry, fluoride and solubility and caries prediction

Stephen H.Y. Wei

Department of Pedodontics, University of Iowa, College of Dentistry, Iowa City, Iowa 52242

Dental enamel consists of millions of enamel prisms tighly packed in a keyhole configuration. The orientation of the enamel crystallites in the central portion of the prism is generally parallel to the c-axis of the prism, but gradually changes as the crystallites approach the periphery of the prism. The cores of enamel prisms are usually more reactive than the peripheral crystallites[1] and enamel dissolution usually begins at the center of enamel crystallites with the formation of etch-pits[2].

Chemically, enamel consists of 96-97% by weight of inorganic material, 0.4 to .8% organic matrix and approximately 3.2 to 3.6% water. The inorganic phase is essentially impure hydroxyapatite of varying chemical composition. Although hydroxyapatite is chemically represented by $Ca_{10}(PO_4)_6(OH)_2$, enamel mineral is usually non-stoichiometric, but the apatite lattice is well retained. The major elements that may be substituted include calcium, phosphorus, carbonate, sodium, magnesium, chlorine, potassium and the minor and trace elements include fluoride, iron, zinc, strontium, manganese and others[3,4,5]

Surface enamel differs considerably in mineral concentration from bulk enamel, and is generally believed to be more highly mineralized, harder, and more resistant to acid dissolution. Surface enamel has much higher concentrations of F, Zn, Fe, Pb, Sn and Cl than subsurface enamel, whereas CO_3, Mg, and Na increase in concentration towards the dentinal-enamel junction. Other constituents such as strontium and copper tend to be more evenly distributed. The impurities can be incorporated in the lattice of the crystallite, and may be located at the Ca/PO_4 or OH sites. Ions may also be adsorbed on the surface, or in the hydration layer of the crystallites, or may even be in the organic matrix. When chlorine and fluoride substitute for OH ions a change in the unit cell dimension is produced which is proportional to the mole percent substitution[6].

Many studies have analyzed the differences in chemical composition between carious and sound enamel, or between subjects who are caries free and highly caries susceptible. Most of the older techniques used acid etching of thick serial sections or bulk enamel and detected significant differences in the calcium and phosphorus concentrations of teeth from caries free and caries immune subjects[7].

Trace Elements and Caries

A tentative classification of the cariostatic potentials of different trace elements has been suggested by Navia[8] as follows:

Cariostatic elements: F,P
Mildly cariostatic: Mo, V, Cu, Sr, B, Li, Au
Doubtful: Be, Co, Mn, Su, Zn, Br, I

Caries inert: Ba, Al, Ni, Fe, Pd, Ti

Caries promoting elements: Se, Mg, Cd, Pt, Pb, Si

Epidemiological studies and animal experiments have suggested that selenium may increase caries susceptibility, but the mechanism of action is not known. On the other hand, molybdenum has a mild cariostatic effect. It has also been suggested that the combined administration of molybdenum and fluoride enhances the cariostatic effect of fluoride, but this has not been convincingly demonstrated.

Fluoride Distribution in Teeth

The relationship of fluoride concentration of drinking water and reduced dental caries has been well established[9,10,11]. Analysis of the enamel fluoride concentration and the drinking water fluoride have usually shown a direct linear relationship[12-15]. The microdistribution of fluoride in teeth has been studied extensively by Weatherall and co-workers[16-19]. Through microchemical analysis of minute enamel samples, it has been shown that:

1. Some fluoride is accumulated in developing enamel and uptake continues post-eruptively.
2. Most of the surface enamel fluoride is acquired prior to eruption, and a smaller amount during the post-eruption maturation. The ability to acquire fluoride diminishes with age.
3. The distribution of fluoride in different regions of the same tooth is very complex and changes throughout the life of the tooth.
4. Abrasion and wear reduce enamel fluoride at the incisal edges and occlusal surfaces.
5. Dental enamel accumulates fluoride much more readily if it is hypomineralized or made porous by the acidogenic activities of bacteria or by some acid treatment.

Relationship of Enamel Fluoride to Caries Inhibition

The ability of fluoride to impart a cariostatic effect to teeth of individuals depends very much upon the genetic and environmental factors operative in the mouth. Depending upon the degree of caries challenge and condition of the enamel, fluoride may or may not be a very strong determinant of caries susceptibility. In a large population, however, an increased fluoride concentration in the sound enamel of the individuals should be accompanied by a decrease in the dental caries incidence. Using the enamel biopsy technique, the fluoride concentration *in vivo* has been correlated to the fluoride in the drinking water. For example, Aasenden *et al*[20] showed that the enamel fluoride concentration in children who live in Salem (F = 1 ppm) was significantly higher than the teeth of children from Hyannis (F 0.1 ppm). The F concentration in enamel at a 2 µm depth averaged 1700 ppm for non-fluoridated communities to 2200-3200 ppm in optimally fluoridated areas to over 4800 ppm in an area with 5 to 7 ppm F[21].

Keene, *et al*[22] showed a tendency for caries-free subjects to have a higher fluoride concentration in surface enamel and a higher exposure to fluoridated water throughout their lives than other subjects who have significantly higher caries experience. Other studies have shown a similar relationship[23].

While it is logical to assume that the fluoride concentrations in enamel would be higher in teeth of subjects who reside in fluoridated communities, the correlation between the fluoride concentration of surface enamel and actual dental caries experience is not clearly established. Using the c log F as a measure of incisor fluoride and $\sqrt{DMFS}$ as the dental caries index, DePaola et al[24] found a correlation coefficient of R=0.4 among 1,447 children from towns with low, optimal and high fluoride in the drinking water. The above transformation results in a linear relationship for caries experience and fluoride in the enamel, but the correlation only accounts for 16% of the variation in the data. Gedalia, et al[26] failed to find a significant correlation between enamel fluoride concentration and DMFT in extracted teeth *in vitro*. Parkins et al[27] did not find a significant correlation between the enamel fluoride concentration of labial enamel in maxillary incisors *in vivo* and the dental caries increment, and Van der Merwe[28] could not establish a significant correlation between DMFT and log F, nor between the DMFT and the degree of enamel fluorosis in a group of African subjects. These confusing findings may be accounted for by the fact that DePaola and others[25,29,30] have shown that there is a very large disparity between the fluoride concentrations in the teeth of individuals and their dental caries experience.

Studies of the effects of topically applied fluorides cast some light on its mode of action. Topical treatment of teeth with fluorides of high concentration produce a high uptake in the enamel. This lasts only for a short period and most of the fluoride is gone within a few days. A high enamel surface fluoride in itself may not be sufficient to inhibit caries. This has been shown by studies utilizing fluoride tablets and rinses of low fluoride concentration where the enamel fluoride is not measurable elevated, and yet there is a definite and significant reduction of dental caries[31]. Comparing the fluoride uptake of a large number of topical fluoride tests, Mellberg[29,30] suggested that an acidulated fluoride would increase fluoride penetration into the enamel and that subsurface fluoride at the depth of 30 to 50 microns was most effective for caries prevention[29].

On sound enamel, topically applied fluorides do not significantly increase enamel fluoride. However, on porous enamel or early incipient caries, a very significant cariostatic effect as well as fluoride uptake is observed[32]. There is increasing evidence to support the hypothesis that post-eruptive fluoride exposures exert as great, if not greater, cariostatic effects than pre-eruptively acquired fluoride[32,33,34]. This observation is supported by clinical data of water fluoridation studies [12], animal studies[35] and clinical trials [36-38]. The positive role of fluoride in promoting remineralization of partially demineralized enamel has been thoroughly reviewed by Silverstone[39]. Other studies have confirmed the clinical observation that topically applied fluorides definitely retard or completely arrest carious lesions[40,41]

Enamel Solubility

It should be stressed that solubility of enamel in acid is not directly related to caries experience, but has been used as one of the parameters to assess enamel resistance to acid dissolution. Studies have shown that certain inhibitors of acid dissolution, such as indium nitrate and lead fluoride, failed to produce any caries inhibition clinically. Enamel of deciduous teeth is more soluble than enamel of permanent teeth.

The solubility of enamel *in vitro* appears to be inversely related to the enamel fluoride concentration, but directly related to the carbonate concentrations.

Regarding the mechanism involved Brown et al[43] have suggested that because the difference in solubility rate between fluorapatite and hydroxyapatite is so small, it is unlikely to be a significant factor in its cariostatic action of fluoride. They propose that the presence of a small amount of fluoride tends to lower the solution pH and the calcium hydroxide activity, and to raise the H_3PO_4 activity thus, altering the rate of diffusion in such a way that the rate of caries formation is diminished and the rate of remineralization is greatly enhanced. Although thermodynamically speaking, fluorapatite should not differ greatly from hydroxyapatite in its dissolution rate. Experimental evidence has shown that fluorapatite has a much lower solubility rate in acid buffer. This may be because a thin layer of calcium fluoride is rapidly formed on the surface which acts as a diffusion barrier and the acid ultimately comes to equilibrium with the new surface phase [44]. The presence of small amounts of fluoride also converts the outer surface of hydroxyapatite to fluoridated apatite with solubility properties of fluorapatite. This may reduce the rate of dissolution by reducing the surface area of the hydroxyapatite available to the acid solution. The dissolution of fluorapatite itself is a potent source of fluoride which will enhance remineralization. High concentrations of enamel fluoride has a bacteriostatic effect, whereas, lower concentrations of fluoride reduce the bacterial acid production by an anti-enzymatic effect[45,46]

In the mouth enamel is covered by bacterial plaque and pellicle. The pellicle consists of high amounts of acidic amino acids and small amounts of basic proteins. The sulfated glycoproteins have a very high affinity for hydroxyapatite and many calcium binding proteins are selectively absorbed on the surface[49]. Tinanoff[38,48] has shown that fluoride mouthrinses have a definite effect on protein absorption on enamel surfaces with some of the cations, such as stannous exerting a major influence. The influence of fluoride on the pellicle or on the microorganisms in plaque as well as the state of fluoride in plaque is still not clear.

Recommendations

While it is possible to perform microchemical analysis of dental tissues to a high degree of precision, such elaborate tests are unlikely of value as clinical caries predictive tests. However, a number of avenues need further research to give better insight into the relationship of fluoride and other chemical components of teeth and dental caries.

1. The history of previous fluoride intake and post-eruptive exposure of teeth to water and foods containing fluoride should be emphasized in the clinical evaluation of caries experience.
2. Clinical and histopathological documentation of the arrestment of caries following topically applied fluorides should be assembled and carefully evaluated.
3. The enamel biopsy technique should be further refined to take multiple overall samples of enamel of posterior teeth, prior to, during and following topically applied therapeutic agents. Emphasis should be placed on assessing differences between sound, incipient caries and frank enamel caries.
4. Multiple correlations of other caries susceptibility tests with chemical parameters of teeth such as fluoride concentration, Ca/P ratios, Co_3, Mg contents, etc., should be performed.
5. Analysis of fluoride and the chemical composition of plaque and pellicle on enamel that is sound, incipient and carious should be continued in order to elucidate the role of fluoride in dental plaque, and its inter-relation with enamel.
6. Using an artificial caries system, the effect of fluoride on an early incipient lesion should be studied with particular attention to chemical changes that will lead to complete dissolution on total remineralization.

LITERATURE CITED

1. Arends, J. and Jongebloed, W.L. 1977. Dislocations and dissolutions in apatites: theoretical considerations. Caries Res. 11:186-188.

2. Jongebloed, W.L., Molenaar, I., and Arends, J. 1976. Anomalous dissolution behavior of hydroxyapatite and fluorapatite single crystals and dental enamel investigated by scanning electron microscopy. Jeol News, 13e, 2:14-19.

3. Brudevold, F. and Soremark, R. Chemistry of the mineral phase of enamel in structural and chemical organization of teeth. Ed. Miles A.F.W. Vol. 11, Academic Press, New York and London, pp. 247-277.

4. Nixon, G.S. 1969. Trace elements content of the hard dental tissues and dental plaque. Caries Res. 3:60-70.

5. Losee, F.L., Curzon,M.E.J., and Little, M.F. 1974. Trace element concentrations in human enamel. Archs. oral Biol. 19:467-470.

6. Trautz, O.R. 1967. Crystalline organization of dental mineral in structural and chemical organization of teeth. ed. Miles A.E.W. Vol. 11, Academic Press, New York and London, pp.165-200.

7. McClure, F.J. 1948. Fluorine in dentin and enamel of sound and carious human teeth. J. Dent. Res. 27:287-298.

8. Navia, J.M. 1972. Prevention of dental caries: agents which increase tooth resistance to dental caries. Int. Dent. J. 22:427-440.

9. Backer-Dirks, O. 1974. The benefits of water fluoridation. Caries Res. 8:2.15, suppl. 1.

10. Dean, H.T., Arnold, F.A. Jr., and Elvove, E. 1942. Domestic water and dental caries: additional studies of the relation of fluoride domestic waters to dental caries experience in 4425 white children, aged 12-14 years, of 13 cities in 4 states. Pub. Health Rep. 57:1155-1179.

11. Hardwick,J.L. 1971. Fluorides and dental health, FORUM MEDICI, No. 13, caries and dental health, pp. 33-43.

12. McClure, F.J. and Likins, R.C. 1951. Fluorine in human teeth studied in relation to fluorine in the drinking water. J. Dent. Res. 30:172-176.

13. Murray, J. 1969. Caries experience of 15 year-old children from fluoride and non-fluoride communities. Br. dent. J. 127:128-131.

14. Scheinin, A., Kalijarvi, E., Harjola, O., and Heikkinen, K. 1964. Prevalence of dental caries and dental health in relation to variable concentration of fluorides in drinking water. Acta. Odont. Scand. 22:229-254.

15. Yoon, S.H., Brudevold, F., Gardner, D.E. and Smith, F.A. 1960. Distribution of fluoride in teeth from areas with different levels of fluoride in the water supply. J. Dent. Res. 39:845-856.

16. Weatherall, J.A., Deutsch, D., Robinson, C., and Hallsworth, A.S. 1977. Assimilation of fluoride by enamel throughout the life of the tooth. Caries Res. 11:85-100.

17. Weatherell, J.A., Deutsch, D., Robinson, C. and Hallsworth, A.S. 1975. Fluoride concentrations in developing enamel. Nature (Lond), 256:230-232.

18. Weatherell, J.A., Hallsworth, A.S., and Robinson, C. 1973. The effect of tooth wear on the distribution of fluoride in the enamel surface of human teeth. Archs. oral Biol. 18:1175-1189.

19. Weatherell, J.A., Robinson, C., and Hallsworth, A.S. 1972. Changes in the fluoride concentration of the labial enamel surface with age. Caries Res. 6:312-324.

20. Aasenden, R. 1974. Fluoride concentrations in the surface tooth enamel of young men and women. Archs. oral Biol. 19:697-701.

21. Aasenden, R., Allukian, M., Brudevold, F., Wellock, W.D. 1971. An <u>in vivo</u> study on enamel fluoride in children living in a fluoridated and in a non-fluoridated area. Archs. oral Biol. 16:1399-1411.

22. Keene, H.J., Mellberg, J.R. and Nicholson, C.R. 1973. History of fluoride, dental fluorosis, and concentrations of fluoride in surface layer of enamel of caries-free naval recruits. J. Pub. Health Dent. 33:142-148.

23. Keene, H.J., Grossman, F.D., Pederson, E.D., Mellberg, J.R. and Nicholson, C.R. 1975. Caries experience and fluoride concentration of surface enamel in dental fluorosis patients. Caries Res. 9:247-250.

24. DePaola, P.F., Brudevold, F., Aasenden, R., Moreno, E.C., Englander, H., Bakhos, Y., Bookstein, F., and Warram, J. 1975. A pilot study of the relationship between caries experience and surface enamel fluoride in man. Archs. oral Biol. 20:859-864.

25. Gedalia, I., Rosenzweig, K.A. and Sadeh, A. 1961. Fluroine content of superficial enamel layer and its correlation with the fluorine content of saliva, tooth age, and DMFT count. J. Dent. Res. 40:865-869.

26. Parkins, F.M., Wei, S.H.Y., and Henderson, W.G. 1975. The relationship of caries susceptibility tests to caries increments. J. Dent. Res. Vol. 54, Abst. #441.

27. Van Der Merwe, E.H.M., Bischoff, J.I., Fatti, L.P., Retief, D.H., Barbakow, F.H. and Friedman, M. 1977. Relationships between fluoride in enamel, DMFT index and fluorosis in high and low-fluoride areas in South Africa. Comm. Dent. Oral Epid. 5:61-64.

28. Aasenden, R., Moreno, E.C., and Brudevold, F. 1973. Fluoride levels in the surface of different types of human teeth. Archs. oral Biol. 18:1403-1410.

29. Mellberg, J.R. 1977. Enamel fluoride and its anti-caries effect. J. Prev. Dent. 4:8-20.

30. Mellberg, J.R. and Singer, L. 1977. Discussion of article by Weatherell et al. Caries Res. 11:101-115.

31. Shern, R.J., Driscoll, W.S., Korts, D.C. 1976. Enamel biopsy results of children receiving fluoride tablets. IADR Abst. #91.

32. Ericsson, S.Y. 1977. Cariostatic mechanisms of fluorides: clinical observations. Caries Res. 11:2-22, Suppl. 1.

33. Horowitz, H.S. 1973. School fluoridation for the prevention of dental caries. Int. Dent. J. 23:346-353.

34. Aasenden, R., DePoala, P.F. and Brudevold, F. 1972. Effects of daily rinsing and ingestion of fluoride solutions upon dental caries and enamel fluoride. Archs. oral Biol. 17:1705-1714.

35. Larson, R.H. 1977. Animal studies relating to caries inhibition by fluoride. Caries Res. 11:42-52.

36. Horowitz, H.S. and Kau, M.C.W. 1974. Retained anti-caries protection from topically applied acidulated phosphate fluorides: 20 and 36 month post-treatment effects. J. Prev. Dent. 1:22-27.

37. DePaola, P.F. and Mellberg, J.R. 1973. Caries experience and fluoride uptake in children receiving semi-annual prophylaxis with and acidulated phosphate fluoride paste. J. Am. Dent. Assoc. 87:155-159.

38. Heifetz, S.B., Mellberg, J.R., Winter, S.J. and Doyle, J. 1970. In vivo fluoride uptake by enamel of teeth of human adults from various topical fluoride procedures. Archs.oral Biol. 15:1171-1181.

39. Silverstone, L.M. 1977. Remineralization phenomena. Caries Res. 11:59-78, Suppl. 1.

40. Hollender, L. and Koch, G. 1969. Influence of topical application of fluoride on rate of progress of carious lesions in children. Odont. Rev. 20:37-41.

41. Hyde, E.J. 1973. Caries inhibiting action of three different topically applied agents on incipient lesions in newly erupted teeth: results after 24 months. J. Canad. Dent. Assoc. 39:189-193.

42. Cutress, T.W. 1972. The inorganic composition and solubility of dental enamel from several specified population groups. Archs. oral Biol. 17:93-109.

43. Brown, W.E., Gregory, T.M. and Chow, L.C. 1977. Effects of fluoride on enamel solubility and cariostasis. Caries Res. 11:118-135, Suppl.

44. Jeansonne, B.G. and Feagin, F.F. 1974. Enamel dissolution in a weak acid containing 0.05, 0.5 or 5.0 mm sodium fluoride. J. Dent. Res. 53:414-417.

45. Jenkins, G.N. 1974. The biochemistry of plaque and caries with special reference to fluoride, Forum Medici, Metabolism and Cariogenicity of dental plaque. p. 20-36.

46. Konig, K.G. 1977. Conclusions and recommendations: in vivo aspects. Caries Res. 11:322-323.

47. Rolla, G. 1977. Effects of fluoride on initiation of plaque formation. Caries Res. 11:243-251.

48. Tinanoff, N., Brady, J.M., and Gross, A. 1976. The effect of NaF and SnF_2 mouth rinses on bacterial colonization of tooth enamel: TEM and SEM studies. Caries Res. 10:415-426.

Discussion of tooth factors and caries prediction chemistry, fluoride and solubility

F.E. Feagin and J.A. Gray

University of Alabama, College of Dentistry, Birmingham, Alabama 35294
The Proctor & Gamble Company, Cincinnati, Ohio

Dr. Wei has shown that at present there is no laboratory test for predicting caries efficiency. We could not agree more. However, it does not mean that these tests do not have utility. Taken collectively they can be useful in selecting candidates for clinical testing. In reality, there is little other choice until such time as mechanisms of action and predictive tests are devised. If nothing else, the present lack of correlation between laboratory tests and actual clinical performance is good reason for the lack of understanding of the mechanism of anti-caries activity of known systems. It is also evident that most in vitro or basic studies are aimed at predicting a reduction in caries rather than an absolute rate of caries.

The use of solubility or dissolution rate measurements for predicting anti-caries activity has previously been reviewed by one of the present authors[1], and little has changed since that review. Such tests provide poor correlation with actual clinical performance, and show many materials as good anti-solubility agents, but with no clinical activity. On the other hand, these tests did lead to the discovery of stannous fluoride[2] and have been very useful, at least in the Procter & Gamble laboratories, for monitoring the efficacy of fluoride products[3].

It has to be an axiom that if caries is caused by the acid dissolution of enamel, then rendering the enamel totally insoluble has to prevent caries. None of the agents presently known will render enamel totally insoluble, and in fact, even the best of such materials, as for instance stannous ion[4] as $SnCl_2$, stop acid attack for only several minutes, impressive though this is. Further, even though many of these agents can arrest surface attack, the undissolved surface is by-passed by the much smaller hydrogen ion leading to subsurface dissolution and white spot formation.

Since white spot formation is really the mode of caries formation, it has been suggested that this type of dissolution is the one that should be studied and Buonocore developed such a test[5]. Although, it appears to be better in correlating with anti-caries activity, at Procter and Gambel, it has still been found to be less than ideal. The test, for example, does not account for the impact of a covering of plaque. A still more realistic test may be needed to simulate all the interference encountered in vivo.

Although much is understood about the mechanism of white spot formation, there are still aspects which need clarification. Better knowledge of these could well lead to better prediction of caries rates, even on an absolute basis. For example, the formation of the sound outer layer needs better definition. Little or nothing is known about the role of carbonate, or other trace elements in white spot development.

One value of any solubility or dissolution measurement is that it can demonstrate the existence of a significant inter-action between the agent under study and dental enamel. Certainly, if the concept being examined calls for such an inter-action and none is found, there is little merit in pursuing work with that particular agent. Furthermore, these tests can often serve as an analytical tool to determine the amount of material that has reacted with enamel and can be used to determine bioavailability of the agent in different systems.

As Dr. Wei has pointed out, fluoride uptake measurements correlate with anti-caries activity only poorly in the case of water fluoridation and not at all in the case of topical applications. Frankly, we do not believe that anyone should be surprised at the poor correlation of fluoride uptake with caries activity because of the variation of fluoride uptake with depth in enamel, soundness of enamel, and access of the enamel site to the fluoride treatment solution, just to mention a few of the problems. Indeed, the uptake of cariostatic levels of fluoride may depend upon the existence of a carious process. Meaningful correlations between fluoride in enamel and caries resistance obviously depend upon determination of fluoride in caries challenged regions of enamel rather than indiscriminate estimations of non-selective tooth structure. This then poses some severe problems for experimentally determining a sound correlation between fluoride uptake and caries activity. However, the fact of even partial correlation is useful and the finding of fluoride in enamel after topical applications is certainly consistent with the concept of the need of its presence for effect on caries activity. Therefore, enamel uptake of any agent is still a logical and worthwhile determination. Although absence of an agent offers pretty fair assurance that lacks utility, its presence is no guarantee of anti-caries activity. Of course, if the activity takes place in plaque, the presence and duration in plaque may be the more valid determination.

Crystal structure and differences in dissolution of different crystal phases of hydroxyapatite are well documented. However, their relationship to caries is still a matter of speculation, and no correlation with caries prediction can be made as yet. One of the present authors has compared artificial white spot formation on enamel with supposedly higher and lower degrees of structural perfection that was obtained from rats and monkey's enamel, and human deciduous teeth. All produced white spots at the same rate as on enamel from human permanent teeth showing that differences in susceptibility of enamel to in vitro caries-like dissolution did not explain the different rates at which caries develops in these teeth. However, it should be noted that the system was not allowed to reach equilibrium, nor did it provide periods of a remineralizing environment such as exists in vivo. This emphasizes the need for test condition that more closely approximate those in vivo.

Small differences in solubility and dissolution rates would be expected to have much greater effects near equilibrium conditions. It is interesting to note, however, that using pH and lactate levels found in plaque along with the white spot rate equations[6], the rate of caries development could be calculated and correlated well with the usual six month period of caries development noted in rampant caries. This approach may provide a basis for determining the absolute caries rate.

The lack of correlation with solubility studies using fluorides and practical observations on caries is probably due to incomplete consideration of all the parameters involved. It seems obvious that explanations for some of the observed solubility behavior are likely to be forthcoming only if the concentrations of calcium, phosphate, fluoride, and hydrogen ions are simultaneously monitored as a function of time both in the solid and solution phases. The resultant understanding of the ionic environment factors that regulate enamel solubility could well provide leads to reliable caries

Fig. 1.

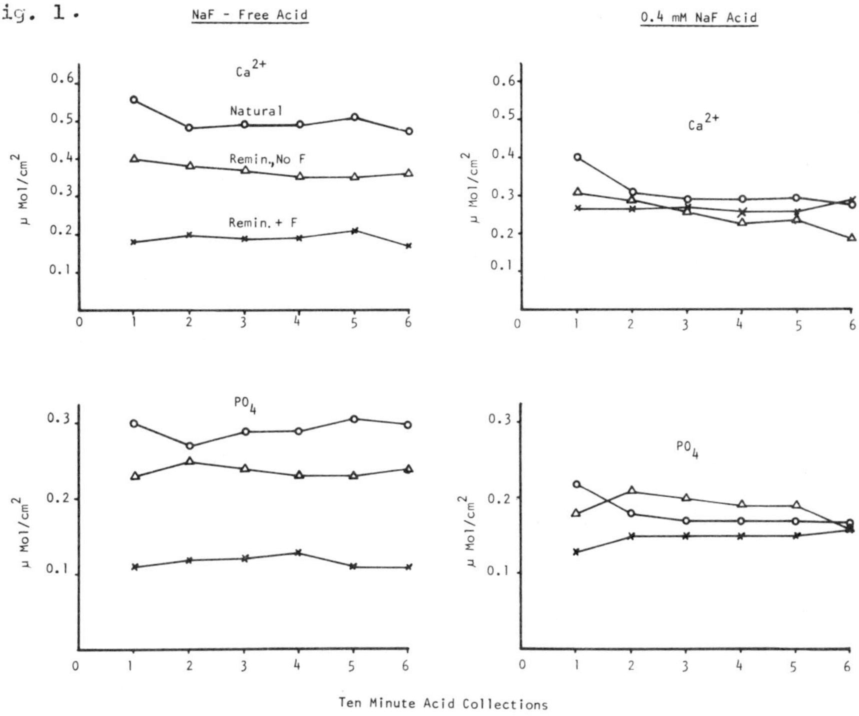

Figure 1. The effect of fluoride in remineralized enamel and in acid on dissolution of surface minerals in laminar flow of acid (10 mM acetic acid, pH 4.5, flow rate 1.2 ml/min., collected at 10 min. intervals).

prediction.

Experiments designed to produce the desired information were carried out on the labial surfaces of bovine incisors that were demineralized, and then exposed to mineralizing solutions containing calcium and phosphorus ions, with or without fluoride. Measurements were made of calcium and phosphorus loss and uptake under different ionic environments of fluorine, calcium, and phosphorus during demineralization, remineralization and a second demineralization.

Figure 1 shows that calcium and phosphorus dissolved in almost constant amounts in each of the 6 samplings of the weak decalcifying acid. Smaller amounts of minerals dissolved from the enamel surfaces remineralized in the presence of sodium fluoride than in its absence. Unexpectedly almost the same amounts of calcium and phosphorus dissolved from natural surfaces and remineralized surfaces in the acid containing fluoride. Figure 2 shows the percentage recoveries of ^{45}Ca from the remineralized surfaces in the collections of acid. Surprisingly, only 15 percent of the NaF remineralized-recrystallized ^{45}Ca was recovered in the NaF-free and acid NaF collections, while most of the calcium dissolved came from the original enamel. The recovery of ^{45}Ca in NaF-free acid from surfaces remineralized in the absence of Na F was reduced by about one-half in each successive, corresponding collection of acid NaF. This showed that the acid NaF reacted rapidly with

Fig. 2.

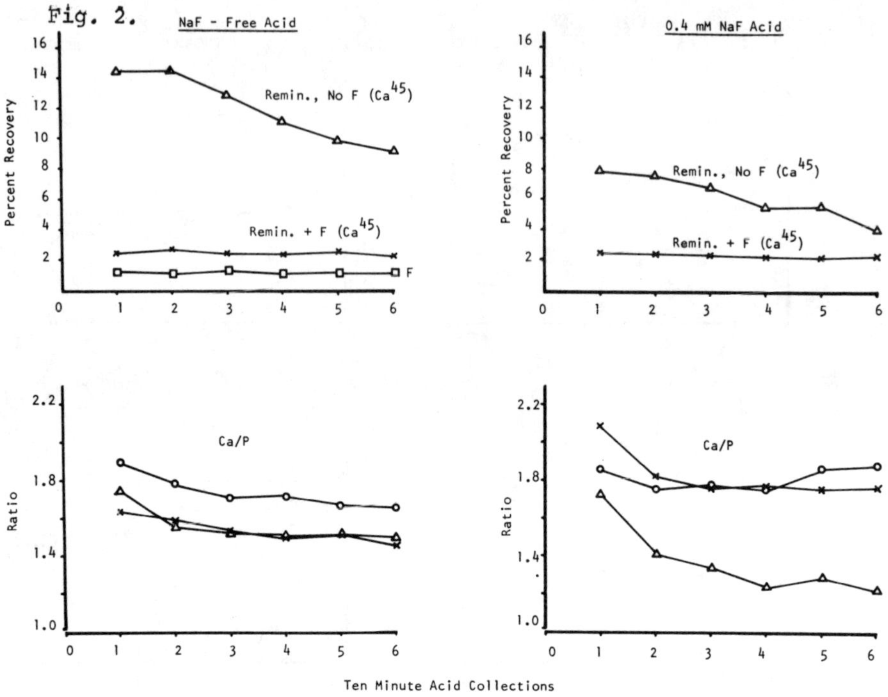

Figure 2. Recovery of ^{45}Ca and Ca/P ratios of minerals dissolved in the collections of acid from surfaces of enamel.

the surface minerals of natural and altered enamel to reduce the dissolution of some fractions of the surface materials. The fluoride in the remineralized surfaces had the same effect on mineral dissolution as sodium fluoride added in the weak acid. The calcium/phosphorus ratios of the minerals dissolved in each collection of acid indicated the composition of the dissolved substances, but they did not correspond with any particular compound which might be expected and certainly did not correspond with any of the acid resistance fractions in the surface minerals. Although the data and its interpretation are incomplete as yet, it certainly indicates that some additional complex factors bear on the mechanism of the fluoride action. These complexities need to be understood before reliable caries prediction based upon fluoride data will be possible.

LITERATURE CITED

1. Gray, J.A. 1968. A critique of enamel dissolution testing for anticariogenic agents. In the proceedings of the American Dental Association Conference on the Clinical Testing of Cariostatic Agents. October, pp. 18-26.

2. Muhler, J.C. 1955. The development of stannous fluoride as an anti-cariogenic agent for topical application by means of a dentifrice. J. Indiana Dent. Assoc. 34:9.

3. Cooley, W.E. 1970. Applied Research in the development of anticaries Dentifrices. J. Chem. Ed. 47:177.

4. Gray, J.A. 1965. Acid dissolution rate of sound and white-spot enamel treated with tin (11) and fluoride compounds. J. Dent. Res. 44:493.

5. Buonocore, N.G. and Gwinnett, A.J. 1967. Chemical, polarized light, and microradiographic study of the effects of various toothpastes on "white spot" formation in vitro . J. Oral Ther. 3:321.

6. Gray, J.A. 1966. Kinetics of enamel dissolution during formation of incipient caries-like lesions. Archs. oral Biol. 11:397.

7. Dean, H.T., Arnold, F.A. Jr., and Elvove,E. 1942. Domestic water and dental caries. V. Additional studies of the relation of fluoride domestic waters to dental caries experience in 4,425 white children, aged 12 to 14 years, of 13 cities in 4 states. Pub. Health Rept. 57:1155.

8. Reed, M.W. 1973. Clinical evaluation of three concentrations of sodium fluoride in dentrifices. J. Am. Dent. Assoc. 87:1401.

9. Englander, H.R., Keyes, P.H., Gestwicki, M., and Sultz, H.A. 1967. Clinical anticaries effect of repeated topical sodium fluoride applications by mouthpieces. J. Am. Dent. Assoc. 75:638.

10. Feagin, F.F. and Gray, J.A. 1977. Remineralization phenomena-discussion. Caries Res. 11:Suppl. 1, 79.

MODERATOR'S SUMMARY OF DISCUSSION OF TOPIC V PRESENTATIONS

It was suggested that since tooth enamel is not an isotropic, homogeneous medium there must be pathways by which caries attack takes place and that knowledge of these and the mechanisms of apatite dissolution at the crystallite level was needed. In response it was pointed out that at the molecular level there is a constant transformation involving different phases of calcium phosphate; according to varying pH and fluoride levels there is a continuous conversion of fluorapatite to dicalcium-phosphate followed in short order by reconversion. It was also noted that in addition to interfering with demineralization fluoride may also operate by promoting remineralization. There was agreement that regardless of a low enamel fluoride level there will be no caries in the absence of a caries challenge, and conversely, that despite a high level of enamel fluoride an overwhelming challenge can cause caries. This means that any attempt to use enamel fluorine alone as a predictor of caries may prove to be a frustrating exercise.

Dr. Mühlemann questioned Dr. Silverstone's claim that a lesion short of the dentine cannot be detected by clinical examination. Noting that there had been a number of comments by various speakers suggesting the inability of clinical examiners to detect a lesion until it was relatively advanced histologically, Dr. Horowitz pointed out that the purpose of epidemologic surveys is not to pick out predicator of decay but rather to identify overt pathology. More collaboration between the histologist and the epidemologist was proposed by Dr. Silverstone as a way of refining diagnostic techniques.

Dr. Mühlemann disagreed with the implication that enamel hardness was related to caries. He cited instances of relatively soft, plaque-free enamel which remained remarkably caries free and also cases of amelogenesis imperfecta where intact soft enamel surfaces seem to be less susceptible to caries than very hard highly mineralized enamel structure.

TOPIC VI

MODELS FOR CARIES STUDY

Moderator:

William H. Bowen
National Institutes of Dental Research
Bethesda, Maryland 20014

Clinical considerations of caries measurement

D.M. O'Mullane

Turner Dental School, Bridgeford Street, Manchester, England

Though many uses for valid caries predictions have been considered, this paper is confined solely to their value in improving efficiency of experimental clinical trials (O'Mullane, 1976). The artificial conditions under which these trials are generally conducted limits their aims to testing the Null Hypothesis of no treatment effect by means of significance tests and estimates of the extent of the effect by means of confidence limits. When criteria for successful achievement of these aims are laid down before the trial starts then it is possible that the efficiency of the current trial designs (Horowitz et al, 1973) could be improved by, for example, reducing their length.

There are two methods of reducing the length of a clinical trial: firstly, the trial can be planned to run for a shorter period in the first place, say one and a half years, or secondly, the data can be analysed as it is collected so that the trial can be stopped as soon as its stated aims are achieved.

Using a sequential t-test (Hajnall, 1961) considerable improvements in efficiency were demonstrated retrospectively in 3 clinical trials conducted by the Dental Health Unit, University of Manchester (Smith and O'Mullane, 1977). In this paper the trials are designated trial A (Rugg-Gunn et al, 1973), trial B (Downer et al,1976), and trial C (Howat, 1977). Even though improvements in efficiency were demonstrated, two assumptions underlying the use of a sequential t-test, the properties of Independence and Identity of Distributions, were violated in the data investigated. By excluding subjects who had an initial DMFS of less than 3, statistical independence of each annual increment for the remaining subjects could be demonstrated. The property of Identity of Distribution of each batch of data (annual increments), however, remains to be solved and will be considered in this paper.

In a sequential t-test the hypotheses tested are as follows:

$$Ho : \mu C = \mu T$$

$$H_1 : \frac{(\mu C - \mu T)^2}{\sigma^2} = \xi^2 \quad \ldots\ldots\ldots\ldots\ldots \quad (1)$$

When calculating ξ^2 it is necessary to state before the experiment begins what is the target percentage reduction considered whorthwhile. In the trials under investigation this was set at 30 percent, in other words:

$$\frac{\mu_C \; - \; \mu_T}{u_C} \quad = \quad 0.3$$

or

$$\mu_C \; - \; \mu_T \quad = \quad 0.3\,\mu_C$$

substituting in (1);

$$\xi^2 \quad = \quad \frac{(0.3\,\mu_C)^2}{\sigma^2}$$

$$= \quad 0.3^2 \;\cdot\; \frac{\mu_C^2}{\sigma^2} \qquad \ldots\ldots\ldots\ldots\ldots\ldots\ldots (2)$$

The assumption of Identity of Distributions demands that the fraction $\frac{\mu_C^2}{\sigma^2}$ (the co-efficient of variation squared) should be constant throughout the trial for each annual increment in the control group. However, this did not prove to be the case in the trial investigated (Table 1). For each trial, the means and standard deviations recorded during the first year are consistently lower than those recorded during the second and third years. It is also apparent that the means and standard deviations of the second year tend to be equal to each other and that they in turn tend to equal those of the third year (identical distributions). For example, in trial A $4.1 \bumpeq 4.0 \bumpeq 4.3 = 4.3$. If this trend could be regarded as consistent, giving a value of unity to $\frac{\mu_C^2}{\sigma^2}$ (Smith and O'Mullane, 1977 it would appear reasonable if the trials were started one year later than those investigated. The average age at base-line of the subjects in the three trials was 11 years and 10 months.

Two interesting questions are posed by the results in Table 1. Firstly, can the consistenly low increment recorded in the first year of the trials be explained? Secondly, are the distributions recorded during the second and third years likely to be repeated for a further year? This second question is important because it is conceivable that a sequential trial, started one year later than previously, could run for more than two years.

There are two factors to be considered when answering these questions:

1. the number of critical teeth or surfaces at risk at the baseline and subsequent examinations.
2. the length of time a surface needs to be exposed to the oral environment before caries develop.

Table 1

Mean annual caries increments of control groups in 3 trials. Initial DMFS $>$ 3. Cavitation into dentine level. Standard deviations in parentheses.

Incremental Period	0 - 1	1 - 2	2 - 3
Trial A	2.2 (3.2)	4.1 (4.0)	4.3 (4.3)
Trial B	0.5 (2.0)	3.0 (2.6)	4.7 (4.0)
Trial C	1.7 (2.0)	3.8 (3.9)	3.1 (2.9)

In an earlier report to this conference (Downer, 1977) it was shown that for the trials investigated, a small group of surfaces ("critical surfaces") on posterior teeth ("critical teeth") accounted for the greater part of the caries increment. Table 2 shows the percentage of these teeth which were erupted at each examination in the 496 subjects who participated in trial C. Figures for the first permanent molars are omitted because all of these were erupted at the baseline examination. Apart from the upper first bicuspids (U4) only 65 percent or less were erupted at the baseline examination. By the end of the second year, over 90 percent of all critical teeth apart from the lower bicuspids (L5) were erupted. These percentages were representative of the other two trials and closely resemble the findings of Todd (1975) who reported on a representative sample of children in England and Wales. From this latter study it can be estimated that in the year prior to age 11 years and 10 months, over 25 percent of the critical teeth listed in Table 2 erupt and only 25 percent of them, approximately, are present in the mouth for more than 1 year when the trials start.

It is important to note when considering these eruption figures that a tooth was defined as erupted when any part of it was visible in the mouth. However, though a tooth may be deemed erupted its critical surfaces may not be truly exposed to the oral environment. Furthermore, two of the critical surfaces (Downer, 1977) were interproximal surfaces and the eruption figures do not take into account the length of time between a tooth first appearing in the mouth and the establishment of contact points. Hence, the eruption figures in Table 2 tend to give an inflated estimate of the percentage of surfaces at risk at each examination.

In considering the length of time taken for a tooth surface to become carious after it has erupted into the mouth, the fate of two groups of surfaces in the control groups are presented; (i) critical surfaces erupted at baseline (Table 3), and (ii) critical surfaces erupting during the first year (Table 4). The figures shown are cumulative percentages, in which caries is defined as cavitation into dentine (Downer *et al*, 1976), and clinical and radiographic scores are combined. In the case of those surfaces which were erupted at the baseline examination (Table 3) it is seen that apart from the occlusal surfaces of upper and lower second molars little

Table 2.

The percentages of five critical teeth which were erupted at each examination. Trial 3. All subjects.

Year	0	1	2	3
Upper 1st Bicuspids (U4)	85	93	97	98
Upper 2nd Bicuspids (U5)	65	79	90	95
Upper 2nd Molars (U7)	49	67	91	98
Lower 2nd Bicuspids (L5)	56	71	86	92
Lower 2nd Molars (L7)	59	77	93	98

Table 3.

The percentage of critical surfaces which were erupted at the baseline examination and which became carious during the trial. Control groups. Cavitation into dentine level (C3+). Clinical and radiographic combined. Trial B and Trial C.

Incremental Period			0		0 - 1		0 - 2		0 - 3	
Trial	B	C	B	C	B	C	B	C	B	C
Surface	No. of surfaces									
U.40	471	400	9.8	5.0	8.7	8.5	15.5	17.0	24.4	25.7
U.50	367	309	12.3	6.8	10.9	9.7	20.1	18.1	27.8	31.4
U.5D	367	309	4.1	3.9	4.6	4.8	9.5	10.0	12.5	16.5
U.7O	271	247	27.3	10.5	29.9	24.3	50.2	49.4	58.7	66.0
L.5D	304	253	5.9	5.1	6.6	9.5	12.2	19.4	16.8	28.1
L.5D	304	253	4.9	1.6	4.9	3.6	9.2	8.7	10.9	11.5
L.70	331	301	35.3	18.3	35.0	27.9	63.1	54.1	70.4	68.1

caries activity was recorded until the end of the second year. At this stage for example 63.1 percent of the 331 occlusal surfaces of the lower 7^s in trial B had decayed. The corresponding figure for the occlusal surfaces of upper second bicuspids was 20.1 percent. For surfaces which erupted during the first year, there were 3 opportunities to examine them during the trials (Table 4). Apart from the occlusal surfaces of upper and lower second molars, little caries activity was recorded until the end of the third year when these surfaces were present in the mouth for an average of two and a half years (Carlos and Gittelsohn, 1965). The figures presented in Tables 3 and 4 confirm that caries, defined as cavitation into dentine, is in general a slow process in most surfaces as reported by Parfitt (1956), Berman and Slack (1972), Backer-Dirks (1961), Marthaler and Wiesner (1973), and Carlos and Gittelsohn (1965).

It would seem, therefore, that the low increment recorded during the first year of the three trials investigated can be explained by a combination of two facts; firstly, a large proportion of the surfaces which contribute to the caries increment were not erupted when the trials started, and secondly, many of those surfaces which were erupted were not exposed to the oral environment for sufficient length of time for caries to develop. In answering the second question "Is the extent and distribution of the caries increment recorded during the second and third year likely to continue for a further year?"; the reply must be in the affirmative. Because of the number of critical teeth which erupt during the first two years of the trials, and the length of time it takes caries to develop, the potential for the development of caries will remain similar to years 2 and 3 during year 4.

In conclusion, therefore, the property of identity of distribution demanded in a sequential t-test is likely to be upheld if the trials start one year later than previously.

Table 4.

The percentage of critical surfaces which erupt during the first year and which become carious during the trial. Control groups. Cavitation into dentine level (C2+). Clinical and radiographic combined Trial B and Trial C.

Incremental Period			0 - 1		0 - 2		0 - 3	
Trial	B	C	B	C	B	C	B	C
Surface	No. of Surfaces							
U.40	48	42	0.0	0.0	0.0	4.8	6.3	7.1
U.50	79	67	1.3	0.0	1.3	4.5	6.3	10.4
U.5D	79	67	1.3	0.0	2.5	0.0	5.1	4.5
U.70	113	82	0.9	4.9	22.1	30.5	46.0	48.8
L.50	75	68	0.0	0.0	1.3	4.4	10.7	7.3
L.5D	75	68	0.0	0.0	1.3	0.0	4.0	2.9
L.70	102	78	0.0	0.0	26.5	25.6	64.7	59.0

LITERATURE CITED

1. Backer-Dirks, O. 1961. Archs. oral Biol., Special Suppl. 6:94.

2. Berman, D.S. and Slack, G.L. 1972. Brit. Dent. J. 134:135.

3. Carlos, J.P. and Gittelsohn, A.M. 1965. Archs. oral Biol. 10:739.

4. Downer, M.C., Holloway, P.J. and Davies, T.G.H. 1976. Brit. Dent. J. 141:242.

5. Downer, M.C. 1977. Proceedings of Workshop on Caries Prediction, Niagara Falls. In Press.

6. Hajnall, J. 1961. Biometrica 48:65.

7. Horowitz, A.S., Baume, L.J., Backer-Dirks, O., Davies, G.N. and Slack, G.L. 1973. Int. Dent. J. 23:506.

8. Howat, A.P. 1977. Caries Res. 11:125.

9. Marthaler, T.M. and Weisner, V. 1973. Helv. Odont. Acta. 17:19.

10. O'Mullane, D.M. 1976. Community Dent. Oral Epidemiol. 4:490.

11. Parfitt, G.J. 1956. Brit. Dent. J. 100:204.

12. Rugg-Gunn, A.J., Holloway, P.J. and Davies, T.G.H. 1973. Brit. Dent. J. 141:242.

13. Smith, V.O. and O'Mullane, D.M. 1977. Proceedings of International Conference on Oral Biology. J. Dent. Res. In press.

14. Todd, J.E. 1975. "Childrens Dental Health in England and Wales, 1973. H.M.S.O., London.

Discussion of clinical considerations of caries measurements

T.M. Marthaler

Department of Cariology, Periodontology and Preventive Dentistry, University of Zurich, Switzerland

In a discussion of Dr. O'Mullane's paper it is important to point out that the sequential design corresponds to a specific aim: to arrive at a decision as quickly as possible. As usual in biometric research, the decision is whether to accept the null hypothesis or not: is it justified to assume a cariostatic effect of a given treatment or not?

This has been a fairly uncommon situation in research on caries prevention. The majority of short-term trials caried out during the last ten years used fluoride as the active agent. The obvious purpose of these trials must have been to estimate the benefits of fluoride, i.e. the efficiency of the fluoride treatment under study. It has been well known for more than ten years that fluoride will reduce the incidence of dental caries when applied frequently enough and in adequate concentrations. When a new fluoride treatment is tested, it is not really a question of the fluoride effect, but of the effectiveness of fluoride under the condition of this treatment. This is also evident from the now frequent cost-benefit analyses, for which the size of the caries reduction must be known with due precision.

The type of design presented by O'Mullane is thus indicated for (entirely) new types of presumed caries-preventive agents or procedures. I don't feel competent to make a great many propositions as to what new method of caries control would be suitable for being tested in sequential trials. I would suggest considering whether it would be interesting to apply sequential design to an old and widespread and widely recommended preventive method, i.e. toothbrushing. Recent findings show that plaque removal as practiced by children at school is not or only slightly effective against dental caries (Horowitz et al. 1977, Silverstone et al. 1977). It is important to decide at what age, and in which situation, the main purpose of using the toothbrush is either to quickly remove food remnants, as suggested by Fosdick's experiment (1950), or else to remove plaque as far as possible.

As to the actual conduct of sequential trials, a great many common practices must be reconsidered.

- What is the ideal patient age at the start? The paper discussed here would suggest that about 80 percent of second premolars and molars should have began eruption (clinical emergence, when any part of the crown projects through the alveolar mucosa).
- How many months should elapse between two subsequent examinations? There are two main reasons for not arranging them too frequently:
  (i) Frequent examinations may mean a considerable workload
  (ii) In short intervals only very few new lesions appear, and it must be assumed that the diagnostic errors may contribute substantially to the variation of the increments.

- The question of sample size is easier to deal with. As the number of children in the trial is increased, the time necessary to arrive at a significant difference shortens.

The proposed type of evaluation may be compared with the usual type that presents results by using the matrix notation of single comparisons. This is done in Table I. The proposed sequential analysis corresponds to coefficients of -1 and +1 for caries counts of two subsequent examinations. The coefficients corresponding to the usual evaluation and presentation of the data is given in the lower part of Table I.

The statistical aspects of the proposed sequential testing procedure may need further investigation. There is ample material available on which the question of independence of subsegment individual increments may be studied.

	Examination			
	1	2	3	4
a) incremental periods 1-2, 2-3, 3-4 (for sequential tests)				
1-2	-1	+1		
2-3		-1	+1	
3-4			-1	+1
b) usual method of evaluation				
after first year	-1	+1		
after second year	-1		+1	
after third year	-1			+1

LITERATURE CITED

1. Fosdick, L.S. 1950. The reduction of the incidence of dental caries. I. Immediate tooth-brushing with a neutral dentifrice. J. Amer. Dent. Assoc. 40:133-143.

2. Horowitz, A.M. et al. 1977. (Abstract 170) Preprinted Abstracts, J. Dent. Res. 56:Special Issue A.

3. Silverstein, S. et al. 1977. (Abstract 169) Preprinted Abstracts, J. Dent. Res. 56:Special Issue A.

Caries research using experimental animals: methods and measurements

H.G. Huxley

National Institute of Dental Research, Auburn Building, Bethesda, Maryland 20014

Introduction

Animal models for any disease process permit experimentation that is not possible using human subjects. In the case of dental caries, rodents and primates are the models I shall discuss. Rats have been the most commonly-used rodents in caries research followed by hamsters. Gerbils and cotton rats have sometimes been used. Relatively little use has been made of mice, and perhaps the genetic control possible with certain pureline breeds remains unexploited in caries research. A comprehensive review of rodents used in caries research, the diets fed and the methods of evaluating caries has been published[1]. Of the primates used as models for caries, macaques have been the most thoroughly studied. Rodents and primates exist as complementary models and should certainly not be viewed as competitors. A review of the procedures applicable to each will make this point clear.

Procedures Applicable to Rodents

The small size and rapid breeding cycle of rodents means that large numbers can be economically obtained, housed and fed. Caries experiments are typically of short duration (2-8 weeks), which makes for a productive model system with sufficient numbers to generate statistically valid data.

On the other hand their small size is a disadvantage. Examination for caries *in vivo* is impractical and unreliable, particularly in rats. Longitudinal experimentation, involving the sacrifice of littermate animals at various times, represents a compromise that derives some justification from observed similarities in caries incidence among littermates[2]. The ability to reliably record caries *in vivo* would significantly improve the model. Techniques for recording plaque *in vivo* have been described[3,4] and shown to be reliable[4]. The small size of rodents is a disadvantage in other respects. Collection of oral secretions is difficult, particularly in younger animals. Biopsy of plaque is possible immediately post-mortem[5]. Biopsy of rat enamel has recently been described[6], though the small size of rat teeth obviously presented problems. In order to have enough sample for microanalysis the biopsy area is extended subgingivally and thus included enamel not subject to the same environmental influences as more coronal enamel. Recording of plaque pH has been made in hamsters using small glass electrodes[7]. Unfortunately the narrow fissures of rat teeth do not admit this electrode. Placement of an antimony microelectrode[8], originally designed to record pH in and around bacterial colonies on agar plates, is possible into rat plaque, and would merit further study.

The ability to alter the oral microbiota of rodents has been exploited in caries research. Notably the availability of germfree and specific pathogen free lines of animals has significantly facilitated research into microbiology of caries. Rodents are relatively omnivorous and will tolerate the addition of a wide variety of agents to the diet or drinking fluid. Methods for monitoring[9] and regulating[10] the feeding behaviour of rodents considerably enhances the validity of dietary experiments.

Procedures Applicable to Primates

The greater size of primates presents advantages and disadvantages. Among the advantages is the ability to conduct a clinical examination analogous to that in man. True longitudinal experimentation is thus possible. The sampling of primate plaque for bacteriological or chemical analysis is relatively simple[11,12] and recording of plaque pH in vivo is feasible[13]. A limited availability of primates, their comparative longevity and greater size and the longer experimental periods employed have generally limited both the number of experiments performed and the number of treatment units per experiment.

One obvious advantage of primates in caries research, as in many other sphere of investigation, lies in the greater confidence in extrapolating results to man. Primates therefore form one part of a logical continuum in the development and testing of therapeutic agents or procedures.

Animal experimentation has provided much information on caries. Some factors, notably the composition of the diet fed and the microbial flora of some dental plaques have been quite thoroughly explored and their influence upon dental caries is recognized and reasonably predictable. This paper discusses two aspects of caries experimentation in rodents that have received much less attention. Firstly, the nature of the preweaning regimen can influence considerably the level of caries in subsequent experimentation. Secondly, the behaviour of individual types of carious lesions is examined as a function of the caries test period. Inferences are drawn about the suitability of criteria commonly used to score caries.

The Preweaning Regime

Evidence exists that the conditions and procedures to which animals are subjected before weaning influence the subsequent caries incidence. Nutritional and other effects are discernible during the rearing of rodent pups. In rats caries incidence bears an inverse relationship to the size of animals at the beginning of and during experiments[14,15]. Protein deprivation during suckling markedly increases caries incidence[16]; this effect may be related to delayed biochemical maturation of the major salivary glands[17]. There is some historlogical evidence that a cariogenic diet of marginal nutritional adequacy affects the development of salivary glands after weaning[18]. Further work is clearly warranted to delineate the effects of various diets upon salivary gland development.

As well as the nutritional sufficiency of a diet offered to the dam whilst suckling, its physical consistency is also of probable importance. Redman and Sweney[19] have demonstrated that suckling rats commence some independent feeding activity from 14 days of age, and that significant quantities of the dam's diet is eaten after 18 days of age. This accounts for the presence of dietary residue in the molar tooth fissures of weanling rats[20]. Observations in this laboratory indicate that some stock pellet residue occurs in the fissures of weanling rats whose dam was transferred from stock pellet to a powdered starch-based diet when the litter was 10 days old. In this instance the stock pellet residue must be derived from the dam's faeces through coprophagy. There are clearly implications for the transmission of various chemical and microbial agents to the oral cavity of the young pups. A much lower incidence of buccolingual caries was noted in rats whose dam was fed stock pellet during weaning rather than a powdered starch-containing diet[21,22]. It is possible that the abrasive pellet diet could have retarded buccolingual plaque formation, with carry-over of this effect into the post-weaning period through ingestion of faeces containing pellet residue. A high fluoride level in enamel occurred when litters were reared on stock pellet[22], and could have contributed substantially towards lowered buccolingual caries incidence.

A need for fuller understanding of the oral environment is highly desirable during the time teeth are erupting. It has been recognized for some time that older animals develop less caries when suitably challenged. Post-eruptive 'maturation' of the enamel is one possible explanation for this phenomenon. More recently it is recognized that large reductions in caries occur by delaying the feeding of cariogenic diet for just a few days [22,23,24]. In this case other influences are probably also at work. Dietary effects upon the developing plaque flora and upon the feeding behavior are likely and require clarification.

The Length of Experimental Period

In early rodent experimentation diagnosis of caries was based upon examination of whole teeth. Latterly microscopic identification of caries has prevailed, with grinding or sectioning of teeth to properly expose lesions. More precise localization of caries and shorter experimental times resulted. Caries in rodents occurs rapidly. Commonly used experimental periods are 2-3 weeks and 8 weeks. Some investigators still conduct longer experiments. It would be reasonable to examine whether comparable treatment results are obtained with different cariogenic periods. In general short-term (2-3 week) and slightly longer (8week) experiments seem to have produced comparable results in the testing of various dietary ingredients. A detailed examination of the question, however, has not been made.

Information on the behavior of different types of lesion would assist in choosing an optimal experimental period. Some results were gleaned from several experiments previously conducted in this laboratory. Littermate Long-Evans rats had been fed cariogenic diet 2056[5] for 1,2 and 3 weeks after weaning. Caries on the buccolingual surfaces of lower left first and second molar teeth was scored by the method of Keyes[25]. Afterwards the lower half-mandibles were serially sectioned, stained, and fissure caries was scored according to König et al[26]. Mean results from 72 litters appear in Fig. 1. By one week nearly maximal numbers of fissure lesions occured (T-lesions). Thereafter the severity of fissure caries increased as evidenced by a higher incidence of moderate (B-) and cavitating (C-) lesions. By contrast the extent of buccolingual caries (SS) did not change significantly over the same period of time, and mean SS scores declined.

The behaviour of caries at single sites was studied further. The original motive behind this research was the need to develop a caries scoring system applicable to single sites on single teeth which would facilitate a direct comparison of plaque and caries at the same locations.

Intact lower jaws from 21 rats fed cariogenic diet 2056 for 3,6,9,13, 17 and 24 days were stained with Schiff's reagent. First and second lower molar teeth on one side were ground buccolingually using a small abrasive wheel mounted in a dental handpiece. Microscopic examination during the entire grinding process permitted recording of 3 parameters in each of five fissures. Parameters chosen were the maximum length of amelodentinal junction that was carious, the maximum penetration of caries into dentine and the maximum area of carious dentine viewed in a saggital plane. Recording of these three parameters onto special score cards permitted their quantitation. The degree of correlation of each parameter with the length of time on cariogenic diet, and with each other, appears in Table 1. The length of carious amelodentinal junction in each of the

Table 1. Correlation coefficients in the regression of length of carious amelodentinal junction, penetration into dentine, and area of carious dentine with time and with each other.

Regression with time	Length	Penetration	Area
Fissure			
Mesial M1+	0.70*	0.78	0.80
Central M1	0.67	0.83	0.83
Distal M1	0.59	0.82	0.80
Central M2	0.74	0.86	0.87
Distal M2	0.74	0.79	0.77
Regression of length with penetration		0.64	
Regression of length with area		0.69	
Regression of penetration with area		0.93	

+M1 = lower first molar, M2 = lower second molar
*All values of are positive and highly significant (0.001)

fissures examined approached a maximum after 13-17 days whereas caries penetration and the area of carious dentine increased continuously. This experiment has certain drawbacks: (1) lesions at different times were in different littermate rats, an example of the simulated longitudinal experiment discussed earlier, (2) the evidence that Schiff's reagent selectively stains caries is indirect, (3) drawing the lesions onto score cards is subjective. Further work, utilizing improved methodology, would be desirable to follow the progress of lesions over a longer period of time.

One interesting implication arises from the results in Table 1. The Keyes system of evaluating rat caries essentially estimates its linear extent. In the original description of the method various grades of caries severity were defined. Latterly, many investigators using the method report only the linear extent of carious enamel. At discrete sites it appears that the linear extent of caries may soon approach a maximum, and thereafter the lesion penetrates into dentine. The omission of severity grade scores accordingly may decrease the sensitivity of the method.

The apparently different behaviour with respect to time of bucco-lingual and fissure caries raises questions about the relatedness of these types of lesions in individual rats fed diet 2056 for 15 days. The frequency of animals with high and low buccal caries extent and high and low incidence of fissure microcavities appears in Table 2. Fisher's test of exact significance was applied to the data arranged as a two-way contingency table. In both strains of rat the probability of the observed data occuring by chance was less than 0.5%. Thus under the experimental circumstances selected, the extent of buccal caries and the severity of fissure caries were related.

Conclusions

The discussion of preweaning regimes draws attention to the importance of this period upon subsequent caries experience. Unfortunately control of many details during this period is denied to investigators who purchase their animals as weanlings. Added impetus is thus given to defin-

Table 2. Frequency of rats exhibiting high or low levels of buccal and fissure caries. All animals were fed diet 2056 for 15 days after weaning.

Buccal caries (Keyes units)	High[a]	High	Low	Low
Fissure microcavities (c-lesions)	High[b]	Low	High	Low
Sprague-Dawley rats	12	0	7	8
Long-Evans rats	20	14	5	19

[a]Buccal caries High 10+ units on first and second lower molars
Low 4- units on first and second lower molars
[b]Fissure caries High 6+ C-lesions in first and second lower molars
Low 2- C- lesions in first and second lower molars

ing the effects upon caries of preweaning variables so that investigators in different laboratories may more readily understand and standardize the animal caries model. Most human teeth are exposed to cariogenic diet continuously during eruption. In short term rodent experiments there is a need to reconcile the opposing demands of emulating the human situation and standardizing the cariogenic period. The role that early introduction of a cariogenic diet plays in determining the ecology of plaque also requires elucidation.

Implications arise from a study of various types of lesions. Firstly there is an obvious need to compare the Keyes and the König et al. scoring systems. Penetration of caries into dentine was the most easily measured parameter that increased continuously over the experimental period studied. This parameter also has considerable biological and clinical significance. It would be of interest to ascertain what relationships exist between the penetration of caries, the degree of demineralization of the tooth tissues, and the severity grade in various caries scoring methods. The anomalous behaviour of buccolingual caries has been studied further and is the subject of a separate communication. Some degree of relatedness of sulcal and smooth surface caries argues for a common aetiology.

LITERATURE CITED

1. Harris, R.S. (ed.). 1968. Art and Science of Dental Caries Research, Academic Press, New York.

2. Marthaler, T.M. 1965. Helv. odont. Acta 9 Suppl. 2:1-71.

3. Mitchell, D.F. and Johnson, M.J. 1956. J. dent. Res. 35:651-655

4. Park, K.C. and Katz, S.J. 1974. J. dent. Res. 53:1346-1350.

5. Huxley, H.G. 1976. Proceedings 'Microbial Aspects of Dental Caries', pp. 773-784. Special Supplement Microbiology Abstracts, Information Retrieval Inc., Washington, D.C.

6. Retief, D.H., Navia, J.M. and Lopez, H. 1977. Archs. oral Biol. 22:207-213.

7. Charlton, G., Fitzgerald, R.J. and Keyes, P.H. 1971. Archs. oral Biol. 16:649-654.

8. Onose, H. and Sandham, H.J. 1976. Archs. oral Biol. 21:291-296.

9. König, K.G., Savdir, S., Marthaler, T.M., Schmid, R. and Mühlemann, H.R. 1964. Helv. odont. Acta. 8:82-96.

10. König, K.G., Schmid, P. and Schmid, R. 1968. Archs oral Biol. 13:13-26.

11. Bowen, W.H. 1967. Path. Bact. 94:55-61.

12. Critchley, P. and Bowen, W.H. 1969. Dental Plaque (ed. McHugh, W.D.), pp. 157-169, E. and S. Livingstone, Edinburgh.

13. Bowen, W.H., Eastoe, J.E. and Cock, D.J. 1966. Archs. oral Biol. 11:833-837.

14. Chung, C.S., Larson, R.H. and Goss, B.J. 1968. J. dent. Res. 47:139-141.

15. Navia, J.M., DiOrio, L.P., Menaker, L. and Miller, S. 1970. J. dent. Res. 49:1091-1098.

16. Menaker, L. and Navia, J.M. 1973. J. dent. Res. 52:680-687.

17. Menaker, L. and Navia, J.M. 1973. J. dent. Res. 52:688-691.

18. Goldberg, M., Lormee, P. and Santa Maria, A. 1976. J. Biol. Buccale 4:123-141.

19. Redman, R.S. and Sweney, L.R. 1976. J. Nutr. 106:615-626.

20. Huxley, H.G. 1971. Archs. oral Biol. 16:1311-1328.

21. Huxley, H.G. 1973. Archs. oral Biol. 18:1543-1547.

22. Navia, J.M. and Lopez, H.J. 1977. J. dent. Res. 56:222-227.

23. Larson, R.H. and Fitzgerald, R.J. 1964. Archs. oral Biol. 9:705-712.

24. Schuster, G.S., Dirksen, T.R. and Morse, P.K. 1977. J. dent. Res. Special Issue B:abstract 337.

25. Keyes, P.H. 1958. J. dent. Res. 37:1088-1099.

26. König, K.G., Marthaler, T.M. and Mühlemann, H.R. 1958. Dt. Zahn- Mund - Kieferheilk.

Discussion of caries research using experimental animals

William W. Briner

Proctor & Gamble Company, 6110 Center Hill Road, Cincinnati, Ohio 45224

Dr. Huxley, in his excellent paper, pointed out the importance of pre-weanling factors on subsequent caries and followed the course of bucco-lingual and fissure caries across time.

Studies on fissure caries in our laboratories generally agree with those of Huxley, and I would like to discuss further the nature and progression of fissure lesions in rats.

Of primary importance is the fact that the susceptibility of the rat tooth to caries is governed, at least in part, by its state of mineralization when challenged by a cariogenic diet in the presence of cariogenic microorganisms. One of the main factors governing the progress of caries in rats is the fact that rat teeth are not completely mineralized when they erupt into the mouth, indeed, they do contain hypomineralized areas. To elaborate on the nature of these hypomineralized areas and their relevance to caries let us first consider the sequence of mineralization of rat molars.

The sequence of mineralization in human enamel has been described by Crabb and Darling[1], and Irving[2] has suggested that the sequence is similar in rats. First, the enamel matrix is deposited; the sequence starts at the cusp tip. Shortly thereafter, a wave of mineralization starts in this matrix and proceeds in an apical direction. These processes continue until the tooth erupts and thereafter if mineralization is not complete. In our laboratories we[3] demonstrated that the sequence in rat molars is similar, except that the tips of the cusps are not capped with enamel as they are in the human molars, and human enamel is thicker. Also areas of hypomineralized enamel (HMA) are common. These are gradually filled in by mature enamel in the sequence described, but in rat molars this is usually not completed in all molars at the time of eruption and continues after the teeth erupt.

We have studied mineralization of rat molars as a function of time. In one experiment animals 22 to 23 days of age were fed a commercial ration (Purina Lab Chow, Ralston-Purina Co., St. Louis, Mo.) and killed at specific time intervals. After death, the molars were stained with silver nitrate and hemisectioned, and the severity of the stained HMA was estimated by the method of Francis[3]. Severity was graded on a four-point scale; zero was no stain and a grade of three was damage (stain) extending into the dentin. No attempt was made to assess the degree of dentinal involvement. In this experiment a decrease in the HMA score indicates mineralization (post-eruptive maturation). The plot, in Figure 1, determined by the method of least squares, shows that the logarithm of the HMA decreased linearly; that is, mineralization increased rapidly at first and then gradually leveled off near completion. There were still HMA's remaining

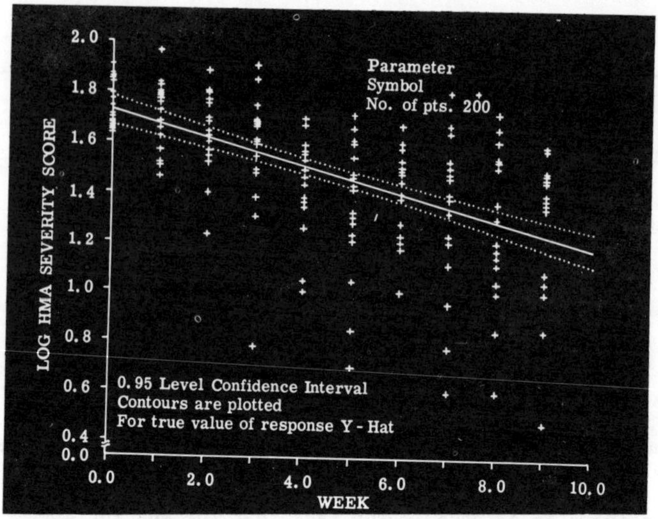

Figure 1. Rate of post eruptive maturation of rat molars. Rats were fed a commercial ration and killed at weekly intervals for nine weeks.

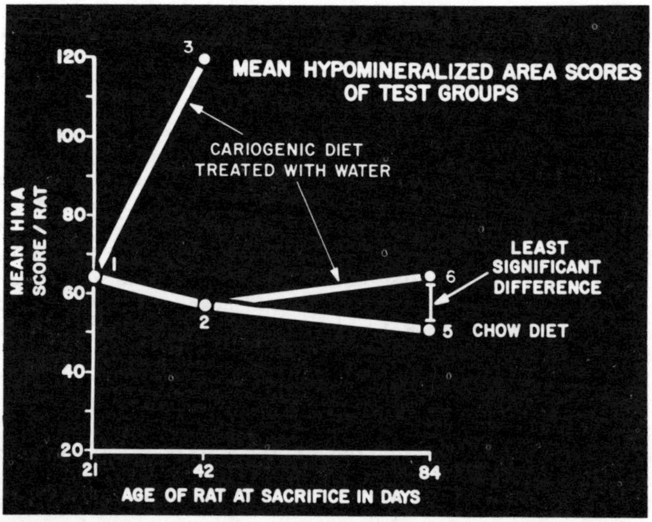

Figure 2. Effect of challenging littermate rats with a cariogenic diet at 21 and 42 days of age.

even after eight weeks.

The relationship between the degree of mineralization and the susceptibility of the teeth to caries demonstrated by challenging littermate rats at 21 and 42 days of age with a cariogenic diet[3]. Figure 2 gives the caries scores of the first molars. It is quite apparent that the older rats whose teeth were more mineralized got less caries than their littermates challenged at an early age. Note that if the HMA scorings at 42 and 84 days had been omitted, one might easily come to the conclusion that the rats challenged at this time did not develop caries.

As confirmation of this finding we investigated the rate of cariogenesis in weanling rats by following the increase in incidence and severity of HMA. Over an eight-day experimental period groups of rats, weaned at 19-20 days were sacrificed at two day intervals for eight days. HMA incidence increased at a rate of about 1 unit per day but HMA severity increased by about 6.5 units per day.

Thus, in young rats the main attack of caries is through extension of preexisting hypomineralized areas rather than the generation of new lesions. It follows that the state of mineralization of the rat molar at the time of challenge, plays a significant role in caries progression. In rat caries experiments, especially ones in which staining methods are used to grade caries, it is necessary to define the state of mineralization of molars at the time of challenge so that the progression of caries is unquestionably documented.

And as a postscript, I certainly do agree with Dr. Huxley in that we need more knowledge about the relationships between "penetration of caries, the degree of demineralization of tooth tissues and the severity grade in various scoring methods."

REFERENCES

1. Crabb, H.S.M., and Darling, A.I. 1962. The Pattern of Progressive Mineralization in Human Dental Ename, Internat Series Mongraphs Oral Biol, Vol 2, New York: Pergamon Press.

2. Irving, J.T. 1973. The Pattern of Sudanophilia in Developing Rat Molar Enamel, Arch Oral Biol 18:137-140.

3. Francis, M.D. 1966. The Effectiveness of Anticaries Agents in Rats Using an Incipient Carious Lesion Method, Arch Oral Biol 11:141-148.

Discussion of caries research using experimental animals

Rachel H. Larson

9310 Fernwood Avenue, Bethesda, Maryland 20034

Dr. Huxley has brought together much valuable information concerning the animal model for the study of caries. It is my purpose to supplement his presentation by a discussion of the importance of providing a consistent and adequate cariogenic challenge in the test animals. By cariogenic challenge we mean the microbial attack on the teeth produced by the interaction between the diet and the oral flora. If sufficiently intensive this challenge will cause carious lesions to develop on the teeth.

Figure 1 is a simple chart in which we show how the level of caries development is determined by the balance between the two forces, cariogenic challenge and animal susceptibility. Animal susceptibility includes not only tooth susceptibility per se, but also any characteristics of the animal which may modify the cariogenic challenge, such as variations in eating habits or salivary flow. Let us look at a few theoretical situations. When high levels of both challenge and susceptibility are present, caries levels will be high, and when both are low, caries will be low or non-existent. However, moderate levels of caries may be obtained by a variety of combinations: low challenge on teeth of high susceptibility, high challenge on teeth of low susceptibility or moderate levels of both.

Some years ago in our laboratory we were able to provide conditions under which the Hunt-Hoppert and Harvard "caries-resistant" strains of rats developed high levels of caries[1,2]. In early studies using the two strains, investigators fed a diet that was incompatible with the development of smooth surface caries, and depended entirely upon the indigenous flora to provide the caries active organisms. Under these conditions the cariogenic challenge was extremely low and caries development was limited to a few small sulcal lesions. In our work the same animals were provided with a combination of diet and oral flora which produced a high cariogenic challenge, and high levels of caries developed on all surfaces of the teeth. These results demonstrate that an adequate challenge must be provided before an animal can be accurately classified as caries-resistant.

Let us look at some of the steps involved in establishing an adequate microbial challenge in the rat. Some workers find that the indigenous flora of the animals fits the needs of their experiments. However, an animal's microflora is constantly changing. Even in barrier-maintained colonies there are changes in the flora with time, most likely due to chance infection. Some breeding colonies are infected with caries-active organisms, some are not. Breeding conditions are rarely, if ever, designed to support a caries-active flora. Such a microflora, if found, is usually the result of chance infection, and may be unevenly distributed. That is, the flora may vary between litters or breeding rooms at a given time as well as at different times. An equally serious, but a different problem also exists.

FIGURE 1.

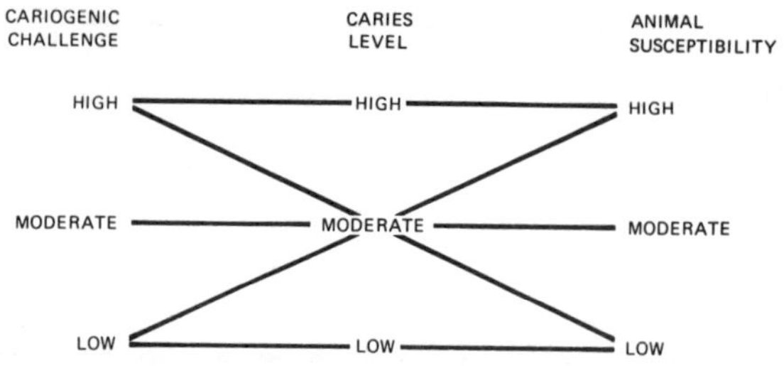

Some breeding colonies have a non-cariogenic flora so well established that implantation of a caries active flora cannot be achieved by usual means.

Rather than accept the uneven quality of animals from commercial sources, some investigators are breeding their own animals. This places an increased burden on staff and space, and is not a foolproof solution. Husbandry is only as good as its weakest link. One of the real needs is an adequate supply of animals suitable for caries research. These"standard" animals would have a good genetic background, tempermentally and physically suitable for caries studies. The breeding diet would be consistent over the years, and nutritionally adquate. The pups would be maintained under specific pathogen-free conditions so that their bacterial flora would consist of only a few non- pathogenic and non-cariogenic types of organisms that would not be incompatible with the implantation of caries active organisms when and if desired.

The original method used to infect test animals[3] with a caries-active flora was by coprophagy that occurs if the yound animals are exposed to older caries-active animals or their feces. A "donor" colony can be maintained for this purpose. Even though it is usually associated with an increased level of caries, fecal infection has the disadvantages of being non-specific and constantly subject to change.

A more consistent procedure for establishing a cariogenic flora to use pure cultures of one or more caries-active organisms, of which S. mutans has been used most widely. This method is also subject to variations. Different S. mutans strains vary in their activity and that of a given isolate may change in vitro. The ideal arrangement would be to provide the animals with a mixed infection of known composition which would produce a "standard" broad range cariogenic challenge, in the "standard" rat. As the caries process is more completely understood, it should be possible to provide a more nearly standard cariogenic challenge in the rodent.

With the wide variates in animals, and infection which have been used in the past, it is not surprising that results of different investigators vary widely and are sometimes in conflict. In a recent co-operative study Larson and co-workers[4] in 6 laboratories, used animals bacterial inoculum, and supplies from the same sources and followed the same detailed protocol. When the teeth were examined by the same person, it was found that the caries levels covered a relatively narrow range and the results of no one investigator were significantly different (P 0.01) from those of all others.

These results support our belief that an attempt should be made to establish a maximinimally "standard" animal model for caries studies, which could be used by all interested investigators. Such a model would use the animals and inoculum which were closest to the ideals previously described, the animals would be fed a standard diet and complete protocol including the method of scoring followed. Even although many studies would require models somewhat different from the "standard", it still would serve as a "bench mark" against which the results of investigations using other models could be measured. The use of such standardized procedures should greatly enhance the animal model as a scientific tool for the study of variables that modify caries development, and could be evaluated for purposes of caries prediction.

LITERATURE CITED

1. Larson, R.H., Keyes, P.H. and Goss, B.J. 1968. Development of caries in the Hunt-Hoppert caries-susceptible and caries-resistant rats under different experimental condition. J. Dent. Res. 47:704-709.

2. Larson, R.H. 1965. Response of Harvard caries-susceptible and caries-resistant rats to a severe cariogenic challenge. J. Dent. Res. 44:1402-1406.

3. Keyes, P.H. 1960. The infectious and transmissible nature of experimental dental caries: Findings and implications. Archs. oral Biol. 1:304-320.

4. Larson, R.H., Amsbaugh, S.M., Navia, J.M., Rosen, S., Schuster, G.S., and Shaw, J.H. Collaborative evaluation of a rat caries model in six laboratories. J. Dent. Res. In press.

Short Papers on Caries Models

The enamel microhardness test

Theodore Koulourides, D.M.D., M.S.

Institute of Dental Research, University of Alabama, Birmingham, Alabama 35294

The microhardness technique has been used since 1908 to measure softening and rehardening of enamel[1,2,3]. This technique entails pressing a diamond or steel indenter, with a preselected weight, against the enamel surface until the indenter is blocked because of the incompressibility of the minerals of the sound enamel. The partial demineralization caused by a carious attack increases the porosity of the subsurface enamel so that the surface has less support and can be penetrated by the indenter to that point at which it encounters the underlying sound enamel. Thus, a change in micro-hardness provides a quantitative approximation of demineralization. More extensive micro-hardness changes in enamel can also be studied by micro-radiography of thin sections. These two complementary techniques are in essential agreement in defining the severity of demineralization. In measuring a "caries" attack, the initial and final micro-hardness test provides an approximation of the thickness of the demineralized layer of enamel, because the resistance of the affected layer to the indenter penetration is considerably less than that of sound enamel. In caries research the micro-hardness test is used to measure the result of mild demineralization and remineralization activities of various fluids as long as the demineralization conditions preserve the integrity of the original test surface, as indicated by the appearance of initial indentations. Compared to the measurements of plaque pH, the micro-hardness measurement represents the magnitude of the integrated acid activity, while pH measures the momentary fluctuations of the plaque acid.

Advantages

1. Sensitivity: The test is applicable only if the dissolution conditions are mild enough so that the original surface is preserved. Such conditions are encountered in natural caries, in *in vitro* systems with acid gels, and in partially saturated acid buffers. The test will detect change in indenter penetration in the range between 0.1 to 20 µm. Beyond that level the test becomes inaccurate either because of collapse of the surface, or because of the difficulty in measuring extremely large indentations under the microscope.

2. Convenience in Experimentation: Because the test is applied directly on the enamel, the investigator can study the effects exerted by various fluid environments on the mineral density conditions under study reflect the magnitude of either the cariogenic challenge or the remineralization activity of synthetic and biological fluids. Because the surface required for each test is small, control and test areas can be evaluated on the same 3 x 5 mm slab.

3. Repeated Evaluation : By assuming that the entire surface is equally affected by the equilibrating fluid, it is possible to perform several series of tests on a single surface. We were able to perform as many as five series of tests on one slab that was subjected successively to three different fluids, such as the fluid of cariogenic plaque, saliva used for remineralizing enamel, and the acid buffer used for testing the enamel resistance after remineralization reactions.

Limitations:

1. Test Planes: Enamel micro-hardness (for accuracy) requires flat surfaces, thus, the accurate testing of the natural tooth surface is very difficult. This limitation has been remedied in our lab by using a micro-radiographic technique for which the test specimen has to be destroyed. In spite of being more elaborate, the micro-radiography test is less sensitive. The lowest range of lesion detection being a "caries" depth of 3-5 μm. The two techniques can be combined to give numerical and pictorial data.

2. Accurate Standardization: In the Intraoral Cariogenicity Test (ICT) the test surface covered with dacron gauze has to be placed exactly flush with the acrylic frame of the prosthetic carrying device. Avoidance of excessive friction between the experimental plaque and the oral soft tissues is critical, since extrusion will diminish the subsequent micro-hardness reading and intrusion will increase it.

3. Subject Selection: Participating subjects must be reliable because their failure to follow instructions will introduce artifacts. In caries studies performed in our laboratory, the micro-hardness test has been used to determine three basic factors: (a) the rate of intraoral cariogenic attack or in vitro attack in acid buffers or acid gels, (b) the rate of remineralization of pre-softened enamel as reflected by the mineralizing activity of synthetic fluids or saliva, and (c) the resistance of the remineralized enamel to a subsequent experimental cariogenic challenge or acid attack. The procedures have been described in several publications [3-8].

In experimental caries studies with the ICT bovine enamel slabs inlaid in prosthetic or orthodontic devices are covered with dacron gauze to enhance microbial retention on the test surface. These assemblies are exposed to pure substrates or foodstuffs under controlled extraoral conditions. In some experiments the subjects were requested to consume a specified diet. An important feature of the ICT for caries studies is the exposure to saliva in the mouth. Two variables are standardized, plaque accumulation using a dacron gauze cover of specified thickness and the resistance of the test enamel by grinding off the outer surface layers of the enamel slabs and polishing them into a flat plane. Control of the effects of patients' oral hygiene practices is achieved by removal of the ICT-carrying appliance during toothbrushing. Control of the effect of cariogenic substrates eaten by test subjects is largely controlled by extraoral exposure of the appliance to sugar solutions. This superimposes the effect of a controlled experimental substrate to that of uncontrolled diet which, as Table I shows, causes some demineralization. Over the past 10 years ICT experiments were carried out repeatedly on 35 subjects. Some typical findings are given in Table I.

Findings Related to Caries Prediction: As a rule, the severity of ICT cariogenesis is predictable for all subjects over a period of weeks, with some subjects being much more active in ICT cariogenesis than others. However a few subjects showed a pronounced shift over periods of months.

1. Among our subjects, only a 27 year old male was caries immune. He had no signs of caries and no fillings. His ICT was negative for the six

Table I.

ICT FINDINGS (7 days, 4 subjects, 4 tests each)
CHANGES IN ENAMEL HARDNESS (penetration)* AFTER
EXPOSURE (10 mts, 4 x daily) TO 3% SUCROSE OR WATER.

Subj.	Expt.	TREATMENT Sucrose	H_2O
		μ	μ
J.R.	1	4.69 (L)	9.52 (R)
	2	5.04 (R)	3.05 (L)
	3	3.78 (L)	0.88 (R)
	4	2.19 (R)	3.00 (L)
	Avg. ± S.E.	3.92 ± 0.64	1.86 ± 0.67
B.F.	1	1.48 (L)	0.53 (R)
	2	1.51 (R)	0.58 (L)
	3	1.59 (L)	0.95 (R)
	4	1.64 (R)	0.42 (L)
	Avg. ± S.E.	1.55 ± 0.04	0.62 ± 0.11
L.P.	1	-0.03 (L)	0.23 (R)
	2	1.30 (R)	-0.03 (L)
	3	0.19 (L)	0.43 (R)
	4	1.43 (R)	0.16 (L)
	Avg. ± S.E.	0.72 ± 0.37	0.20 ± 0.09
C.W.	1	0.05 (L)	0.01 (R)
	2	0.04 (R)	0.16 (L)
	3	0.88 (L)	0.36 (R)
	4	0.05 (R)	0.00 (L)
	Avg. ± S.E.	0.25 ± 0.21	0.13 ± 0.08
TOTAL Avg. ± S.E.		1.61 ± 0.40	0.70 ± 0.24

* Based on before and after measurements of 3 indentations.

months that he participated in our experiments. With extraoral sucrose supplements, he exhibited extremely low ICT cariogenicity. In microbiological studies, we were unable to isolate S. mutans or lactobacillus from the ICT gauze or from his interproximal samplings. We interpreted these results as indicative that he was truly caries immune since his diet and oral hygiene were average.

2. One of our highly cariogenic subjects (with full-upper and a partial-lower denture) was diagnosed as diabetic. During a hospitalization, while she was on a strict low-carbohydrate diet, her ICT caries approached zero.

3. One subject developed pronounced ICT caries during the stress of her mother's terminal illness. Shortly after the mother's demise the subject returned to an ICT non-cariogenic status. The patient maintained that her oral hygiene and dietary habits were unchanged during the period of stress.

4. Frequent exposure of the test enamel to 3% or 10% sucrose solutions increased ICT caries in all subjects. Exposure to 3% sucrose for 10 minutes, 4 times daily, doubled the baseline caries attack. The effect of 10% sucrose was more pronounced, but was not statistically different. Addition of 1 ppm fluoride to the sucrose solution eliminated its effect and increased the acid resistance of sample enamel. Among the various substrates tested, xylitol was outstandingly non-cariogenic.

5. When exposed directly to saliva, surfaces without the dacron-gauze microbial shelter did not develop ICT caries.

6. A combination of fluoride applications and ICT challenge increased the resistance of enamel to future challenge more than when either of them was used alone.

7. Treatment of the ICT plaque with chlorohexedine twice daily eliminated the experimental cariogenesis.

The above observations indicate positive responses of the ICT test to (1) the caries free (immune) status, (2) sucrose and xylitol supplementation, (3) the presence of fluoride in the sucrose supplements or in topical applications, (4) diet regulation, (5) stress, and (6) antibacterial treatment. With the exception of the stress effect, which may be controversial, all observations were predictable according to our knowledge of caries etiology.

Since the test enamel surfaces can be considered standard, the individual's ICT cariogenicity varies in relation to some unknown factor, perhaps their diet or the composition and/or flow rate of their saliva. This serves to emphasize the principal advantage of this test, namely that it is carried out in the presence of natural saliva and includes this factor in the caries findings. This saliva factor assumes great importance when caries is viewed as the result of alternating demineralization-remineralization activities rather than as a simple demineralization effect. Although the microhardness technique as applied in the ICT is a convenient method for a study of specific etiological factors of caries in the human mouth, it is not practical to use it for large scale epidemiological studies of caries prediction.

Experiments with the ICT have strengthened the belief that during the caries attack there is an inter-action between mineral dissolution and enamel remineralizing activities. If we consider the first as the environmental stress, and the second as the tooth defense, incipient caries exhibits features of enamel adaptation to stress, involving mainly mineral turnover. This dissolves the easily soluble mineral components from the enamel and deposits from the surrounding fluid its most insoluble ionic components. The inter-action can be described as a two-phase cycle consisting of alternating phases of demineralization and the remineralization. Each cycle can change the resistance of enamel to stress. In optimal conditions of mild stress (in terms of duration and frequency of challenge), and appropriate composition of the parent fluid (especially the presence of fluoride) remineralization would increase the resistance of demineralized enamel to a level that would withstand the caries challenge that initiated the initial demineralization. However, under different circumstances the same challenge could produce open cavities. Thus, caries prediction is an elusive interplay of two factors, the cariogenicity of the individual and the unknown local resistance at the high risk areas.

The ICT has been used to study individual factors as they affect the magnitude of either the cariogenic challenge or the resistance of experimental enamel. It is believed that the findings in ICT studies will lead to a better understanding of the natural carious process and that resultant deductions could be made useful for caries prediction.

LITERATURE CITED

1. Head, J. 1912. A study of saliva and its action on tooth enamel in reference to its hardening and softening. J.A.M.A. 59:2118-2122.

2. Caldwell, R.C., Gilmore, R.W., Timberlake, P., and Pigman, J. 1958. Semi-quantitative studies of in vitro caries by micro-hardness tests. J.D.R. 37:301-305.

3. Feagin, F., Koulourides, T., and Pigman, W. 1969. The characterization of enamel surface demineralization, remineralization, and associated hardness changes in human and bovine material. Archs. oral Biol. 14:1407-1417.

4. Koulourides, T., Phantumvanit, P., Munksgaard, E.C., and Housch, T. 1974. An intraoral model used for studies of fluoride incorporation in enamel. J. Oral Path. 3:185-195.

5. Koulourides, T., Bodden, R., Keller, S., Manson-Hing, L., Lastra, J., and Housch, T. 1976. Cariogenicity of nine sugars tested with an intraoral device in man. Caries Res. 10:427-441.

6. Manson-Hing, L.R., Keller, S.E., Feagin, F.F., and Koulourides, T. 1972. Microradiographic comparison of artificial caries systems. J.D.R. 51:929-933.

7. Manson-Hing, L., Keller, S., Bodden, R., and Koulourides, T. 1973. Effect of sucrose with 1 ppm fluoride on experimental cariogenicity in humans. IADR Abst. #579.

8. Keller, S., Manson-Hing, L., Lilley, V., and Koulourides, T. 1975. Enhancement of fluoride effectiveness by cariogenic priming of human enamel. IADR Abst. #L308.

Caries-like lesions using acid gels

Leon M. Silverstone

Division of Cariology, College of Dentistry, University of Iowa, Iowa City, Iowa 52242

Although organic acids are generally accepted as the principal destructive agents in caries, enamel exposed to such acids *in vitro* shows changes which differ histologically from the structural changes seen in enamel caries (Silverstone, 1966). For example, the dark zone at the advancing front of the lesion and the relatively unaffected surface zone are not produced using dilute lactic acid alone. Therefore, although the initiation of caries must be associated with the presence of acid, or acids, in the immediate environment of the tooth caries it is unlikely to be a simple process of demineralization. The presence of plaque must modify, in some way, the acid attack in order to produce the characteristic changes in enamel seen in early caries.

Using a technique employing viscous gelatin gels acidified with one of a number of organic acids, it has been possible to simulate caries histology accurately *in vitro* (Silverstone, 1966, 1967). When the gels were employed at a gelatin concentration of 10-20%, lesions created in enamel with one of a number of organic acids appeared indistinguishable from natural caries when examined by polarized light and microradiography(Silverstone, 1967). Under these conditions, not only were all of the classic zones of the small carious lesion produced *in vitro*, but the advancing fronts of such lesions followed irregular courses in the enamel. The most critical single factor in determining rate of attack on the enamel was the concentration of the gelatin - there being an inverse relationship between concentration and rate. Transport of ions both to and from the enamel interface may be restricted by the physical bulk of the gel, its concentration of calcium ions and also, perhaps, by the charge of the macromolecule. In this way the acidified gel may be regarded as a simple *in vitro* model of the plaque/enamel interface.

Thus, since acid alone produces lesions devoid of either a surface zone or dark zone, the two zones created in gelatin enamel caries as a result of remineralization (Silverstone, 1973), indicates that the acid-gel technique provides an environment ideal for remineralization phenomena to occur. This production of enamel, lesions *in vitro* which are indistinguishable from enamel caries demonstrates the significance of remineralization in formation of the small carious lesion and provides a further example of the dynamic processes involved in lesion formation.

Surface Zone Phenomenon in Enamel Caries

One of the important characteristics of caries of human dental enamel is that the greatest degree of demineralization occurs at a subsurface level. Thus, the small enamel lesion remains covered by a surface layer which appears relatively unaffected by the attack. When a small carious lesion in enamel is examined with the polarizing microscope after imbibition with a medium having a refractive index remote from that of the enamel, water for example (n = 1.33), the porous subsurface enamel is seen to be positively birefringent whereas the surface zone retains its negative birefrigence. Thus, even though the subsurface region of the lesion has been demineralized to a stage exhibiting a pore volume of 25% or more, the surface zone remains relatively unaffected having a pore volume of between 1 and 5% (Silverstone, 1968). This relatively unaffected surface zone is also identifiable on microradiographs where it is seen as a radiopaque zone, approximately 30 μm in depth, sharply demarcated from the radiolucent subsurface region of the lesion.

To date, many workers have suggested that the formation of a relatively unaffected surface layer overlying the small lesion of enamel caries was closely associated with the special properties of surface enamel. Chemical studies by a number of workers have shown that if the original enamel surface was removed, then the remaining enamel was more susceptible to acid demineralization. The greater resistance of the surface enamel to carious dissolution has been explained as being due, in part at least, to its higher degree of mineralization compared with subsurface enamel (Thewlis, 1940; Brudevold, 1948; Hals et al., 1955). This, together with a higher fluoride and lead content (Isaac et al., 1958) and perhaps a greater amount of insoluble protein in the surface enamel (Darling, 1958) may account for it being less soluble than subsurface tissue as shown by acid-etching studies (Sullivan, 1954).

Several workers have removed part of the natural enamel surface prior to in vitro experiments with artificial caries systems in order to see if a surface zone would form superficial to the lesion on the new enamel surface. Sperber and Buonocore (1963) showed by microradiography that when a tooth was abraded prior to their studies with various acid buffers, a lesion could be produced that still had a greater mineral content at the surface than at its subsurface region. Gray and Francis (1963) also showed that a relatively well mineralized layer could be produced superficial to a demineralized region on abraded enamel. The studies of Von der Fehr (1967) showed that a well-mineralized surface layer could be created on abraded enamel, overlying heavily demineralized regions, in vivo as well as in vitro. All of the above lesions were examined by microradiography showing a radiopaque surface layer superficial to a more radiolucent subsurface region. Using an acidified gel technique, Silverstone (1968) produced lesions on artificially abraded enamel surfaces which had up to 500 μm of surface enamel cut away prior to experiment. The lesions created on these surfaces still showed well mineralized surface layers. When examined in water with polarized light, a negatively birefringent surface zone was observed overlying the more heavily demineralized subsurface region.

Therefore, these results suggest that the 'special' physical and chemical properties of surface enamel, relative to subsurface enamel, are not entirely responsible for the presence of a well-mineralized surface zone above the small carious lesion. The probability is that the surface zone remains intact and well mineralized because it is a site where calcium and phosphate ions, released by subsurface dissolution, or from the saturated solution in plaque, become reprecipitated into the surface enamel. The high fluoride concentration of surface enamel, presumably released at the initiation of solution of outer enamel, would also favour precipitation. The special properties of surface enamel relative to subsurface enamel would be responsible for maintaining the surface zone from demineralization for longer periods.

These experiments therefore support further the concept that the formation of the carious lesion is due to a dynamic series of events rather than one of simple demineralization. It would appear therefore that the surface zone of enamel caries is thus a manifestation, in part at least, of remineralization.

To date, only lesions produced in vitro with the acidified gel technique demonstrate surface zones indistinguishable from the surface zone in enamel caries. That is the surface zone appears negatively birefringent when the section is examined in water with the polarizing microscope. Thus, the surface layer has a pore volume of less than five per cent. In many cases the surface zone still exhibits negative birefringence when the section is examined dry in air. In such lesions, the surface zone has less than one per cent pore volume in spite of the subsurface region being demineralized to a stage exhibiting a pore volume of twenty-five per cent and more. The presence of a radiopaque surface layer on microradiographs can not be used to give a quantitative estimation of the degree of breakdown of the surface versus subsurface region. Thus, if the surface layer had a pore volume of thirty per cent, and the subsurface region forty per cent, this would still manifest as a radiopaque surface layer on a microradiograph. Thus, the most important criterion for a surface zone being indistinguishable from that in caries is that it must exhibit negative birefringence in polarized light after imbibition with water.

The Dark Zone of Enamel Caries

The dark zone at the advancing front of the lesion has been regarded as a breakdown stage successional to the translucent zone and preceding the body of the lesion. It has always been difficult to explain why in the first zone of enamel caries, the translucent zone, relatively large pores are found whereas in the succeeding stage of breakdown, the dark zone, a micropore system is found in addition to the large pores. Darling et al. (1961) explained the micropores in the dark zone as being the result of demineralization or the 'opening' up of specific sites in the tissue which were not attacked in the first zone of breakdown. However, in experiments in which carious lesions were exposed to synthetic calcifying fluids in vitro, (Silverstone, 1967b; Silverstone and Poole, 1968; Silverstone, 1977) an area previously identified as the body of the lesion had, after experiment, taken on the histological characteristics of the preceding stage, the dark zone. That is, the dark zone has increased significantly in width, spreading from its original site at the advancing front of the lesion back towards the enamel surface. If some of the relatively large pores of the body of the lesion could, in effect, become the minute ones of the dark zone, then this could indicate that the micropore system of the dark zone may not be formed by a simple process of demineralization. Thus, the zone may not be a stage in the sequential breakdown of the tissue as was previously thought. The micropores may be formed by 'remineralization' whereby either the size or the accessibility of the large pores is reduced by the deposition of material. The results from in vitro studies suggest that mineral deposition could account for the 'closing down' of the original pores created as a result of demineralization, such as are found in the translucent zone, although in vivo organic material might also contribute. If this is the case, then this lends further support to the concept that the carious process in enamel is a dynamic one with phases of demineralization, rather than a more simple process of continuing disolution. In this way, the variation in distribution and width of the dark zone over the advancing front of the enamel lesion may be explained as functions of the efficacy of the 'remineralization' process. Only the acidified gel technique has so far created lesions in enamel in vitro which show dark zones as a regular feature of their advancing fronts.

LITERATURE CITED

Brudevold, F. 1948. A study of the phosphate solubility of the human enamel surface. J. dent. Res. 27:320-329.

Darling, A.I., Mortimer, K.V., Poole, D.F.G., and Ollis, W.D. 1961. Molecular sieve behaviou of normal and carious human dental enamel. Archs oral Biol. 5:251-273.

Gray, J.A. and Francis, M.D. 1967. Physical chemistry of enamel dissolution; in Sognnaes Mechanisms of hard tissue destruction. 213-260. Am. Ass. Advancement of Science (Publication No. 78), Washington.

Hals, E., Morch, T., and Sand, H.F. 1955. Effect of lactate buffers on dental enamel in vitro observed in polarizing microscope. Acta odont. scand. 13:85-122.

Isaac, S. Brudevold, F., Smith, F.A., and Gardener, D.E. 1958. Solubility rate and natural fluoride content of surface and subsurface enamel. J. dent. Res. 37:354-363.

Silverstone, L.M. 1966. The primary translucent zone of enamel caries and of artificial caries-like lesions. Br. dent. J. 120:461-471.

Silverstone, L.M. 1967. Observations on the dark zone in early enamel caries and in artificial caries-like lesions. Caries Res. 1:261-274.

Silverstone, L.M. 1967. The histopathology of enamel lesions produced in vitro and their relation with enamel caries. Ph.D. thesis Bristol.

Silverstone, L.M. 1968. The surface zone in caries and in caries-like lesions produced in vitro. Br. dent. J. 125:145-157.

Silverstone, L.M. and Poole, D.F.G. 1968. Modification of the histological appearance of enamel caries after exposure to saliva and a calcifying fluid. Caries Res. 2:87-96.

Silverstone, L.M. 1973. The structure of carious enamel, including the early lesion; Oral sciences reviews, No. 4: (Munksgaard, Copenhagen) Dental enamel, pp. 100-160.

Silverstone, L.M. 1977. Remineralization phenomena. Cariostatic Mechanisms of Fluoride. (Ed. W.E. Brown and K.G. König), Caries Res. 11 (Suppl. 1) 59-84, S. Karger, Munchen.

Sperber, G.H. and Buonocore, M.G. 1963. Enamel surface in white-spot formation. J. dent. Res. 42:724-731.

Sullivan, H.R. 1954. The formation of early carious lesions in dental enamel. J. dent. Res. 33:231-244.

Thewlis, J. 1940. The structure of teeth as shown by X-ray examination. HMSO Spec. Rep., Series 238.

Von der Fehr, F.R. 1967. A study of carious lesions produced in vitro in upbraded, exposed and F-treated human enamel surfaces with emphasis on the X-ray dense outer layer. Archs oral Biol. 12:797-814.

The orofax

Basil G. Bibby

Eastman Dental Center, 800 Main Street East, Rochester, New York 14605

Several procedures will produce caries-like lesions *in vitro*, and are useful for providing information on the caries resistance of teeth or for comparing the effects of chemical agents on the demineralization of enamel. Unfortunately their ability to record differences between the caries susceptibility or resistance of individual subjects is at this time quite limited. We have devised a method which we believe has potential usefulness of that sort, and which can be used to detect and quantitate some of the factors that have bearing on the caries attack in individual subjects. These are the caries modifying factors in an individuals saliva or that of the foods that he is eating. It is an improved form of what other investigators have called an 'Artificial Mouth' to which, for simplicity and identification, we have given the name 'Orofax'.

Most procedures for producing *in vitro* caries have used bacterial culture media which, of course lacks some of the physical chemical properties of saliva and supports different and non-oral types of bacteria. Previous methods that have used human saliva have done so only in a preliminary way and none seems to have made an effort to provide a flow of saliva of the sort that occurs over teeth in the mouth; nor do they seem to have taken steps to prevent the changes in the physical properties of saliva that occur when it is stored.

Much basic study has been done in the preservation of perishable foods, human tissues, tissue fluids and microorganisms.

No corresponding studies have been made of saliva but the information from tests on somewhat similar fluids suggested that rapid freezing to -78°C would be desirable and that storage at that temperature and rapid thawing was likely to preserve the greatest numbers of salivary microorganisms and prevent precipitation of the mucin. Figure 1 shows that that method gave good results in bacterial preservation. When thawed it also gave a clear unclotted fluid that did not clog small apertures as other stored saliva tends to do.

The way in which we now use saliva is to collect it by paraffin stimulation expectorating directly into a long storage tube packed in dry ice in a well insulated container. So that the bacterial content of the saliva will not be too much depleted by continuous secretion, collections are made at least two hours after a meal in amounts of about 50 ml at each session. The storage tubes with their frozen saliva are later transferred to the Orofax apparatus (Figure 2) where they serve as saliva reservoirs.

The Orofax apparatus consists of a cold chamber to keep the saliva frozen until it comes in contact with the thermostat controlled thawing element onto which the frozen saliva tube descends as saliva melting proceeds.

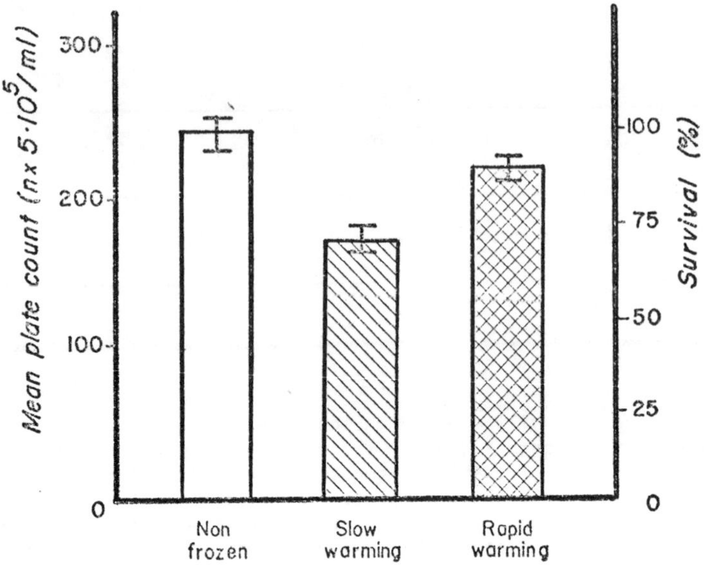

Figure 1 Effect of Thawing Procedure on Survival of Salivary Bacteria Cooled Rapidly to -78°C

The thawed saliva flows down a surrounding collecting tube, during which time it is warmed, to be delivered drop by drop onto the underlying test specimens. To distribute the saliva in appropriate amounts over a number of tooth samples, each drop of saliva as it falls breaks a photoelectric beam to activate an electric circuit which rotates a Carousel slide projector that carries the attached specimen tray to the next position. We have found that one drop of saliva for each specimen each 10 minutes is satisfactory for plaque formation and 'caries' production.

To study plaque formation blocks of enamel mounted in wax are first exposed to a heavy inoculation with plaque material suspended in whole saliva and then to a flow of saliva. Forty-eight hours gives a very definite plaque that thickens somewhat up to ninety-six hours. These have the appeearance and physical properties of the plaque developing on human teeth and ferment sucrose to depress their pH to as low as pH4.

To study caries, carbohydrate is held in contact with the enamel under a flow of saliva. This is done either on enamel blocks, on which carbohydrate is held in a small open ended tube, or on enamel laminates consisting of enamel sections mounted between plastic coverslips. In this latter method the enamel edges are held in contact with a gauze partition on which the test carbohydrate is placed and onto which the saliva drops fall. The enamel sections in their laminates can be removed and examined under polarized light to determine the extent of demineralization that has occured since the previous examination. Thus a quantitative comparison of the caries producing effects of foods can be obtained or a comparison made of different salivas using the same carbohydrate substrate.

In areas somewhat related to the purpose of this conference the Orofax has been used, to date, to study plaque formation in several salivas and also to compare the 'caries' production by about 20 foods. Selected findings on the cariogenicity of some foods, given in Table 1, show a gen-

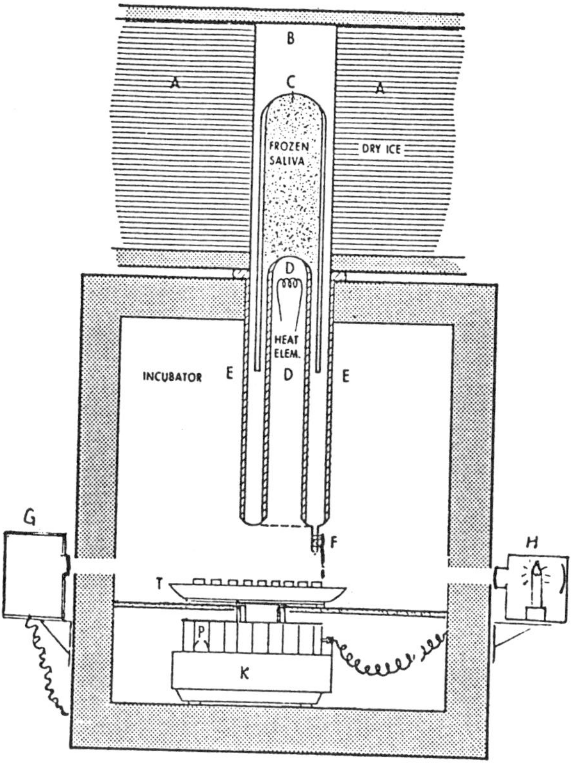

Figure 2

The Orofax Apparatus

A. - Low Temperature Chamber. B. - Cold Core of Chamber. C. - Resevoir tube of frozen saliva. D. - Heating element for thawing saliva. E. - Jacket to collect thawed saliva. F. - Outlet for saliva and light screen. G. - Photo-Electric Relay System, Exciter Lamp Unit. H. - Photo-Electric Relay System Receiver. J. - Thermostat. K. - Kodak Carousel Slide Projector. P. - Plastic stops in slide compartment to stop Carousel rotation. T. - Specimen bearing Rotary tray of Carousel elevated on plastic collar passing through floor of incubator chamber.

eral parallelism to the caries produced in rats in tests in the König-Hofer automatic feeding apparatus. Other results were not as satisfactory.

We feel that some further experience or perhaps some refinements of techniques may be needed to reduce the technical demands of the Orofax procedure. More correlations with animal caries or in vivo test in human subjects are needed before Orofax findings can be considered reliable caries predictors.

Table 1 'Caries' Rankings in Orofax and Rat Caries

	Orofax	Rat Caries
Diet MIT 200	1.0	1.0
Milk Chocolate	0.22	0.41
Dark Chocolate	0.44	0.82
Graham Crackers	0.84	0.80
Potato Chips	0.89	0.86
Fudgies	1.33	1.22
Caramels	1.51	1.19

LITERATURE CITED

1. Yaari, A. 1973. Experimental caries system using thawed saliva. Thesis, University of Rochester.

2. Yaari, A., Bibby, B.G. 1976. Production of plaques and initiation of caries *in vitro*. J. Dent. Res. 55:30.

Plaque-pH-telemetry

H.R. Mühlemann and Th. Imfeld

Dental Research Institute, Zurich, Switzerland

Biotelemetry in general enables direct and continuous measurements of biological phenomena without disturbing the process to be evaluated. Measured data may be conveyed to the recording equipment by wireless transmission (radio-telemetry) or by means of direct connection (wire-telemetry).

In 1965 and 1966 Graf and Muhlemann (4,5) first announced radio-telemetry of plaque-pH from the interdental area. Miniaturized glass electrodes, and for a short period also antimony electrodes, (6) were used to measure H^+ion activity with potential freedom from experimental artifacts in otherwise fairly inaccessible places of the oral cavity. Since 1965 valuable experiences and innumerable data have been accumulated. Reviews were published in 1969 (3), 1971 (8) and 1977 (7). All these studies have shown the reliability and reproducibility, the quality and accuracy of the pH-telemetric system for the investigation of human plaque-pH behaviour.

Thus telemetry has become an important tool for assessing pH-changes both of dental plaque and oral fluid in response to any kind of food or drug.

The construction and use of telemetric partial prostheses has been described in detail in 1977 (7). A diagram of the electronic circuitry is given in figure 1. As shown in figure 2 the electrodes with their tips embedded in perforated tooth crowns are set to reach the artificial interdental spaces created by the perforated tooth crowns in the prostheses and the volunteer's abutment teeth.

The test prostheses with clean pH-electrodes are inserted and the subjects are asked not to alter their eating habits. With the single exception of water rinses they are to refrain from all oral hygiene measures. The prostheses are not removed during the test period of 3 to 7 days thus allowing an undisturbed growth of plaque over the tips of the electrodes. pH-changes resulting from acids formed in interdental plaque when exposed to fermentable carbohydrates can be recorded with good reproducibility and analysed statistically when experimenting with 3- to 7-day-old bacterial deposits. pH-changes of mixed saliva by dietary acids, e.g. citric acids added to candies, can also be measured with the same pH-sensor if clean and not covered by plaque.

Some prostheses are equipped with two pH-electrodes. Using a prosthesis with an interdentally orientated electrode which is plaque-covered and a plaque-free lingually orientated pH-sensor submerged in mixed saliva, it is possible to record simultaneously:

- acid formed by plaque coating the interdental sensor
- acid formed by the total oral microflora (dental plaques and micro-organisms on the dorsum of the tongue, etc.) which lowers the salivary

Figure 1.

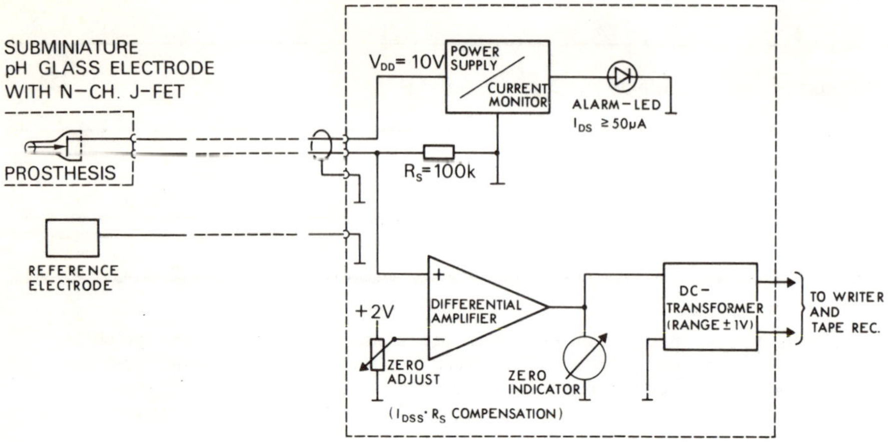

Figure 1. Schematic diagram of pH-wire telemetry electronic circuitry with FET-inpedance converter.

pH at the site of the lingual sensor, and
- dietary acid contacting the clean electrode directly during ingestion.

Another method for the assessment of the glycolytic activity of dental plaque was described by Frostell in 1970 (2). It is mainly used in Great Britain (9). The pH of plaque samples collected from the teeth before and after the ingestion of carbohydrates is measured in vitro.

A reevaluation of these classical in vitro plaque pH-studies in the light of plaque pH-telemetry reveals that the latter is yielding far more detailed information on pH-changes in plaque with regard to the acidogenicity of foods.

Plaque pH is influenced by several factors that are assessed to differing degrees by the two methods. The most significant ones are presented in Table I.

A final assessment of the acidogenicity and potential cariogenicity of marketed foods, drugs and sugar substitutes (7) should preferentially be performed under in vivo conditions with plaque pH telemetry. In vitro measurements are only indicators of substrate fermentability.

pH-telemetry today is utilized on a statistical base similar to pH-measurements on collected plaque [10]. Plaque pH telemetry can only be performed on adults and not on children. Apparently this is only a theoretical disadvantage because it has never been shown that plaques collected in adults and in children behave differently when exposed to fermentable carbohydrates.

LITERATURE CITED

1. Brunner, K., Gabathuler, H., Schneider, Ph. 1974. Multi-channel oral wire telemetry. Helv. odont. Acta. 18:83.

2. Frostell, G. 1970. A method for evaluation of acid potentialities of foods. Acta Odont. Scand. 28:599.

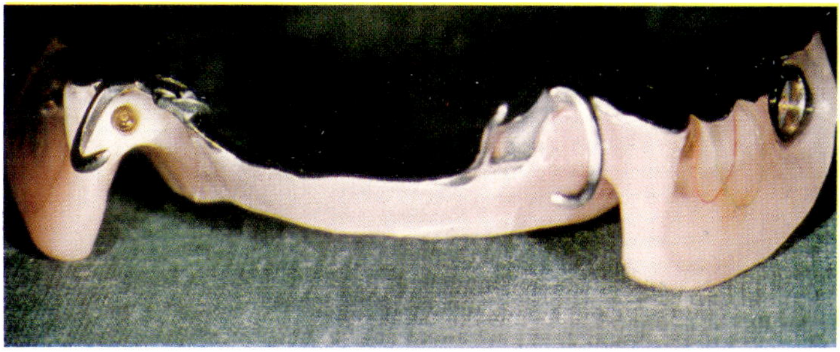

Figure 2. Prosthesis with interdental pH-sensor.

Table 1 Comparison of plaque pH telemetry and pH-measurements of collected plaque.

Influencing Factor	pH-telemetry	Collected plaque
- Permeation of plaque by carbohydrates	Adequately assersed	Permeability characteristics destroyed by sampling procedure
- Buffer activity of plaque environment	All dynamic changes adequately assessed	Not assessed
- Dietary carbohydrates containing protein and fat	Effects on pH adequately assessed	Possible contamination of collected plaque and non-physiological interference with pH
- Dietary acids permeating the plaque	Discrimination between dietary and glycolytic acids possible	No discrimination between dietary and glycolytic acids
- Oral clearance time of dietary carbohydrates	Continuous clearance curve possible	Not possible

3. Graf, H. 1969. Telemetrie des pH der Interdentoplaque. Med. Habil., Zürich.

4. Graf, H., Mühlemann, H.R. 1965. Glass electrode telemetry of pH changes of interdental human plaque. J. dent. Res. (Abstract) 44:1039.

5. Graf, H., Mühlemann, H.R. 1966. Telemetry of plaque pH from interdental area. Helv. odont. Acta. 10:94.

6. Hassel, Th. M. 1971. Construction of micro-antimony electrodes for use in radio telemetry of plaque pH. Helv. odont. Acta. 15:50.

7. Imfeld, Th. 1977. Evaluation of the cariogenicity of confectionary by intra-oral wire-telemetry. Helv. odont. Acta. 21:1 in Schweiz. Mschr. Zahnheilk. 87:437.

8. Mühlemann, H.R. 1971. Intra-oral radio telemetry. Int. dent. J. 21:456.

9. Rugg-Gunn, A.J., Edgar, W.M. Geddes, D.A. and Jenkins, G.N. 1975.

The effect of different meal patterns upon plaque pH in human subjects. Brit. dent. J. 139:351.

10. Imfeld, Th., Hirsch, R.S., Mühlemann, H.R. 1978. Telemetric recordings of interdental plaque pH during different meal patterns. Brit. Dent. J. in press.

In vivo experimental human caries

W.M. Edgar

Markham Laboratories, University of Newcastle on Tyne, Newcastle, England

The Experimental Human Caries technique introduced by von der Fehr, Loe and Theilade in 1970 is a method of studying, quickly and cheaply, the initiation of caries-like changes in the enamel surface *in vivo*. It has therefore been employed to test a variety of known or potential anticaries agents and procedures. In addition, however, it can also be extended to basic studies of the interactions between host, diet and plaque in an attempt to identify the circumstances under which caries initiation occurs.

The Experimental Caries Index

The experimental model depends upon the visual "Caries Index" (Table1) described by von der Fehr (1961). This is a subjective index of changes in the optical properties of enamel and most of the appearances are not seen by the naked eye, and unless the enamel is dried very thoroughly before viewing. Scoring of teeth *in vivo* is normally carried out with a stereo-microscope at X15 or X16 magnification and with optimum lighting conditions.

Table 1.

Caries Index (Fehr, 1961)

0	Surface appears intact
1	Limited greyish tinge, with or without accentuated perikymata
2	Perikymata well accentuated, in some areas confluencing into greyish-white spots
3	Pronounced white decalcification

Intermediate scores 0.5, 1.5 or 2.5 given to lesions that do not fit one of the above stages.

The grades of the Caries Index (C.I.) were shown to be linearly related to the porosity of the underlying enamel and to the depth of the lesion (Fehr, 1966). This relationship is, of course, crucial to the validity of interpretation of changes in C.I. as reflecting de- or remineralization between the C.I. and other tests for initial caries formation, such as hardness testing and birefringence measurements (discussed by Dr. Koulourides and Dr. Silverstone in this Conference) requires further study.

The higher grades (2.5, 3.0) of the index probably relate to the clinical picture of a "white spot" lesion and thus, to conventional criteria for caries diagnosis, but lower grades whose descriptive criteria refer to special conditions of dryness, lighting and magnification, are not seen in normal clinical examination. However, with thorough drying and adequate lighting, the unaided eye is capable of detecting changes in the appearance of enamel at a level which can be related to the lower grades of the C.I. (Edgar, Jenkins, and Rugg-Gunn, unpublished). Table 2A gives a description of a new Index based on naked-eye observations under these conditions, and in Table 2B, the frequency distribution of scores for the sound enamel surfaces awarded by the C.I. using X15 magnification and by the new "Naked-eye Index", shows a high degree of correlation between the two indices.

Table 2.

"Naked-eye" Index and Correlation with Cl

A. "Naked-Eye" Index (Edgar *et al*, unpublished)

0	Normal enamel
1	Slight pearly-grey opacity
2	'Speckled' grey-yellow area
3	Diffuse white area
4	Well-defined white spot, shiny surface
5	Chalky white spot, loss of surface sheen

B. Bivariate frequency distribution of C.I. and "Naked Eye" Index scores

		"Naked Eye" Index				
		0	1	2	3	4 + 5
	0	12	1	1		
	0.5	21	4	6		1
Caries	1.0	8	6	12	1	
	1.5	2	5	11	1	
Index	2.0	1		5	4	1
	2.5			1	3	7
	3.0		1	1	1	11

Spearmand rho (r_s) = 0.74; $p < 0.001$

The ordinal nature of the C.I. scores raises doubts as to the alidity of employing standard statistical tests depending upon normally istributed continuous data. In practice, the values of C.I. are usually veraged over the whole mouth and these mean C.I. data may not depart excesively from the conditions required for parametric tests. However, due aution in testing is required to avoid invalid conclusions, and often the spects of the results being tested may require the use of non-parametric tatistics.

he "Experimental Human Caries" method

The application of the C.I. to the rapid production of reversible aries-like changes *in vivo* is analogous to similar work in the field of eriodontal disease. In the original work of von der Fehr (1970), volunteer ubjects refrained from oral hygiene for 23 days; during this time they onsumed their normal diet, but half of them increased the frequency of xposure of their plaques to fermentable carbohydrates by rinsing with a 0% sucrose solution 9 times each day. In these latter subjects (Sucrose roup) the mean C.I. in the buccal/labial enamel of the anterior and preolar teeth rose during the 'no oral hygiene' period, while in the controls ho did not rinse with sucrose, the mean C.I. was virtually unchanged.

After this 'no oral hygiene' period the subjects resumed their normlly high standard of oral hygiene, and rinsed their mouths daily with a olution of 0.2 per cent NaF. This treatment reversed the changes in C.I. that the mean C.I. values approached those recorded pre-experimentally. his reversal of the induced C.I. increment is essential for the ethical cceptability of the method, and has been confirmed in all studies of this ind.

This first report (Fehr *et al*, 1970) as well as describing the method, lso highlighted the role of plaque, and of the frequency of exposure to ermentable carbohydrate, in the induction of caries-like changes in these ormally caries-resistant sites. Subsequent studies indicated that when the evelopment or activity of plaque was suppressed by chlorhexidine or toothrushing (Loe, von der Fehr and Schiott, 1972), or by augmented activity of e lactoperoxidase-thiocyanate system of saliva (Hugoson *et al*, 1974) the ncrease in C.I. was largely prevented even when the subjects rinsed 9X per y with sucrose solution.

Levine (1975) used the method to study, not the induction, but the gression of caries-like lesions. Fifteen subjects underwent an induction ase without oral hygiene and with sucrose rinsing, and after 21 days the .I. increment was recorded. On resuming oral hygiene, 8 of them rinsed rice daily with an experimental remineralizing fluid. This group showed a re rapid fall in C.I. during the following 8 weeks than did a control oup who rinsed with a 0.5 per cent NaF solution in widespread use in caries evention.

Preliminary studies in our laboratory (Jenkins, Geddes, and Cooke, 73; Geddes, Edgar, and Jenkins, 1975) confirmed the earlier results (Fehr *al*, 1970) showing a rise in C.I. during the 'no oral hygiene' period, but re in conflict in showing no difference between the control subjects nsuming a normal diet and the sucrose rinsing group. This result was later investigated using further developments in technique including the reducon of the 'no oral hygiene' period to 14 days (Edgar and Jenkins, 1977). e latter study confirming the results of the original report (Fehr *et al*, 70), but emphasising that under the conditions of the experiment, individls' susceptibility varied.

The use of the method to test the effectiveness of a potential antiries agent (calcium glycerophosphate) was described by Geddes *et al* (1975).

The results of this trial showed that glycerophosphate (at 1% in the sucrose rinse) did not prevent the rise in C.I. during the 'no oral hygiene' period. Following this negative result, the effectiveness of a proven cariostatic procedure (topical application with 2% NaF solution) was assessed (Edgar et al, 1975). While the results were encouraging in showing a tendency for topically applied Na F to reduce the rise in C.I. during the 'no oral hygiene' period, thus, validating the method as a model for tests of caries, the trend was not statistically significant.

Photographic recording of C.I.

Because of the difficulty in avoiding the possibility of bias in the assessment of C.I. when the observer is aware of the stage of the experiment during the microscopic examinations the advantage of scoring C.I. from photographic records (used without success by Fehr et al, 1970) led us to develop a method for photographing the C.I. appearances in black-and-white and colour slides (Edgar, Jenkins and Rugg-Gunn, 1976). With adequate standardisation of lighting and exposure, colour photography proved to give satisfactory records from which C.I. data could be scored, all data being recorded at the end of the experiment with the photographs randomised to avoid bias.

The bivariate frequency distribution of the scores awarded using the direct (microscopic) method and from photographs, for each tooth surface in a baseline examination of 9 subjects (Edgar, Jenkins and Rugg-Gunn, unpublished) are shown in Table 3. The association between the two scores is highly significant by Spearmans test ($r_s = 0.81$; p 0.001) indicating that the photographic appearance is closely related to the index criteria described for the direct method.

Table 3.

Bivariate frequency distribution of scores from direct (microscopic) and photographic recording of C.I.

		Photographic Recording						
		0	0.5	1.0	1.5	2.0	2.5	3.0
	0	3	8	1				
	0.5	2	22	1	1			
Direct	1.0	2	9	8	4			
	1.5		5	7	5	2		
Recording	2.0		1		6	2		1
	2.5				2	3	2	1
	3.0				1	3	4	6

Table 4. Repeatability of C.I. Scoring by Direct and Photographic Method. (3 subjects scored in triplicate)

A. Direct	Mean C.I. Score	B. Photographic Mean C.I. Score
Exam. 1	1.20	0.99
2	1.12	0.99
3	1.15	1.00
Analysis of Variance between examinations	F = 0.316 p 0.25	p 0.99
	Reliability co-efficient 0.945	0.997

The repeatability of scoring by one examiner using the two methods (Table 4A and 4B) showed that the mean score for triplicate examinations of 72 tooth sites in three subjects did not differ significantly, and the reliability co-efficient (Winer, 1962) was in excess of 0.94 indicating that random error in scoring by either method was of negligible importance.

The Experimental Caries Method in Studies of Caries Susceptibility

In a parallel study of the C.I. changes in enamel during the 'cariogenic' (no oral hygiene and sucrose) period in relation to the concomitant development of plaque on the same enamel surfaces (Edgar, Rugg-Gunn and Jenkins, 1977) the increase in C.I. was found to be related to the apparent thickness of the overlying plaque. Some plaque-covered areas of enamel did not, however, show a rise in C.I., pointing to the variability between subjects and between different tooth sites in the same subjects, in the conditions necessary for the induction of caries. Identification of these conditions by detailed examination of the enamel and plaque awaits further study, but some indication of between-subject variation in the susceptibility to changes in C.I. is given by the finding that in the group not rinsing with sucrose, in some subjects a rise in C.I. occurred during the 'no oral hygiene' period, presumably because of the fermentable carbohydrate present in their diet (Jenkins et al, 1973; Edgar and Jenkins, 1977), an observation which is confirmed by the data of von der Fehr et al (1970). The increased susceptibility of one such subject could be related to the acidogenicity of the plaque, associated with a low salivary flow rate, while other parameters (quantity and chemical composition of the plaque; amount and frequency of dietary carbohydrate) were not related in this subject.

Ethical Considerations

The possible hazards to the dentitions of subjects participating in experiments of this type have been recognised by all workers. It is essential that the induced lesions and concomitant gingival disease should be fully reversible on resuming good oral hygiene procedure together with fluoride mouthrinsing, a point also discussed by Horowitz (1976). In our work, we have observed the following rules:

1. All subjects are informed volunteers. Only dental students, who are able to comprehend fully the possible hazards of the experiment, have been used as subjects. So that no element of coercion might influence their decision to volunteer, subjects have been drawn from year-groups no longer taught or examined by the experimenters, and have been unpaid.

2. A thorough dental examination is carried out before the volunteers are accepted into the trial, and any whose caries rate or gingival index is

high is excluded, as are subjects with soft tissue conditions including opercula over erupting 3rd molars. Any necessary dental treatment is carried out, and the subject is given instruction in oral hygiene so that his gingival index before the experiment approaches the optimum.

3. After the experiment, subjects are followed up for 3 years. The C.I. is rescored, and clinical and radiographic caries diagnosis carried out.

In no case has any subject who has participated in such an experiment required the filling of more than 2 newly attacked surfaces during the 3 year follow-up period, and no gingival condition has been created which did not resolve within 48-72 hours of resuming oral hygiene, nor has any evidence been found of a permanent increase in C.I. in the areas of enamel where lesions developed during the trial.

In view of the daily fluoride mouthrinsings carried out by our subjects, and the insight they receive into the relationships between plaque, caries and periodontal disease, we believe that they may well be in a better state of dental health after participating in the experiment than they were before.

The Value of the Method in Caries Prediction

In examining data for those subjects who have been assessed by one examiner and have participated in 14 day experimental caries trials, no relationship between initial mean C.I. score and subjects DMF score has been found. This is perhaps surprising, but may be explained by the incorporation in the C.I. data of lesions present initially which are not the result of caries - for example, it may be difficult to exclude developmental anomalies and the white marks of idiopathic or fluoride mottling. An additional explanation may be that any pre-carious lesions which occur would be likely to have progressed to cavity formation in these young adults; thus, in a high-caries subject the lesions would have been filled and the enamel surfaces in which they occurred excluded from the assessment of C.I.

However, the rise in C.I. during the experimental period in sucrose rinsing subjects has also been found in our laboratory to show no relationship with their DMF although Loe et al (1972) state without giving details that such a relationship exists. The explanation of this is less clear, but many possibilities exist. The multifactorial nature of caries makes it unlikely that the same conditions of cariogenicity persist for the number of years between the occurrence of the first cavity and the subject's participation in the experiment. Furthermore, crude DMF data do not distinguish between caries in different sites, and pit and fissure lesions may develop in conditions which for morphological and other reasons are not found on adjacent smooth surfaces. We do not have sufficient data on the relationship between the rise in C.I. and the free smooth surface DMF scores to judge whether or not a significant association occurs.

This lack of association with caries experience data makes the use of C.I. assessments in prediction of caries for clinical purposes questionable, although the results presented by Dr. Klock yesterday might suggest that C.I. scores might be valid predictors of caries incidence. The imposition of a cariogenic regime in such a context is clearly unacceptable. The main value of the techniques of C.I. scoring and the induction of lesions in volumteer subjects will remain the testing of potential anti-caries agents or procedures at a level intermediate between the laboratory and the clinical trial; and equally usefully in the exploration of the conditions necessary for the inter-action of plaque, enamel and diet to lead to the predictable development of lesions which may be interpreted as the initial stages of caries.

LITERATURE CITED

1. Edgar, W.M., Geddes, D.A.M., Howell, R.A., Jenkins, G.N. and Rugg-Gunn, A.J. 1975. Experimental caries in man. II The effect of topically applied NaF solution. Proceedings IADR Abst. #S76.

2. Edgar, W.M., Jenkins, G.N. and Rugg-Gunn, A.J. 1976. Experimental caries in man. Comparison of visual and photographic recording. J. Dent. Res. 55:Special Issue B, B84.

3. Edgar, W.M., Rugg-Gunn, A.J. and Jenkins, G.N. 1977. Correlation between the distribution of caries-like changes in enamel, plaque distribution and enamel surface morphology. Caries Res. 11:115-116.

4. Edgar, W.M. and Jenkins, G.N. 1977. Variations between subjects in experimental human caries trials. Preprinted Abstracts, 24th Congress of ORCA, Megeve, Hungary. Abst. #74.

5. Edgar, W.M., Jenkins, G.N. and Rugg-Gunn, A.J. Unpublished observations.

6. Fehr, F.R. von der. 1961. The effect of fluorides on the caries resistance of enamel. Acta odont. Scand. 19:431-442.

7. Fehr, F.R. von der. 1966. The caries inhibiting effect of acid-phosphate-fluoride tested by the gold plate technique. Adv. Fluor. Res. 4:121-135.

8. Fehr, F.R. von der, Loe, H. and Theilade, E. 1970. Experimental caries in man. Caries Res. 4:131-148.

9. Geddes, D.A.M., Edgar, W.M. and Jenkins, G.N. 1975. Further studies on experimental caries in man. Caries Res. 9:315.

10. Geddes, D.A.M., Edgar, W.M., Jenkins, G.N., Howell, R.A. and Rigg-Gunn, A.J. 1975. Experimental caries in man. I.Methods and calcium glycerophosphate trial. Proceedings IADR Abst. L54.

11. Horowitz, H.S. 1976. Ethical considerations of study participants in dental caries clinical trials. Community Dent. Oral Epidemiol. 4:43-50.

12. Hugoson, A., Koch, G., Thilander, H. and Hoogendoorn, H. 1974. Lacto-peroxidase in the prevention of plaque accumulation, gingivitis and dental caries. (III) Effect of mouthrinses with amylo-glucosidase and glucoseoxidase in the model system of experimental gingivitis and caries in man. Odont. Revy. 25:69-80.

13. Jenkins, G.N., Geddes, D.A.M. and Cooke, J.A. 1973. Reinvestigation of experimental caries in man. J. dent. Res. 52:967.

14. Levine, R.S. 1975. An initial clinical assessment of a mineralising mouthrinse. Brit. dent. J. 138:249-253.

15. Loe, H., Fehr, F.R. von der and Schiott, C. Rindum . 1972. Inhibition of experimental caries by plaque prevention. The effect of chlorhexidine mouthrinses. Scand. J. dent. Res. 80:1-9.

16. Winer, B.J. 1962. Statistical principles in experimental design. Section 4.5, p.124, McGraw-Hill, New York.

Short Papers on
New Techniques for Caries Detection

Detection of early carious conditions by ultrasound

Sidney Lees

Forsyth Dental Center, 140 The Fenway, Boston, Massachusetts 02115

Mineral loss from enamel may be the result of direct surface dissolution or etching, or that seen in the "white spot" precursor of caries in which there is more demineralization on the subsurface than surface layers. We recognize a third condition in which, in addition to mineral loss from both layers, there is a redisposition of amorphous material on the surface. Despite these distinctions there is subsurface depletion in all situations which is detectable by ultrasonics. Unlike microradiography the ultrasonic technique does not destroy the tooth specimen and will detect mineral loss from the moment it begins. To indicate its advantages and limitations, some basic concepts of the ultrasonic method will be described.

Ultrasonic waves are propagated through a medium by the elastic distortions induced in the medium and the velocity of propagation is determined by the longitudinal elastic modulus and the density:

$$c = \sqrt{\frac{K}{\rho}} = \text{longitudinal sonic velocity}$$

$$k = \text{longitudinal elastic modulus}, \rho = \text{density}$$

At an interface between two media there is a reflection if the acoustical impedances of the two media differ, where

$$z = \sqrt{K\rho} = c\rho = \text{acoustical impedance}$$

As seen in Figure 1, the tooth surface exposed to air or liquid exhibits a change in acoustical impedance, so an echo can be observed. The subsurface layer has density and elastic moduli different from the intact enamel, so there can be a second echo from this layer. But if the subsurface layer is thin compared to the sonic pulse length, the two echoes will overlap and only one somewhat distorted echo is observed. It is possible at least in theory to determine the properties of the subsurface layer from various kinds of information in addition to the modified sonic pulse. Several theoretical possibilities have been explored, but we have not yet had the opportunity to evaluate any of them.

In our experimental arrangement there are two ultrasonic transducers, one monitoring the tooth-liquid interface from the tooth side, and the other from the liquid side (Figure 2). The echo patterns are shown in Figure 3, one from each transducer. Each pattern shows two echoes, one used as a reference and the second from the tooth-liquid interface.

If the tooth surface is etched away, the echo pattern moves away from the transducer and the interval between the reference and tooth surface

Figure 1.

ULTRASONIC REFLECTION AT THE ENAMEL-LIQUID INTERFACE

LIQUID (Water) c = 1.5 mm/μsec, Z = 1.5 x 10^9 kg/sec-m^2

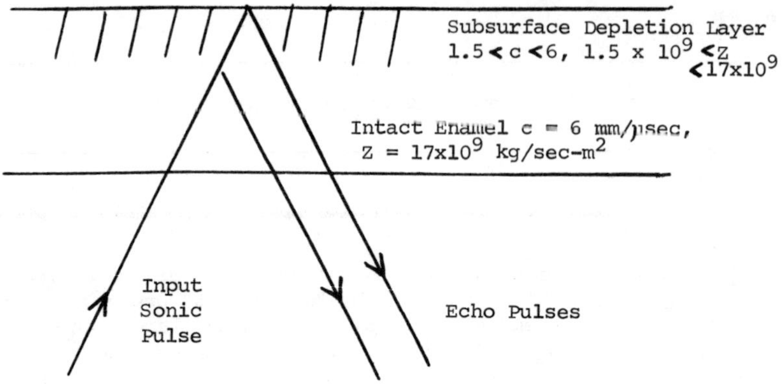

Figure 2.

TWO TRANSDUCER ARRANGEMENT AND TEST CELL

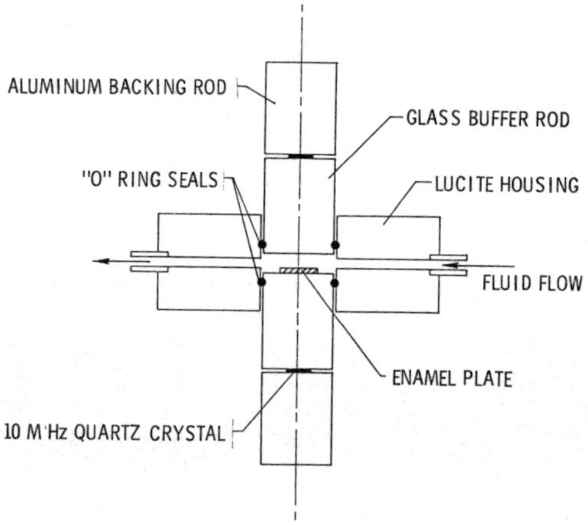

echoes increases. The contrary is true for the tooth side echo patterns. Careful instrumentation using sampled data digital techniques makes it possible to measure time differences with an uncertainty less than 10^{-3} of the total interval, or under certain operating conditions much less. In dynamic processes where a continuous change is underway and least square curve fitting can be applied it is possible to reduce the uncertainty to an equivalent of no more than 0.1 microns.

Figure 4 shows some results for surface etching with hydrochloric acid of different concentrations flowing over a prepared plate of bovine incisor enamel. It is to be noted that the data begins almost at zero time when the experiment started, that the range of displacement is in microns and the time scale in minutes. In other experiments at lower acid concentration (higher pH) the time scale extended to a few hours. There are two lines for each acid concentration, one from the tooth side (with squares),

Figure 3.

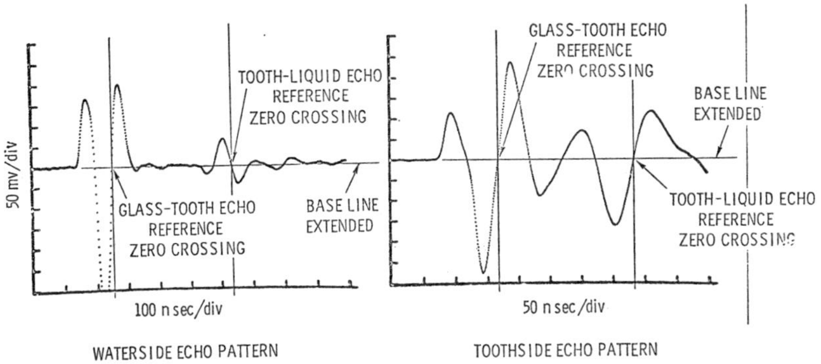

Figure 4.

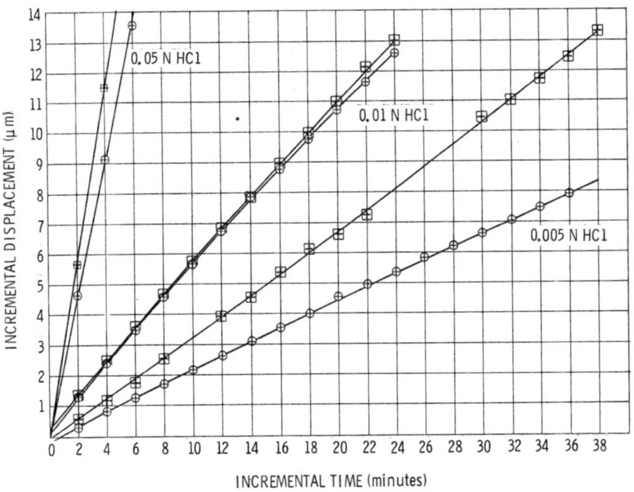

and the other from the liquid side (with circles). The slope of each line indicates the etch rate.

The divergence of the two lines is interpreted to mean that the liquid side echo comes from the top of the subsurface depletion layer, while the tooth side echo comes from the bottom of this layer. The divergence indicates that the layer increases in thickness as time progresses even while the outer surface is being depleted. By plotting the data a least squares straight line was found which gave an expression for the etch rate as a function of acid concentration:

$$E = 43\ N^{0.92}\ \text{microns/min.}$$

where E = etch rate, N = acid concentration in normality for a flow rate of 25 ml/min. at 27° C. The velocity over the tooth surface is estimated to be of the order of 0.25 mm.min.

Experiments on a subsurface lesion in which the depth of the demineralized zone was about 14 microns gave the ultrasonic records for both acid and tooth sides of the interface that are shown in Figure 5. The acid side record did not remain constant, but instead showed the growth of a deposit on the surface apparently up to 2.5 microns. The acid side echo is unambiguous since the sonic velocity of water is well known. The tooth side echo is not so readily interpretable so the decrease in the time of flight, the primary measurement, is shown instead of displacement. The magnitudes of the two displacements are significantly different. The acid side curve shows a rapid rise for the first 250 minutes after which the curve levels off. The tooth side curve descends steeply for the first 300 minutes, and then continues to descend more moderately. The surface displacement detected by the acid side transducer was interpreted to be due to a deposit or precipitate forming on the surface.

Scanning electron micrographs that were obtained of the tooth surface after the test was completed, showed a thin amorphous-like layer on the surface. When the depth of the demineralized zone was calculated from flight (2.27 nsec) and 0.5 sonic velocity in enamel (3 um/nsec) a figure of 6.8 microns is obtained. That this is far less than the observed zone thickness of 14 microns verifies our hypothesis that the displacement of the echo is due to changes in the acoustical properties of the layer rather than a true surface displacement. The echo appears to come from some level within the demineralized zone. The reduction of the theory to numerical results requires additional measured quantities, and yet to be developed, data reduction techniques.

The capability of ultrasonics to sense an attack on the tooth surface so quickly; to measure such small changes while the experiment is underway; to detect and measure layer thickness to a fraction of a micron and to be able to distinguish the type of attack from the onset makes it possible to carry out a wide variety of experiments. It is of special interest that the same sample can be subjected to a variety of conditions in succession. In all situations there is a change in the acoustical properties of the subsurface which can be correlated with observable changes in the physical properties of the layer together with the characteristics of the process inducing the change as determined by scanning electron microscopy, micro-

Figure 5.

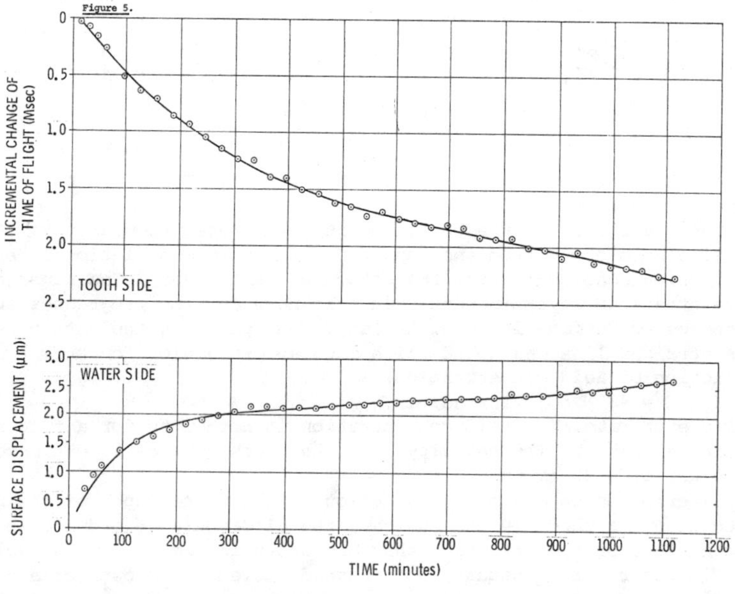

radiograph, or microchemical analysis. In other words the ultrasonic technique permits continuous monitoring of the enamel surface which, at the termination of the test, is not destroyed, and is still available for study by other methods.

This advantage can be used to relate changes of the tooth surface associated with bacteriologically induced or purely chemical processes, to observed changes in the ultrasonic echo patterns; to monitor dissolution and remineralization ultrasonic echo patterns while both processes are underway; to subject the tooth surface to a succession of conditions which alternate dissolution and remineralization, and to observe how the rates of the two opposing processes vary with induced changes in the tooth surface and the depth of penetration.

The high resolution capability of our ultrasonic technique requires great mechanical stability as well as stability in the performance of the ultrasonic system itself. This is provided by the mechanical, electrical and system design of the apparatus and, in large part, by its method of use. We employ differences between an internal reference and the test surface so that by keeping the tooth sample fixed with respect to the internal reference surface the sources of mechanical instability are minimized. These restrictions and the need of a controlled temperature environment to minimize variations of elasticity have, to date, required all experiments to be performed in a test cell or "artificial mouth". In this respect the ultrasonic technique is much like other high resolution instrumentation.

To reiterate, it can be claimed that in spite of some physical limitations the digital ultrasonic technique has several potential advantages. It makes it possible to study conditions that induce caries at the earliest possible stage and to monitor the process while it is underway. Perhaps the system's most powerful capability is its flexibility whereby the immediate effect of changing the environment can be observed. The sensitivity of the technique makes it possible to shorten the duration of experiments limited only by the chemical dynamics. The structure of the experimental arrangement permits other experimented procedures to be used simultaneously, thereby aiding in the interpretation results.

Fluorescent dye-uptake as an aid to early diagnosis of incipient carious lesions

H.R. Rawls, K.Q. Robert, E.L. Zimmerman, III, and W.D. Owen

Dental School, Louisiana State University, and Southern Regional Research Center, New Orleans, Louisiana 70119

At present, the commonly used *clinical* methods for detecting caries are inadequate for reliable diagnosis of lesions until demineralization is well underway (Downer and O'Mullane, 1975; Downer, 1975; Radike, 1968). By the time a reliable diagnosis can be made, the damage is often irreversible and restorative methods may be necessary to effectively prevent further progress of such lesions. Likewise, in epidemiological surveys and in clinical trials of possible new caries therapies, researchers have been limited to observing the disease, *in vivo*, only after it reaches the "white spot" stage of development. Because about two years are required for a lesion to reach the cavitation stage (Backer-Dirks, 1966), clinical trials are invariably long and costly.

Accurate diagnosis at a sufficiently early stage would allow clinical trials to be shortened and thus make possible the evaluation of new preventive treatments that otherwise might not be considered. Community dental health programs and epidemiological studies would also benefit. Early detection might well help the practicing dentist to more effectively employ topical fluoridation, and in the future, remineralization and sealant procedures. (Robinson et al, 1976; Buonocore, 1975)

We have attempted to develop a method to aid in the diagnosis of caries at the earliest stages. It has been tested *in vitro* and to a limited extent in monkeys with promising results. In this paper the technique is described and its potential uses in research and in clinical practice are indicated.

We have attempted to develop a method to aid in the diagnosis of caries at the earliest stages. It has been tested *in vitro* and to a limited extent in monkeys with promising results. In this paper the technique is described and its potential uses in research and in clinical practice are indicated.

Our approach was to take advantage of the fact that an increase in enamel porosity is the first physical manifestation of a caries attack, and to develop a fluid which could be strongly taken up (imbibed) by carious enamel at a very early stage. A fluorescent indicator dissolved in the carrier fluid could then be deposited within the lesions. After removal of the excess fluid, examination with an ultraviolet lamp would allow an examiner to see the fluorescent indicators which were retained at the sites of increased enamel porosity. Approximately 100 different combinations of solvents, surfactants, and fluorescent indicators were evaluated and three most promising were chosen for more extensive evaluation. These three "caries-diagnostic formulations" (CDF) are designated as follows: CDF-1: ethanolic solution that produces yellowish-green fluorescence; CDF-2: aqueous solution that produces red fluorescence; 3: propylene glycol solution that produces yellowish-green fluorescence.

The three candidate fluorescent CDF were found to disclose the sites of natural "white spot" lesions, pits and fissures, cracks and frank lesions on extracted teeth. In many cases fluorescent spots appeared where there was no other clinical evidence of a lesion. About 20 such spots were tested for their microhardness and all were found to be substantially softer than the surrounding enamel. Poorly adapted restoration margins were also found to be detectable using the CDF technique.

Artificial lesions are detectable as well. Extensive experiments were conducted using lesions which were induced by exposure to pH 4.5 buffer (0.1M acetate) solution for varying lengths of time. Both detection sensitivity and detection specificity were determined as a function of lesion severity. Time of exposure to acid buffer was used as a means of varying lesion severity.

In the method of evaluation, artificial lesions were randomly placed at specified sites on the smooth surfaces of sound molars. Five 4th year dental students were asked to identify the sites of the lesions and to assign a number from 0 to 9 according to their confidence in the identification. Half of the sites contained no lesions and were control sites. If an examiner is completely sure that a given site contains no lesions, he assigns it a zero ranking. If he is only 10% sure that a site contains a lesion, he assigns it a ranking of 1—and so on until he is completely sure (90-100%) that a lesion is present and he assigns a ranking of 9. This is a 2-decision, forced choice, experiment and results in data which can be evaluated by statistical decision theory (Green and Swets, 1966). The percentage of correct responses at each confidence level are plotted against the percentage of incorrect responses at each level of confidence. This results in an observer-unbiased function known as a receiver-operating-characteristic (ROC) curve. Figure 1 shows a ROC curve for 2-hour lesions (2 hours exposure to acid buffer).

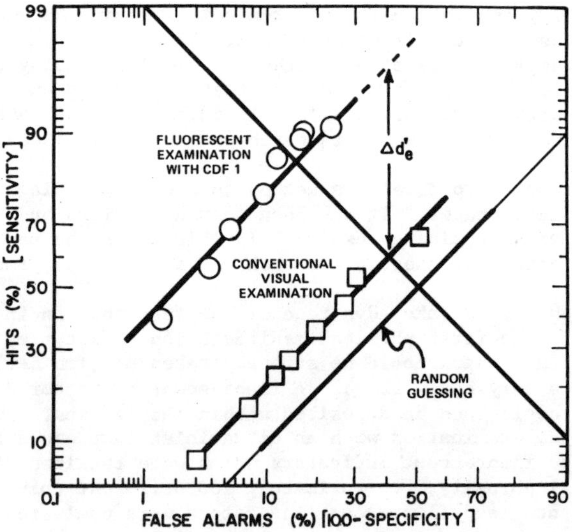

Figure 1. ROC curve for 2-hour artificial lesions plotted on double probability coordinates. The positive diagonal line is the line along which observations will be made if examiners are purely guessing. The vertical distance from the positive diagonal is a measure of detectability, d'_e.

Each point on the ROC curve is the result of each of 120 observations by each of the 5 examiners. Thus each point represents 600 total observations. The closer an ROC curve approaches the left and upper sides of the diagram, the greater the detection sensitivity and specificity (i.e., the more infallible an observation becomes).

Similar experiments were conducted in which 4-hour, 6-hour, 8-hour and 10-hour lesions were used. As the severity of the lesions increased, the fluorescent detectability increased and remained highly sensitive and specific. The sensitivity and specificity of conventional (unaided visual) diagnosis also increased with increasing lesion severity but did not become equal to the fluorescent method until lesions were used which had been exposed to 10 hours or longer of acid buffer treatment. The average lesion-detectability improvement for these experiments is shown in Table I.

AVERAGE IMPROVEMENT ($\Delta d'_e$)

	(EXPERIMENTAL)			(THEORETICAL)
FORMULA	WEIGHTED MEAN	±	S.D.M.	S.D.M.
CDF-1	1.42	+	0.22	0.18
CDF-2	0.66	+	0.17	0.16
CDF-3	0.56	+	0.31	0.18

Table I. Observed improvement in diagnostic efficiency over the conventional method due to the use of fluorescent CDF diagnostic dental aids on artificial early carieslike lesions, averaged over five levels of lesion-severity bracketing the "threshold" of conventional detectability.

The best results were obtained with CDF 1. This formulation has been subjected to extensive safety evaluations in animals and has been found to be non-toxic and non-irritating to mucous tissue. It does not stain sound enamel and leaves only a light yellow stain on carious enamel. This yellow stain disappears in a day or two. The taste has been adjusted so that it is readily tolerated in the mouth, but is slightly unpleasant so as to discourage young patients from swallowing it.

A fluorescent method for detecting interproximal lesions has also been developed. Radiography is relatively insensitive and detects lesions only after they are well beyond the stage where conventional visual observation could detect them if they were located on a buccal or lingual type of surface (over 120 hrs. of in vitro demineralization are required to reach the detectability threshold). Using in vitro experiments on extracted teeth, it was found that certain interproximal lesions can be detected by using a CDF. However, the more advanced but subradiographic lesions are often heavily stained. This staining masks the fluorescent indication of the CDF and sometimes prevents detection.

Since it is capillary forces which draw the fluorescent fluids into a lesion, it should be possible to reverse this and to draw the fluorescent indicators back out of a lesion and allow them to be detected with ultraviolet light. A material which would serve to "blot" or "wick" the indicators out of a proximal-surface lesion could serve this function. Finely divided powders are such materials.

Several powdered materials were tested for use in this way. The powder was suspended in a volatile carrier liquid, such as ethyl alcohol. A drop or two of this suspension was then applied to the contact point between teeth. The carrier liquid evaporates and leaves a layer of powder which can then draw out the fluorescent indicators. The powder layer acts similarly to a thin-layer-chromotography layer. In the ideal case the indicators would migrate through the powder layer sufficiently to become accessible to direct visual detection under UV illumination, but remain close enough to the lesions from which they were withdrawn to serve to identify their locations.

It was found that when this method (fluorescent indicators followed by a powder "developer") was used, approximal lesions could be detected with a high degree of sensitivity and specificity compared to conventional radiographic methods. These experiments were carried out with extracted teeth having natural, subradiographic lesions. In half the cases tested the lesion was mounted next to a sound tooth surface; in the other half, two sound surfaces were mounted next to each other and served as controls. Figure 2 shows the results plotted as ROC curves.

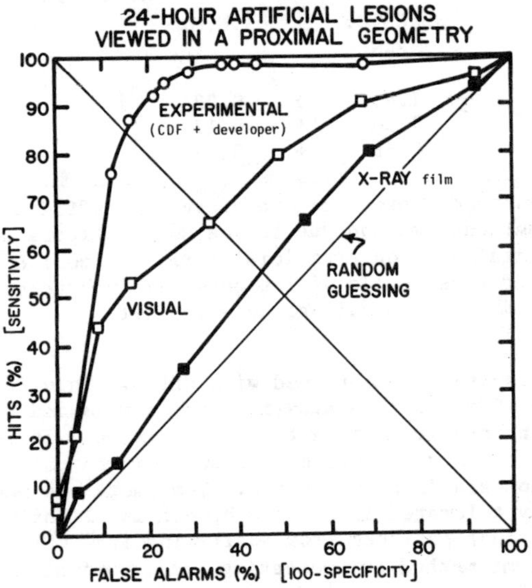

Figure 2. ROC curves comparing the detectability of 24-hour artificial lesions by four different methods.

In other, more limited experiments, the fluorescent indicator/powder developer combination was tested in a rhesus monkey. Fluorescent spots were seen to develop at the sites of clinically obvious lesions when CDF 1 was applied. When CDF 1 was followed with a powder developer, fluorescent material was seen to be drawn into the powder layer and a much enhanced fluorescence was observed. Dampness was found to affect fluorescence development and the ability of the powder layer to remain intact and to withdraw the fluorescent indicator solution. However, cotton rolls and warm air were found to sufficiently control dampness.

On the basis of *in vitro* studies, the fluorescent caries-diagnostic technique has been demonstrated to have great promise as an aid in diagnosing caries at the very earliest stages. However, the technique has only been fully developed for use on smooth surface lesions on accessible surfaces. Preliminary studies indicate its potential for adaptation to approximal surfaces. The CDF method should also be capable of detecting occlusal lesions, but will perhaps require some alteration to adapt it to this diagnostic situation.

The preliminary work with monkeys indicates that the best of the three experimental formulations, CDF 1, is taken up by carious lesions *in vivo* and causes fluorescence to develop at clinically identifiable lesions. Together with the *in vitro* results, this result justifies clinical investigations to determine the *in vivo* diagnostic efficacy of the CDF method. Lesions on smooth enamel surfaces (which provide the simplest diagnostic case) should be studied first, and later occlusal, and then approximal surfaces. Such investigations must await FDA clearance. At present FDA clearance has been granted to conduct "phase one" studies, which have the primary purpose of evaluating safety in humans.

The CDF + developer technique requires further laboratory development and subsequent *in vitro* evaluation before clinical trials are warranted. Powder developers show good promise for use in extending the CDF technique to approximal lesions, and will probably also be useful in assessing occlusal surfaces. The preliminary experiments demonstrate the feasibility of the use of powder developers, and justifies the further development and refinement of this extension of the CDF technique.

Lesions probably develop as a result of imbalances between demineralization and remineralization processes. Thus lesions that are in a very early stage of development may appear to spontaneously reverse and disappear. The CDF method is expected to detect all lesions at a very early stage, but cannot be expected to predict which lesions will ultimately develop to the cavitation stage. Thus, great care would have to be taken in interpreting a CDF examination for its caries predictive value.

LITERATURE CITED

Backer-Dirks, O. 1966. Posteruptive changes in dental enamel. J. Dent. Res. 45:503-511.

Buonocore, M.S. 1976. Nature of adhesion in the use of adhesives in dentistry. C.C. Thomas, Springfield, Ill., pp. 405-413.

Downer, M.C. and O'Mullane, D.M. 1975. A comparison of the concurrent validity of two epidemiologic diagnostic systems for caries evaluation. Community Dent Oral Epidemiol 3:20-24.

Downer, M.C. 1975. Concurrent validity of an epidemiological diagnostic system for caries with the histological appearance of extracted teeth as validating criterion. Caries Res. 9:231-246.

Green, D.M. and Swets, J.A. 1966. Signal detection theory and pscho-physics. Wiley, New York.

Radlike, A.W. 1968. Criteria for diagnosis of dental caries. Proc Conf on clinical testing of cariostatic agents. Am Dent Assoc, Chicago, October, pp. 87-88.

Robinson, C. et al. 1976. Arrest and control of carious lesions: a study based on preliminary experiments with resorcinol-formaldehyde resin. J. Dent. Res. 55:812-818.

Detection of occlusal caries by measuring the electrical resistance

George E. White, Anthi Tsamtsouris, David L. Williams

Department of Oral Pediatrics, Tufts University School of Dental Medicine,
1 Kneeland Street, Boston, Massachusetts 02111

Dentists lack the proper means for detecting early caries. Early detection may permit curative rather than restorative procedures and might shorten the time required for clinical trials.

The method of diagnosing caries by measuring electrical resistance was first proposed by Pincus[1] using direct current (DC) of up to 300 microamperes. Mayuzumi, Suzuki, and Sunada[2] studied the electrical resistance and the degree of caries susceptibility and concluded that teeth having a low electrical resistance had a high susceptibility to dental caries. Those that showed resistance of over 600,000 ohms almost all had no caries and had a low susceptibility to caries. In contrast, teeth with resistance of under 250,000 ohms either had actual dentinal caries or the teeth suffered caries subsequently, regardless of the sound clinical appearance of pits and fissures at the time of examination.

Von Dobrenic and Jelenik[3] confirmed the general conclusion of Mayuzumi, *et al.* and stated that "the investigation of electrical resistance offers possibilities for a test aimed at the detection of the pre-carious lesion." Our[4] preliminary data demonstrated a correlation of tooth conductivity with tactile examination criteria of caries.

The specific purpose of the present cross-sectional study was to detect the presence or absence of occlusal carious lesions in human teeth *in situ* both with a resistance measuring instrument, developed by ABCOR, Inc* and with conventional clinical examination and to compare the findings to those given by histological examination.

The instrumentation we used differed somewhat from that described previously[4]. The use of a Morse 23 explorer for the probe tip and modification of the signal to a battery operated oscillator (180 Hertz) necessitated a change in amplifier calibration. In this study, 4×10^6 ohms was used as the dividing point for carious and sound categories. This reading was then noted by the recorder (5 volts).

The cross-sectional clinical evaluation involved 62 children, aged ten to fourteen years. These subjects were children whose bicuspids needed to be extracted for orthodontic purposes. After obtaining parental consent the children's teeth were examined in the Oral Pediatric Department. The examinations were made after drying and isolation with cotton rolls using a number 5 mirror and a new number 23 dental explorer. To insure that the probe was not dulled, each explorer was discarded after approximately 50 examinations. Radiographs were not used because they are of little value in the diagnosis of incipient carious lesions in the occlusal surface.

The examiners (Drs. Tsamtsouris and White) used written criteria selected for the diagnosis of the carious lesions.[5] Their examination

*Wilmington, Massachusetts

standards were calibrated on 25 patients prior to beginning the study and as an additional check on both intra-examiner and inter-examiner variability each examiner re-examined approximately one-half of his own subjects and one-half of those previously examined by the other examiner when the subjects returned to the clinic for the removal of the remaining becuspids. The study proper consisted of two examinations at a one week interval. Assistants were used to record the findings.

The conventional caries examination was performed first since these data were regarded as more subjective. Thereafter the measurements of electrical resistance were made. This was done in the distal pit, center fissure and the mesial pit of the test bicuspids. To avoid examiner bias the investigators were rotated when making these measurements. The validity, sensitivity, specificity and inter- and intra-examiner reproducibility were determined for the instrument on test teeth. Values were compared for the same tooth surface measurement taken at the same time by two dentists or at different times by one dentist. Using the students 't' test no significant difference was found between the dentists during measurements made on 1,023 tooth surfaces. After extraction the teeth were cleaned of debris, washed with tap water, and immediately stored in individual containers at -20° C.

For the histological examination for caries the teeth from the freezer were washed, and the lingual cusp was removed using a high speed dental drill to expose the central fissure. After further washing the specimens were placed in murexide stain for 36 hours[6,7] and then examined for caries using dental loupes of 3X magnification. The entire procedure was done without reference to data from the clinical or instrument examinations.

The results of the clinical, resistance, and histological examinations are given in Table 1 and 2. It is evident that the electrical resistance instrument can locate the same carious lesions as are found in a routine dental examination (7) and that the instrument is much more sensitive.

An excellent correlation (r=0.965) was found between the instrument finding and murexide stained lesions in the sectioned teeth. The lower correlation (r=0.466) with the explorer as compared to the stain is due to the lower sensitivity of the former method (sensitivity of explorer 0.146 and sensitivity of instrument 0.896).

Our overall findings were that, if the positive murexide stain of the extracted teeth is diagnostic for dental caries, the instrument was

TABLE I

FINDINGS ON CARIES BY HISTOLOGICAL, CLINICAL AND INSTRUMENT METHODS

Histological Finding	Clinical (Explorer)	Resistance Instrument	No. of Teeth
+	+	+	7
+	-	+	36
+	+	-	0
+	-	-	5
-	+	+	0
-	-	+	3
-	+	-	2
-	-	-	39

TABLE II

CARIES FOUND BY STAIN (S) VS. INSTRUMENT (I) VS. CLINICAL EXAM (C)

S \ I	+	-
+	43	5
-	3	41

$r = 0.965$(1)
Sen. = 0.896
Spec. = 0.932

S \ C	+	-
+	7	41
-	2	42

$r = 0.466$(1)
Sen = 0.146
Spec. = 0.955

I \ C	+	-
+	7	39
-	2	44

$r = 0.496$(1)
Relative Sen. = 0.152
Relative Spec. = 0.957

(1)Pearson

(1) much more sensitive than the clinical (explorer) detection of carious lesions, and (2) the instrument findings were as specific as clinical methods for carious lesions.

Sensitivity: In the seven cases of clinically positive caries findings those made by the instrument also indicated that a carious lesion was present; a finding that was validated by the murexide stain. More importantly, there were 36 instances of negative clinical findings and positive instrument findings that were validated as carious by the murexide stain. Of 44 teeth that were negative to both examinations five gave a positive staining reaction.

Restorations, on an area of a tooth not being examined, did not interfere with the instrument determination. Neither was it affected by adjoining amalgam restoration, except at the amalgam-enamel junction. Actual contact with a metal restoration gives a false 'carious' reading due to the high conductivity of the metal.

Reproducibility was occasionally difficult with the instrument because of its high sensitivity. Some of the resulting variability could be blamed on difficult examiner techniques such as attempting to place the probe in the same location for repeated trials. Moisture contamination from saliva, dental plaque, or respiration by the subject also diminished sensitivity of the instrument and hampered reproducibility.

Specificity: The specificity of the instrument findings can be assumed since the same false positive rate was found as the clinical examination. The false positive error of the instrument occurred in three instances out of 44 negative staining cases. This is likely a result of moisture contamination by either saliva or dental plaque. The error of three cases out of 44 was comparable to the clinical false positive rate of two cases out of 44. Significantly there were no cases found in which the clinical examination and the stain were positive for caries and the instrument was not. Further supportive data of the specificity of the instrument is seen in the finding of 39 instances where the clinical examination, instrument and stain all agree on a negative finding.

Experimental noise that could conceivably have an effect on the electrical resistance of the teeth are: trace moisture contamination, electrode explorer pressure and developmental faults. While these factors are the subject of an ongoing study, they were not noted to affect the examination of 1,023 tooth surfaces by both dentists in the present study.

It is noteworthy that while the clinical examination agreed with the findings of the murexide staining in 49 out of 92 cases or 54.3%, the instrument agreed with the findings of the murexide staining in 84 out of 92 cases or 91.3%.

Summary: A resistance measuring instrument has been developed and tested which is more sensitive and as specific for detection of occlusal carious lesion detection than the traditional clinical examination. Clinical examinations were made of recently erupted bicuspid teeth and resistance values were recorded at three points along their occlusal fissure. The teeth were extracted, sectioned along the fissure, and stained with murexide and examined for initial carious lesions.

In 36 instances the instrument revealed the presence of carious occlusal lesion that could not be detected clinically, but was shown to be present by the murexide stain.

LITERATURE CITED

1. Pincus, P. 1951. A New Method of Examination of Molar Tooth Grooves for the Presence of Dental Caries. Journal of Physiology. 113:13-14.

2. Mayuzumi, Y., Suzuki, K., and Sunada, J. 1964. A Method of Diagnosing Incipient Caries in Pits and Fissures by Measuring Electrical Resistance, Journal of Dental Research. 43:431.

3. Von Dobrenic, M. and Jelinck, E. 1969. Versuch der Entdeckung Prakarioser Lasionen durch Messung des Elektrischen Widerstandes der Zahnhartgewebe, Deutsch Zahnarztliche Zeitschrift. 24:16-21.

4. Williams, D.L., Tsamtsouris, A. and White, G.E. Electrice Resistance Correlation with Tactile Examination on Occlusal Surfaces, Journal of Dental Research, in press.

5. Radike, A.W. 1968. Criteria for Diagnosis of Dental Caries, pp. 87-88, in Proceedings of the Conference on the Clinical Testing of Cariostatic Agents.

6. Keyes, P.H. 1944. A Method of Recording and Scoring Gross Carious Lesions in the Molar Teeth of Syrian Hamsters, Journal of Dental Research. 23:439-451.

7. Navia, J.M. and Harris, R.S. 1969. Longitudinal Study of Cariostatic Effects of Sodium Trimetaphosphate and Sodium Fluoride when Fed Separately and Together in Diets of Rats, Journal of Dental Research. 48:183-191.

An ultraviolet photographic technique for the early detection of carious lesions

I. Kleinberg, R. Chatterjee, A. Domokos, C.R. Castaldi, M. Fain and F. Chebib

Sch. Dental Medicine, State Univ., New York, Stony Brook, NY, and Sch. Dental Medicine, Univ. Connecticut, Farmington, CT, USA ; Fac. Dentistry, Univ. Manitoba, Winnipeg, and Alphametrics, Ltd., Winnipeg, Canada

Mirror, probe and x-ray examination is the traditional method of scoring for dental caries and the difference between two scores carried out at different times gives a measure of the caries increment. Even under the best circumstances, this method is an inaccurate procedure (DePaola, 1967) largely because of the difficulty of being able to identify or measure the early caries lesion. Because most clinical trials for dental caries are carried out on children or young adults who still have most of their tooth surfaces intact, the early lesion necessarily comprises a large percentage of total caries score (Backer-Dirks, 1963).

Human tooth enamel and dentin both fluoresce under ultraviolet light and lose this fluorescence when they become carious (Benedict, 1928; Hartles and Leaver, 1953; Francis and Meckel, 1963). Francis and Meckel (1963) developed an ultraviolet photographic technique based upon this phenomenon which enabled them to monitor caries lesion formation in extracted teeth in vitro. When we began our studies in this area, it became apparent that fluorescence or loss of fluorescence was not sufficiently sensitive for the detection of the early caries lesion. We found, instead, as will be described in this report, that differences in ultraviolet absorption and reflection, particularly at shorter ultraviolet wavelengths, was a much more sensitive procedure for early carious lesion detection.

When demineralization of the enamel occurs during caries lesion formation, the spaces formerly occupied by calcium phosphate become filled with plaque and with pellicle material derived from the oral environment. Because the deposited material contains substances,such as protein, that absorb photons in the ultraviolet portion of the electromagnetic spectrum and the calcium phosphate which makes up most of the healthy enamel tissue does not, visualization of lesions in their earliest stages becomes possible. This is evident from the visible and ultraviolet photographs in Figures 1 and 2 which demonstrate in extracted teeth and teeth in vivo the difference in appearance of the same cleaned tooth surfaces under the two types of illumination. If visible filters are used to permit only the transmission of ultraviolet light, little or no differences are seen. However, if ultraviolet filters are used to permit transmission only of the visible light, the early lesion either cannot be seen or can only be seen with considerable difficulty. Tests such as this, made it quite clear that the differences seen in Figures 1 and 2 are mainly due to variation in the ability of tooth surfaces to absorb and reflect ultraviolet radiation and not to differences in fluorescence or loss of fluorescence.

The studies of Tiede and Chomse (1934), Hartles and Leaver, (1953), and Armstrong (1963) indicate that the blue-fluorescing material in enamel and dentin is part of the organic component of these tissues and may be peptide

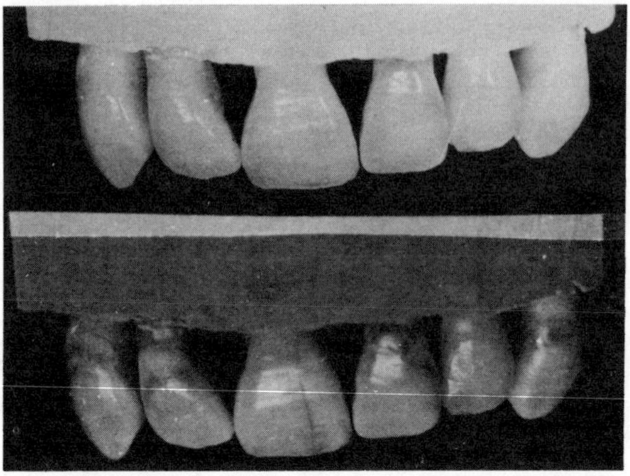

Figure 1. Anterior teeth *in vitro* under visible light (upper set) and ultraviolet light (lower set).

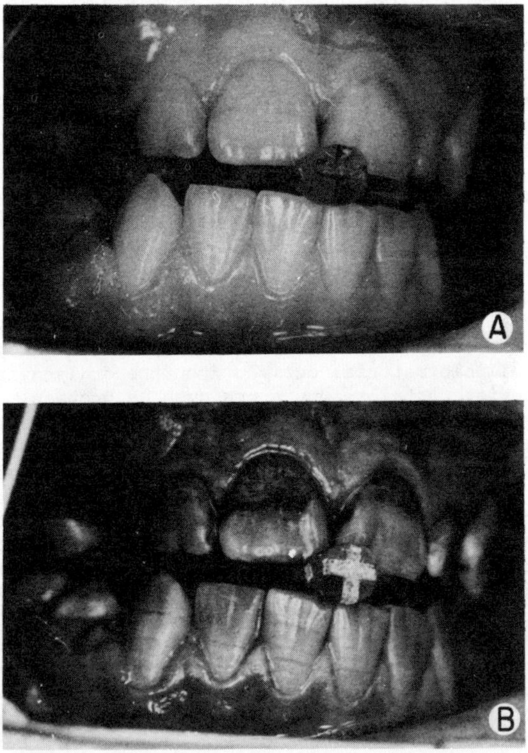

Figure 2. Anterior teeth *in vivo* under visible and ultraviolet light. Upper set of photographs (A) was taken under visible light, the lower set (B) is of the same teeth with ultraviolet light.

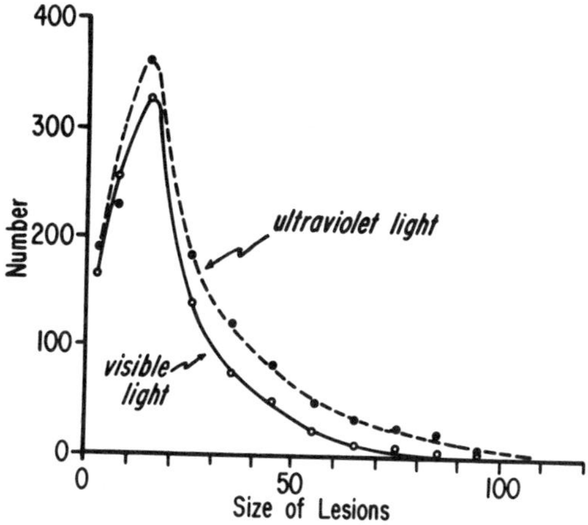

Figure 3. Distribution of sizes of lesions observed by various examiners under visible and ultraviolet light.

in nature. On the other hand, Glasser and Fonda (1938) believe that the fluorescence is linked to the mineral component of the tooth, since calcium phosphate in certain crystal states will also fluoresce, as for example when it is heated to 400°C after the organic material is destroyed. In either case, during the caries process, both the organic and mineral components of enamel and dentin are destroyed or altered. The calcium phosphate is lost or re-deposited in a crystal form other than that laid down in the original tissue; the organic portion may be lost by enzymic degradation, or become covered by non-fluorescing deposits of calcium phosphate or organic material such as pellicle.

We initiated a study to compare how well examiners could detect lesions by probing with dental explorers under visible and under ultraviolet illumination. Ten sets of extracted maxillary and mandibular incisors and canines were set up as in Figure 1. Seven examiners, using sharp probes then examined the 120 teeth on each of four different occasions, twice using ultraviolet and twice using visible light. Examiners were instructed to diagram the lesions on teeth outlined on graph paper. The cavity size in relative units were determined from the areas as measured with a planimeter; lesions were grouped according to size and a distribution curve drawn (Fig.3) Although the curves in Figure 3 are similar in shape, they show that more lesions can be detected under ultraviolet than under visible light and that the lesions appear larger. The similarity of the shape of the two distribution curves is a reflection of the "stage in caries progression" of the teeth examined. In other words, if the sample had contained teeth with a larger number of advanced and a smaller number of initial lesions (equivalent to a later stage in caries development), the peak would have been located more to the right.

The frequency of reversal of diagnosis and the error of diagnosis under visible and ultraviolet illumination was then evaluated by arbitrarily dividing each diagrammed tooth into mesial, middle, and distal thirds. Both negative and positive reversals from the two independent examinations with each light source were scored (Backer-Dirks, 1961) and the results are shown in Table 1. The number of reversals were similar for visible and ultraviolet light but because the number of lesions detected with ultraviolet light was more, the error in determining the caries score will be less.

Table 1.

Diagnosis of Sound and Carious Surfaces
Under Visible and Ultraviolet Light

Non-reversals	Visible	Ultraviolet
Sound	651	555
Caries	240	351
Reversals		
Sound to caries	47	45
Caries to sound	64	51
Total surfaces	1,002	1,002

Although scoring under ultraviolet illumination was more sensitive than under visible light, the increased sensitivity was not sufficient to warrant the extra effort necessary to protect both examiner and patient from the long exposure to ultraviolet radiation resulting from this approach. Like the mirror and probe examination under visible light, scoring under ultraviolet illumination was tedious and subjective, and therefore, prone to significant scoring error. The much lesser sensitivity of this method than ultraviolet absorption photography is due to the fact that the human eye is sensitive to visible, but not to ultraviolet light. As a result the eye can detect differences due to fluorescence, but it cannot see differences due to ultraviolet absorption and reflection. To meet this problem a camera with the ultraviolet transmitting properties of a quartz lens was developed to our specifications by Alphametrics, Ltd. (Winnipeg, Canada). The camera and its components are shown in Figures 4 and 5.

The camera has a special lens which uses only quartz and fluorite elements to achieve high resolution between 200 and 1,000 nm without refocusing. Photographs can be made either with ultraviolet or visible light illumination. The ultraviolet source is a low pressure mercury vapor lamp; several small tungsten bulbs serve as the source of visible illumination.

A barrier filter wheel located in front of the lens enables selection of 254 or 365 nanometer narrow band pass, as well as Wratten 2A fluorescence filters. This makes it possible to isolate and photograph fluorescence absorption phenomena. Exposure times are electronically controlled. An interchangeable camera back system makes it possible to use 35 mm single lens reflex, polaroid sheet film, 120 roll film and motorized large magazine 35 mm camera backs.

Special mouth pieces were developed for use with the dental camera. The labial-buccal tooth surfaces are the easiest to photograph. However, by using a mouthpiece with a mirror assembly, the lingual and occlusal tooth surfaces can also be reached. The mouth pieces come in different sizes and are designed for easy removal from the camera to enable sterilization.

An opportunity presented itself to use the ultraviolet camera technique in a clinical study designed to determine whether caries activity was related to plaque calcium, phosphorus and ash levels which parameters have been shown earlier to be inversely related to the caries susceptibility of the incisor teeth (Kleinberg et al, 1971; Ashley, 1975). The two year study embraced one group of 71 adolescents, aged 12-14, and a group of 51 adults aged 19-26. Caries prevalence and increment were determined by mirror, probe and x-ray examinations. The clinical examination was of the whole mouth and was carried out following a careful rubber cup prophylaxis by a hygienist and using a disclosing solution. Scoring was carried out by each of 2 examiners at the beginning, and 6, 12, and 24 months after the start of the study. At the beginning of the study and at the 12 and 24 month exam-

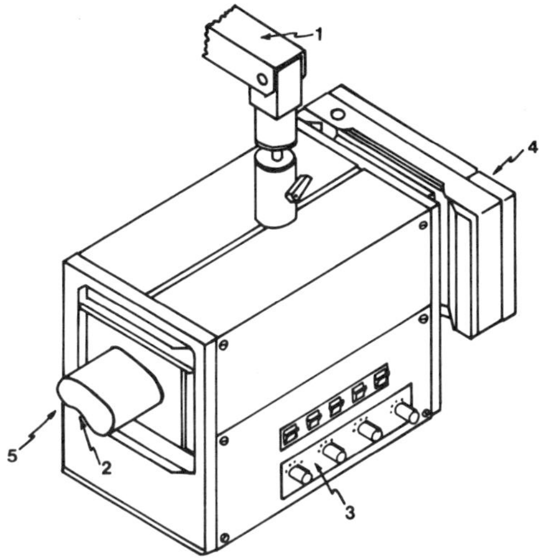

Figure 4. Schematic diagram showing the exterior of the ultraviolet dental camera. 1-suspension as on dental x-ray machines; 2-removable mouthpiece attachment; 3-panel with controls for selecting ultra violet or visible modes, wavelength and filters, exposure time, focus, and normal or automatic modes; 4-removable camera back 5- main body of camera. The power supply is a separate unit and is not shown. (taken from U.S. Patent Publication No. 3,971,954; August, 1976).

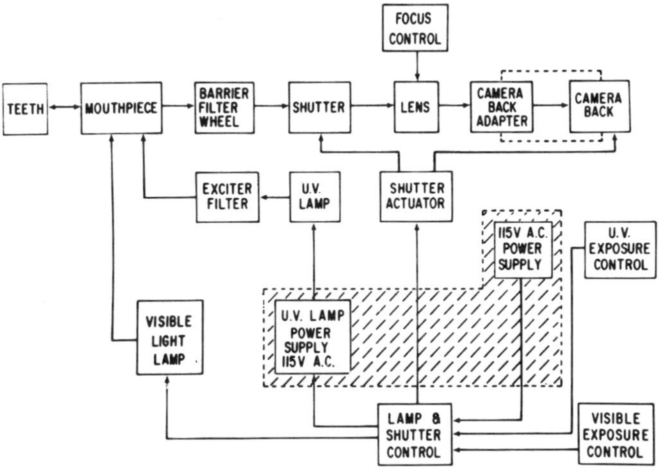

Figure 5. Schematic diagram showing the functional components of the ultraviolet camera. Ultraviolet or visible radiation passes through the mouthpiece to the patient and is then reflected back through the barrier filter wheel which controls the radiation that passes through the lens to the camera back. (Taken from U.S. Patent Publication No. 3,971,954; August, 1976).

Table 2.

Caries scoring* of the adolescent and adult subjects in each of the four examinations.

	Restorations	Early Lesions	Late Lesions	X-ray Lesions
Examination I (0 months)				
Adolescents	0.02 ± 0.00(8)	0.42 ± 0.04	0.07 ± 0.01	0.14 ± 0.02
Adults	0.26 ± 0.06	0.24 ± 0.05	0.14 ± 0.03	0.09 ± 0.03
Examination II (6 months)				
Adolescents	0.02 ± 0.00(9)	0.30 ± 0.04	0.09 ± 0.02	0.13 ± 0.02
Adults	0.28 ± 0.06	0.21 ± 0.04	0.16 ± 0.04	0.08 ± 0.02
Examination III (12 months)				
Adolescents	0.02 ± 0.00(9)	0.30 ± 0.04	0.13 ± 0.02	0.14 ± 0.02
Adults	0.31 ± 0.06	0.19 ± 0.04	0.12 ± 0.03	0.06 ± 0.02
Examination IV (24 months)				
Adolescents	0.10 ± 0.03	0.22 ± 0.04	0.16 ± 0.04	0.24 ± 0.05
Adults	0.32 ± 0.04	0.17 ± 0.01	0.12 ± 0.03	0.13 ± 0.03

* Number of lesions scored per subject for the incisor teeth including the cuspids.

inations, photographs were taken of the anterior teeth under ultraviolet light,and for comparison, under visible light. The mirror and explorer examinations made at the various examination periods revealed no increments of caries in the incisor teeth (although the plaque chemistry was indicative of it-Table 2). However, caries was found in the ultraviolet photographs in amounts that correlated with the evidence of caries revealed by the plaque analyses.

Examination of the individual ultraviolet photographs of each subject who remained in the study for the full 2 years showed that there was an increase in some cases, no changes in others and clearly a reversal in others The ultraviolet photographs enabled differentiation between a true reversal, and one due simply to examiner error. In a typical case (Figure 6) ultraviolet photography detected caries in a maxillary left lateral incisor one year after the study started, but it was not until the end of the 2 year period that the lesion became evident by visible light and was recorded by mirror and probe examination.

Reliability of caries diagnosis was higher with the ultraviolet than the visual method. Of the 528 surfaces examined by each examiner, between the first and second set of ultraviolet photographs (one year increment), diagnoses were opposite on only two occasions, whereas between the first and third examination period (two year increment), this occurred only once. We attribute much of this good agreement to the fact that it is a more precise procedure to compare photographs, and decide whether or not there is a difference than to determine whether a change has occurred from differences between caries scores made at 6 to 24 month intervals by mirror and probe examination (cf. DePaola, 1967).

Among the findings of our study that deserve emphasis is that although there was only slight development of caries lesions in both the adolescent and adult group, that small increase was seen quite readily by ultraviolet photography. Because lesions can be detected at an earlier stage in their development by ultraviolet photography than by mirror and probe examination, it is apparent that ultraviolet photography can simplify the determination of caries increment at least on tooth surfaces accessible to this technique.

Examination of caries experience by mirror and probe, x-ray or even ultraviolet photography only measures the effects of the disease entity, dental caries. It does not measure whether a person is going to develop lesions. For this it is necessary to be able to measure the susceptibility of the individual to lesion formation i.e. parameters of the disease process itself. This was done in the present study by the analyses of plaque calcium and phosphorus which, as has been pointed out elsewhere (Kleinberg et al, 1971), serves as an indicator of caries activity. Significant inverse relationship was found between plaque calcium and phosphorus levels and the development of early, ultraviolet-detected caries.

Absence of correlation in the present study of caries increment by mirror and probe examination with the plaque variables measured can be attributed to the fact that the caries attack rate was so slow that the increment, because of the large error associated with its determination, could not be determined by mirror, probe and x-ray examination. However, because the increment could be determined accurately and readily by ultraviolet photography, it was possible to show a highly significant correlation.

Although at the present time restricted to the more accessible surfaces of the dentition, the use of ultraviolet photography for the determination of caries increment, despite this deficiency, holds considerable promise, since presence of caries lesions on the accessible surfaces such as the anterior teeth is an indicator of the presence of caries lesions in the remainder of the mouth. Not only does this mean that fewer subjects and shorter times of testing can be used to explore the efficacy of an agent or procedure in a clinical trial, but most important and worthy of further exploring is the use of caries increment measurement by ultraviolet photography as an early warning of future serious damage. If sufficiently early, it could alleviate the need, in many cases, for a caries susceptibility test.

Finally, in many clinical studies, reversals have been suspected and have often been attributed to errors of diagnosis at the time of mirror and probe examination. The present results with ultraviolet photography show that lesion reversals do take place and most important they suggest that, if suitable therapeutic agents are developed to effect remineralization, then the progression of carious lesions to a stage requiring restoration by a dentist might be avoided.

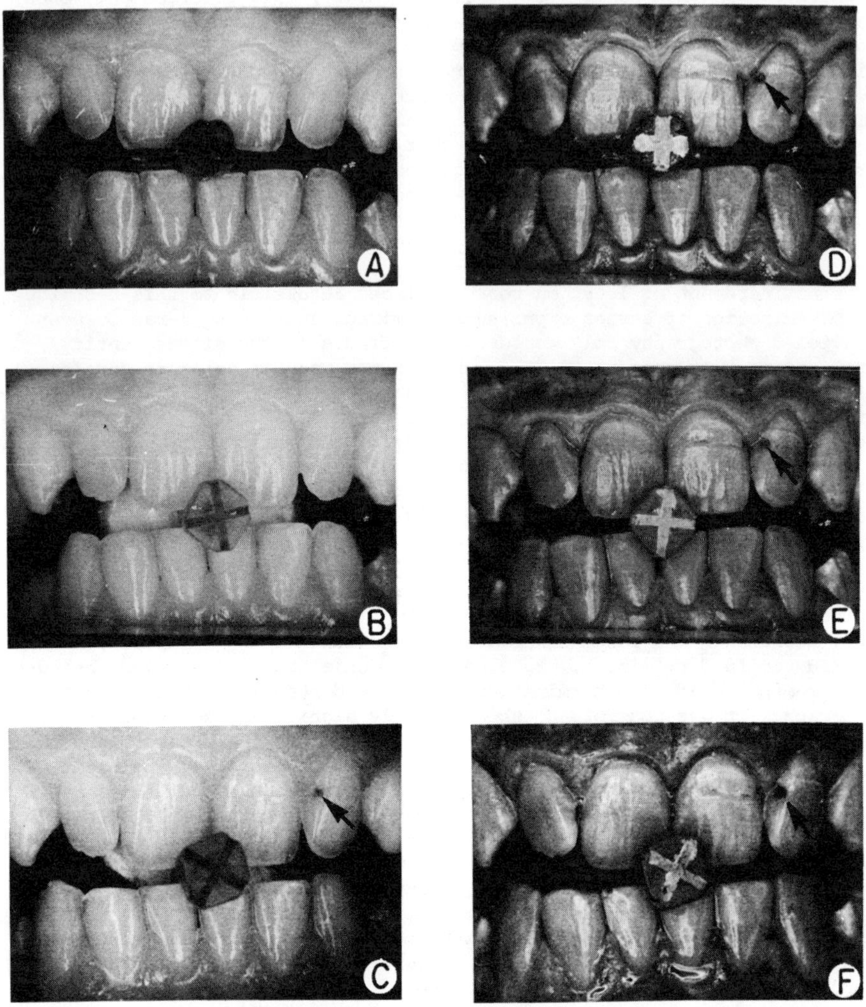

Figure 6. Photographs under visible and ultraviolet light of caries progression in anterior teeth over a two-year period. Figures A,B, and C show the 0, 12- and 24-month visible results while Figures D, E, and F show the corresponding ultraviolet results. Note the lesion on the mesial surface of the maxillary left lateral incisor indicated by the arrow.

LITERATURE CITED

Armstrong, W.G. 1963. Fluorescence characteristics of sound and carious human dentine preparations. Archs. oral Biol. 8:79-90.

Ashley, F.P. 1975. Plaque calcium and phosphorus levels in human dental plaque-variations according to site collection. Archs. oral Biol. 20:167-170.

Backer Dirks, O. 1961. The present study of caries prevention by fluorine-containing dentifrices. In Caries Symposium Zurich. Mühlemann, H.R. and König, K.G. (eds) Huber, Berne, pp. 37-46.

Benedict, H.C. 1928. A note on the fluorescence of teeth in ultra-violet rays. Science 67:442.

DePaola, P.F. 1967. Examiner inconsistency in clinical caries research. J. oral Therap. Pharmacol. 4:200-204.

Francis, M.D. and Meckel, A.H. 1963. The in vitro formation and quantitative evaluation of carious lesions. Archs. oral Biol. 8:1-12.

Glasser, J. and Fonda, G.R. 1938. The fluorescence of double salts of calcium phosphate. J. Amer. Chem. Soc. 60:722.

Hartles, R.L. and Leaver, A.G. 1953. The fluorescence of teeth under ultra-violet irradiation. Biochem. J. 54:632-638.

Kleinberg, I., Chatterjee, R., Kaminsky, F.S., Cross, H.G., Goldenberg, D.J., and Kaufman, H.W. 1971. Plaque formation and the effect of age. J. Periodont. 42:497-507.

Tiede, E. and Chomse, H. 1934. Ber. dtsch. chem. Ges. 676:1988 cited in Biochem. J. 1953. 54:632.

Clinical-visual and radiographic grading of dental caries

T.M. Marthaler

Dental Research Institute, Zurich, Switzerland

In surveys and experiments carried out in Switzerland, a fairly elaborate system of grading caries lesions has been used. The clinical-visual and radiographic grading system is shown in Tables I and II. What type of additional information is obtained from this kind of detailed grading?

Table I. Clinical-visual examination for dental caries

	Pits and fissures	Smooth surfaces
Grade 0:	No changes indicating caries	
Grade 1:	Yellow or slightly brown	White spot, vertical extension < 2 mm
Grade 2:	Dark brown or black	White spot, vertical extension ≥ 2 mm
Grade 3:	Small cavity	
Grade 4:	Cavity with smallest diameter of the opening > 2 mm	

According to Marthaler (1966)

Table II. Examination for caries on radiographs of the buccal segment

Grade 0:	No radiolucency
Grade 1:	Translucence visible in the outer half of the enamel layer
Grade 2:	Translucence visible in the inner half of the enamel layer
Grade 3:	Translucence visible in the outer half of the dentine
Grade 4:	Translucence visible in the inner half of the dentine

According to Marthaler (1966)

Example 1. In approximately 150 children, oral hygiene levels have been assessed 12 to 18 times during a 3-year study period. A selection was made of children who either repeatedly showed abundant amounts of plaque or, by contrast, only minimal amounts of plaque. Results regarding caries counts are shown in Table III. On the level of D(3-4)MF tooth and surface counts which exclude pre-cavity lesions, no difference could be found between the low-hygiene and the good-hygiene groups. However, the number of white spot lesions was considerably (and significantly, $P < 0.01$) smaller in the good hygiene children as compared to the low-hygiene group.

Table III. Comparisons of DMF experience in children with either bad or good oral hygiene during a 3-year study period. Age 14

	Low Hygiene Level	High Hygiene Level	T,	P_t
Number of children	41	45		
Counts disregarding Grades 1 and 2				
D(3-4)MFT	5,658	5.177	0.73	>0.1
D(3-4)MFS	10.805	9.511	0.92	>0.1
Counts of Grades 1 and 2*				
D(1-2) Smooth surfaces	2.073	0.844	2.77	<0.01

Unpublished material, examinations made in 1976
*buccal and lingual surfaces on second molars and labial and approximal surfaces of canines and incisors

Example 2. In 1963, supervised toothbrushing exercises performed at school 6 times a year were introduced in the Canton of Zürich. The fluoride applied thereby and in the fluoride dentifrices used at home as well as other beneficial factors (such as less frequent sugar intake between meals, better oral hygiene, etc.) have reduced dental caries levels by more than 50% when statistics are based on cavities. Radiological findings are given in Table IV. The number of radiolucencies limited to the enamel, D(1-2)S, has remained constant while the deeper lesions were reduced from 9.62 to 3.65. These data show that there was an inhibiting effect on initiation as well as on progression of carious lesions.

Table IV. Radiolucencies of varying depth in 1963, when a preventive program was started, and in 1975, after 12 years of preventive activities, 24 surfaces at full eruption. Age 14

	1963	1975
Sound surfaces	5.59	11.26
D(1-2)S, enamel lesions	7.84	8.14
D(3-4)MFS, dentinal etc.	9.62	3.65

Data from Marthaler (1977)

Example 3. After initial examination, 47 children were given appointments at the school dental clinic for 20 preventive sessions. At the end of the year the children were re-examined. Initial and final states of caries predilection sites were studied by using transition matrices. Of a total of 519 initially sound free smooth surfaces of molars, only 25 developed a small (Grade 1) and 7 a large white spot (Grade 2). On the other hand, the majority of white spots initially present had disappeared (Table V).

Table V. Free smooth surfaces on posterior teeth, transition matrix of 47 children with intensified prevention during 1 year (16 visits to school dental clinics)

First Exam	Second Exam: Sound	D(1)	D(2)	D(3-4)F
Sound	487	25	7	0
D(1)	116	38	9	1
D(2)	31	7	11	2
D(3-4)F	5*	0	0	10

*Five obvious recording errors
Unpublished material, examinations 1974-75

The transition matrix presenting radiographic findings (Table VI) shows a fairly stable picture. In all rows and columns, the diagonal frequencies, counting surfaces with the same caries grades at the initial and final examinations, were highest. Of the five dentinal lesions which developed, four were seen in the inner half of the enamel, and the fifth was seen in the outer enamel at the initial examination. None of the initially sound surfaces developed a dentinal lesion, but new decalcification was seen in the outer enamel of 13 surfaces and in the inner enamel of 5 surfaces.

Table VI. Surfaces on radiographs, transition matrix of 47 children with intensified prevention during 1 year (16 visits to school dental clinics)

First Exam	Second Exam			
	Sound	D(1)	D(2)	D(3-4)F
Sound	448	13	5	0
D(1)	19	20	11	1
D(2)	9	5	10	4
D(3-4)F	1*	1	0	36

For footnotes see Table V.

Example 4. Example 3 is not typical because the intense preventive program inhibited further development of carious lesions. Example 4 (See Table VII) shows data from 59 children examined at ages 15 and 24 (Germann 1977). The deeper the radiolucency had penetrated at age 15, the higher was the probability of penetration of the radiolucency into the dentine until age 23 (Grades 3,4 or filled). This would be expected for radiographic data since even small radiolucencies are known to correspond to a considerable loss of mineral, and often to cavity (Marthaler and Germann, 1970).

Discoloration of fissures is obviously an uncertain precursor to later cavitation, since it is sometimes due to discolored material in the fissure or at its entrance while the enamel might be unaltered. However, the transition matrix (Table VII, Fissures and pits) validates the idea that fissures and pits which at age 14 appeared discolored upon inspection were more likely to develop cavities than those appearing free of any visible change.

The lower part of Table VII shows that if on smooth surfaces a white spot was present at age 15, development of a cavity during 9 following years was more probable than on initially sound smooth surfaces (sound = without any symptoms of early carious demineralization).

This long-term longitudinal study supports the hypothesis that white spots and brown fissures as detected by inspection are precursors of clinical caries. The study of lesions not having developed yet into cavities thus provides valuable information.

The examples given may illustrate the additional information which may be obtained by grading of carious lesions and subsequent analysis by transition matrices in follow-up studies. A further illustration is given in Fig. 1 of the paper by Grondahl et al. (1977). In view of the fact that caries activity in many developed countries is decreasing, the study of early lesions and their development into cavities becomes more important. Dental treatment is often at a high level and the D(M)F count at the cavity level may be a (M)F count in many children. This would mean that the epidemiologist is counting fillings only under such circumstances, the diagnosis having been made by the dentist in charge of the treatment. Early lesions at the pre-cavity levels have the advantage that they are less interfered with by dental treatment.

Table VII. Transition matrices of caries predilection sites of 59 subjects examined at age 14 (1965) and at age 23.

Initial Grade	Initial number of sites	Final Grade after 9 years 0	1	2	3+4+F(F)*	3+4+F	Extr.
0	428	179	56	47	146(99)	34%**	0
1	280	30	37	49	164(128)	58%	0
2	149	3	1	7	138(111)	93%	0
3*	348	1	1	0	346(312)	-	0
Fissures and pits of molars and premolars							
0	357	180	51	30	96(93)	27%	0
1	168	47	20	24	77(64)	46%	0
2	181	11	6	34	130(112)	72%	0
3*	560	2	1	6	551(540)	-	0
Free smooth surfaces of molars and premolars							
0	1297	1031	81	95	90(70)	7%	0
1	100	57	9	21	13(6)	13%	0
2	33	6	2	14	11(6)	33%	0
3*	57	2	2	7	40(35)	-	0
All surfaces of incisors and canines							
0	2402	2059	110	66	159(134)	7%	8
1	37	16	7	5	9(6)	24%	0
2	40	2	4	11	21(17)	52%	2
3*	153	3	2	1	146(133)	-	1

*3+4+F: denotes all sites with a Grade 3 or 4 or with a filling; the number of filled sites at the final examination is given in parentheses.
**146 as percentage of 428

In earlier work, a discriminant function has been used for computing individual caries predictors (Marthaler 1968). Some 30 percent of increment variance was accounted for when pre-cavity lesions were considered in the predictor.

LITERATURE CITED

Germann, B. 1977. Kariesbefall und Zahnverlust in der Altersspanne 14 bis 23 Jahre, eine Longitudinalstudie an 59 Probanden. Med.Diss. Zürich.

Gröndahl, H.G., Hollender, L., Malmcrona, E., Sundquist, B. 1977. Dental caries and restorations in teenagers. II. A longitudinal radiographic study of the caries increment of proximal surfaces among urban teenagers in Sweden. Swed. Dental J. 1:51-57.

Marthaler, T.M. 1966. A standardized system of recording dental conditions. Helv. odont. Acta 10:1-18.

Marthaler, T.M. 1968. On the use of discriminatory analysis for constructing strata in clinical caries increment studies. Helv. odont. Acta. 12:66-71.

Marthaler, R.M., Germann, M. 1970. Radiographic and visual appearance of small smooth surface caries lesions studied on extracted teeth. Caries Res. 4:224-242.

Marthaler, T.M. 1977. Dental caries 12 years after introduction of a preventive program-Preliminary report from seven communities. Helv. odont. Acta 21:63-68. In: Schweiz. Mschr. Zahnheilk. 87:823-828

MODERATOR'S SUMMARY OF DISCUSSION OF TOPIC VI

A common criticism raised by many speakers was that few investigators had attempted to determine whether the technics employed are detecting early carious lesions. It was also suggested that some of the lesions examined were enamel defects unrelated to dental caries. It was agreed that one or two approaches, particularly that detecting changes in enamel resistance, held some promise and that a longitudinal study being carried out should help to determine the validity of this approach.

TOPIC VII

CORRELATION OF MEASUREMENTS

Moderator:

William H. Bowen
National Institutes of Dental Research
Bethesda, Maryland 20014

Aspects of design and data evaluation in population studies

R.G. Schamschula, B.L. Adkins, Helen M. Agus, D.E. Barmes and G. Charlton

Dental Research Institute, 2 Chalmers Street, Sydney, Australia

Population studies of caries etiology, as distinct from clinical trials, aim to identify variables influencing odontolysis and to define their roles and interactions *in vivo*. The scope of such studies is increasing through advances in analytical and computer technology and the availability of multi-variate methods of statistical analysis. Today, the human oral environment can be defined in terms of many parameters, with high precision. Resultant data may comprise variables diverse in their biological nature, yet interconnected in the pathogenesis of caries.

My intention is to discuss selected problems encountered in multi-factorial caries studies from the viewpoint of the dental investigator working in collaboration with the statistician. In particular, I propose to deal with aspects of experimental design and data evaluation which appear to influence the correlation of independent variables with caries experience.

Reference will be made to studies in three populations, on which most of our experiences are based. The first study (1-3) was a three-year longitudinal investigation of 20 diverse intraoral parameters in relation to the prevalence and incidence of caries in 400 Australian schoolchildren, aged 9 years at the first examination. The second study (4-6) was limited to a single determination of 10 inorganic constituents of plaque, related parameters, and caries prevalence in 72 eleven year old schoolchildren in New South Wales, Australia. In the third study (7) associations between the prevalence and severity of caries and over 80 oral variables were examined in 300 primitive New Guineans aged 12-24 years, against a background of racial, socio-economic, dietary, nutritional and geochemical characteristics. In each study subgroups were exposed to contrasting levels of environmental fluoride.

Longitudinal or cross-sectional design? Most biological values vary with time. The ideal way to determine the relationship between odontolysis and an oral variable which is subject to time-related variation would be continuous monitoring of that variable over an extended period. This is rarely possible even for a single parameter. The next best alternative is to carry out repeated determinations to establish the average status of each variable in relation to the development of carious lesions during the period of observation. Longitudinal observations also have the potential to indicate changing trends of values with the development of lesions, and therefore provide a more realistic basis for caries prediction than cross-sectional data. Whereas longitudinal studies require far greater resources than the prevalence approach, the returns are also proportionately greater.

Initiation or progress of lesions? The etiological background of the initiation and progress of lesions may be substantially different. To test this contention, we have introduced into the New Guinea study (8) a self designed index indicating the severity or destructiveness of lesions. DMFS and DMFT were very closely correlated with each other, but less so with the severity score (Table 1).

Table 1.

Correlation coefficients between DMFT, DMFS and Severity score values. New Guinea Study, n=301.

	DMFT	DMFS
DMFS	0.98	-
Severity score	0.56	0.54

The intraoral variables examined in New Guinea could be grouped according to the area of etiological relevance: those reflecting the properties of enamel or plaque or saliva, or miscellaneous variables. As part of preliminary analyses, some 80 variables, approximately equally divided between the four groups, were submitted in free competition to multiple stepwise linear regression analyses (MSLRA) against DMFT, DMFS and the severity score as dependent variables in turn. Table 2 shows the division between groups of the first 10 independent variables which entered the analyses against the three dependent variables.

Table 2.

Distribution of first ten independent variables which entered MSLRA-s vs. DMFT, DMFS and the Severity score, between areas of etiological relevance. New Guinea Study, n=292.

Independent variables	Dependent variables		
Ares of relevance	DMFT	DMFS	Severity score
Enamel properties	4	4	2
Plaque properties	5	5	2
Saliva properties	1	1	5
Miscellaneous	-	-	1

DMFT and DMFS, which indicate the number, and by inference the initiation of lesions, are primarily associated with enamel and plaque related variables, whilst variables connected with saliva assume importance with regard to the score indicating the progression of lesions. Apart from obvious etiological implications, it is clear that the choice of variables for prediction should depend on whether the number of progression of lesions is to be predicted.

Homogeneity of the population studied. A constant feature of our studies was the increase in the strength of association between individual caries experience and the oral variables measured, singly or collectively, within progressively smaller natural sample divisions. Thus, using the same parameters, higher simple or multiple correlation coefficients were reached for town or village aggregates of subjects than in Village Groups, or in turn, over the whole sample. Examples are shown in Tables 3 and 4. Discriminant analyses also produced better results within smaller groups of subjects than overall. We feel that this is a manifestation of progressively increasing geochemical, other environmental, socio-economic and in New Guinea racial, homogeneity.

Table 3.
Multiple correlation coefficients between DMFT (dependent variable) and identical sets of independent variables related to plaque per geographical area and overall. Australian Study.

	n	Step no.*	R	P<
Area I	25	6	0.66	0.10
Area II	26	8	0.74	0.05
Area III	21	3	0.77	0.01
Area I + II + III	72	4	0.50	0.001

* at 'critical' F level

Table 4.
DMFS regressed on identical sets of independent variables. Correlation coefficients at the third step for the whole sample and within Village group 1 and constituent villages. New Guinea Study.

Overall

R = 0.48 n = 292 P < 0.001

Village group 1

R = 0.65 n = 38 P < 0.001

	Village 1	Village 2	Village 3
R	0.82	1.0	0.90
n	15	9	14
P	< 0.001	< 0.001	< 0.001

Apart from these wider aspects, sample homogeneity also deserves consideration from the viewpoints of independent variables and the dentition. Two widely recognized factors exert dominant opposing influences on individual caries experience; fluoride and carbohydrates. It is mostly overlooked that unless the effect of these two factors is neutralized, or happens to be uniform, the role of less influential variables selected for study may be partly or completely obscured. Figure 1 illustrates the point using artificial data, but the underlying principle is based on firm epidemiological evidence. It is universally accepted that population means of caries experience rise progressively with decreasing fluoride levels in water, particularly under 1 ppm (9,10). In an area, where the fluoride content of water varies between 0.5 and 0.2 ppm, or there is comparable variation in environmental exposure to fluoride from other sources, at the age of 13 years local means of the DMFT score may differ by ± 2-3 units from an area mean of 5 units because of fluoride effect. We have demonstrated such differences between neighboring village groups in New Guinea. In each group there was a positive correlation between plaque quantity and DMFT and inverse trends between plaque quantity and variables reflecting fluoride exposure.

This example is idealized in Figure 1 to illustrate the consequences of ignoring a dominant variable. The relationship between DMFT and plaque quantity is perfect (r = 1.0) at each level of fluoride exposure. If fluoride had not been considered and the 12 pairs of values were analysed as a single sample, the r value would drop to 0.58 and the new slope would misrepresent the change in DMFT for unit change in plaque quantity. Since the very same problem exists with respect to all operating interdependent variables, in reality the situation is much more complex.

In the experimental sense and at the population level, the problem can be alleviated if contrasts with regard to major variables are recognized and the sample selection or data analysis is carried out accordingly. However, no complete remedy can be offered, especially at the individual level,

FIGURE 1

LINEAR REGRESSIONS OF DMFT ON PLAQUE QUANTITY WITHIN GROUPS EXPOSED TO IDENTICAL LEVELS OF FLUORIDE AND OVERALL (MODEL)

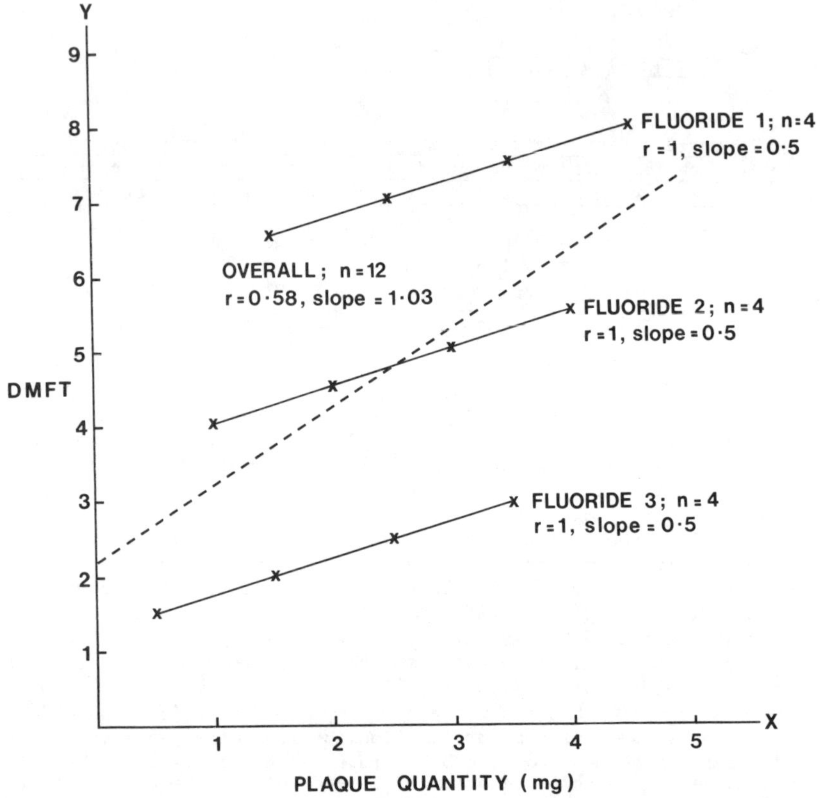

MSLRA :	Dependent variable	DMFT
	Independent variables	Plaque quantity
		Fluoride

n	Step	R
12	2	1·0

for two reasons: 1. We are only beginning to explore the patterns of interdependence between variables which influence caries. 2. Even where the effect of a variable on an association can be identified - as in the case of some known determinants of caries - the extent of the effect is difficult to determine. In particular, there are no firm criteria for weighting the protection conferred on an individual at a given exposure to fluoride or the risk imposed by a certain intensity of carbohydrate challenge. Development of such criteria would be of infinite value in caries prediction and prevention.

In looking at statistical means for alleviating the problem, the variables used in our ideal example were submitted to MLRA which produced a multiple R value of 1.0, restoring the perfect correlation. In other instances the improvement will depend on the configuration of the data. The constraints imposed by the real life situation still exist.

With regard to the tooth surfaces sampled, individual variation in caries risk, vested in the surfaces, must be recognized and if possible catered for:

1. Major variations in morphological features such as the presence or absence of pits and fissures, their shape and depth and the prominence of a surface are associated with different levels of risk. Attention to detail and common genetic background of subjects help to make valid intercomparisons.
2. The decreasing probability of a tooth surface becoming carious with time elapsed since eruption (beyond the first few years) is recognized although the underlying biology is not understood. However, heterogeneity can be reduced by considering subjects with similar tooth age.
3. Lack of proximal contact reduces caries risk sharply. Since spaced proximal surfaces can not be considered in the same etiological context as the majority, which are in contact, they should be excluded from the sample.
4. The presence or absence of microdefects, hypoplasia or hypocalcification needs to be noted. As a minimum precaution it should be established whether or not results relating to defective surfaces correspond to those obtained for intact surfaces. Our findings indicate that certain types of microdefects strongly predispose to caries.
5. Attrition and abrasion may moderate caries. The rates vary with many factors, such as dietary patterns, cultural habits and cleansing techniques, and should be considered where their relevance is apparent.

Seeking maximum contrast between variables under examination, and maximum homogeneity regarding major determinants not explicitly studied at the individual level, are corner stones of population studies of caries etiology. Awareness of possible unexpected but operating sources of heterogeneity helps to avoid pitfalls which often arise from comparing non comparable subjects. Figure 2 shows a simple example of the latter point using means of DMFS and age in subgroups of our New Guinea sample, where mean ages differed for reasons beyond our control. Over the whole sample there is an inverse association between DMFT and age. In this case the anomaly is obvious and the expected trend prevailed within groups. However, less apparent but important sources of heterogeneity may be very difficult to detect.

Form of relationship between variables. The most widely used tool for the study of associations between individual caries experience and pertinent variables is regression analysis. This approach only measures the extent to which variables are linearly related. Biological considerations suggest that this is rarely so. It would be reasonable to expect that threshold and saturation levels exist for most variables. The principle is illustrated in Figure 3, which implies that under a certain intensity of acid attack no damage occurs and beyond a level no further damage is possible. We can offer experimental support for threshold levels; in four out of six population groups where we have examined the relationship between individual caries experience and the fluoride content of plaque, inverse

FIGURE 2

RELATIONSHIP BETWEEN MEANS OF
CARIES EXPERIENCE AND AGE
NEW GUINEA STUDY

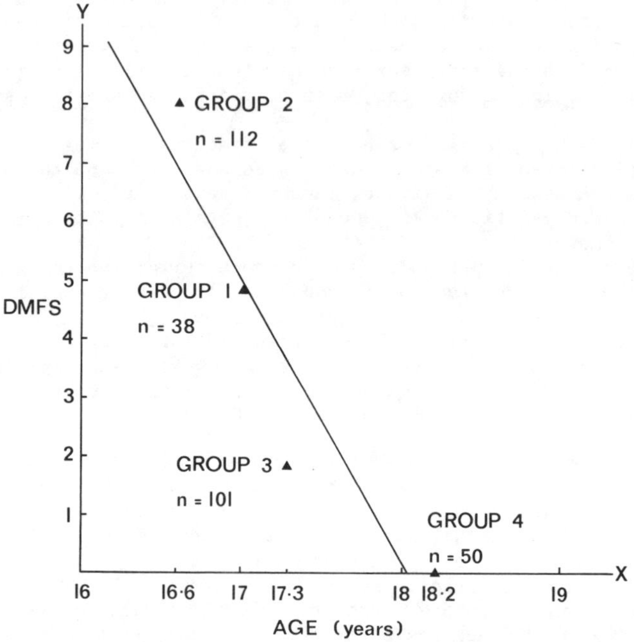

associations were demonstrated. The other two groups were resident in fluoride deficient areas and had the lowest mean plaque fluoride levels. However, present knowledge concerning the forms of associations between caries experience and its determinants or between the latter is practically non existent. Advances in this field would make possible linearization of relationships by appropriate transformation, with consequent improvements in the strength of associations.

Caries prediction using bivariate and multiple linear regressions. Susceptibility or resistance to caries are not absolute terms. The extent to which a person may be susceptible or resistant is determined by the interaction of many factors. Therefore, high correlations based on individual data can only be expected between any one influencing variable and manifestations of the disease if one or more of the following conditions apply: 1. The variable is dominant to the extent that in comparison the effect of other factors is negligible. 2. The sample is approaching homogeneity in all respects except the variable under examination. 3. The variable reflects the joint effect of operating determinants. For these reasons consistency of results must rate at least equal to the strength of association. In fact, we were more impressed with r values of 0.29, 0.33 and 0.30 ($P < 0.0005$ in each case) obtained in the three years of our first N.S.W. study between DMFS and salivary buffering capacity, than we would have been with twice the size of coefficients on a single occasion.

FIGURE 3

POSSIBLE FORM OF RELATIONSHIP
BETWEEN CARIES EXPERIENCE AND CHALLENGE

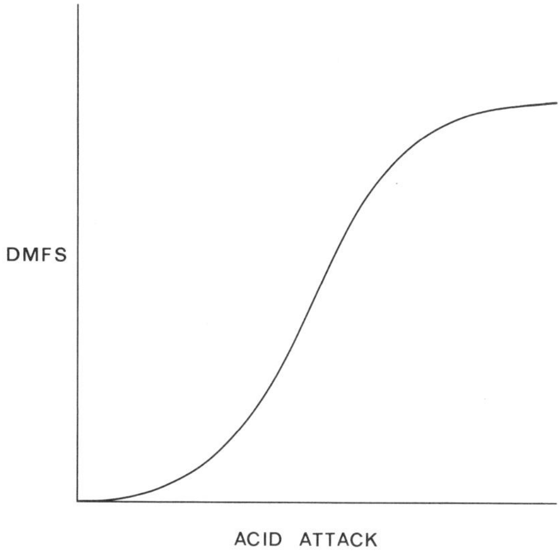

By regressing several independent variables simultaneously against an expression of caries experience, the coverage of operating variables and consequently the proportion of variation explained can be increased. Some practical points concerning this approach deserve consideration: 1. In MLRA-s as the number of subjects: number of variables ratio decreases, the probability of obtaining a high R value increases and it is possible to reach a meaningless R value of 1.0 using irrelevant variables. 2. Intercorrelated variables reflect each other's effect; the little improvement of R when several members of such a group enter the process involves sacrifice in the significance level. Moreover, in free competition with interrelated variables the effect of a variable closely correlated with caries may not become apparent. However, variables can be classified according to their correlations with the dependent variable, with each other and on biological grounds. Submitting marker variables representative of their class to final analyses facilitates wide coverage of etiological areas and meaningful use of the information contained in the data.

Ranking of variables. Given that a set of variables of substantial collective caries predictive capacity has been identified, the question may be asked: is it possible to attach a relative importance to each? In the statistical sense the answer is affirmative, in that, attributes such as strength of association with caries experience, direction of slope, contribution to multiple regression and discriminant power may form bases for ranking variables. However, it would be wrong to equate statistical importance with biological activity. Consider the following example: If the effect of fluoride on caries experience were examined in a group free of plaque, there would be no possibility to observe an effect since caries would not occur in the absence of microbial contact with teeth. This argument extends to non zero quantities. Thus, if one were to find that DMFT and fluoride in enamel were correlated at $r = -0.4$ and DMFT and plaque activity at $r = 0.3$, slopes being equal, it should not be construed that fluoride is more important than plaque activity. Since interaction means that one factor conditions the effect of another, it would be more appropriate to ask: what protection could be attributed to a certain exposure to fluoride at a given intensity of plaque mediated challenge? Exploration of interactions in this context is a major task which remains to be accomplished.

From the etiological point of view, maximum contrast between variables examined, comparability of tooth surfaces and homogeneity of operating determinants of caries not explicitly studied, are fundamental requisites for successful caries prediction. Longitudinal observations result in a better overall estimate of the relevance of a variable than measurement at one point in time. Different sets of variables may assume importance in the initiation and progress of lesions. Work is needed to define the true forms of relationships between caries experience and its determinants, interdependence patterns of factors influencing odontolysis and the relative importance of casually related sets of parameters operating in interaction. Attempts to rank the casual importance of variables in isolation are unlikely to succeed. Population studies where the former points are kept in mind are the best means known for testing the in vivo validity of laboratory based concepts of the pathogenesis of caries.

LITERATURE CITED

1. Schamschula, R.G. and Charlton, G. 1971. A Study of Caries Etiology in New South Wales School Children. The Streptococcal Flora of Plaque and Caries Prevalence. Aust. Dent. J. 16:77-82.

2. Charlton, G., Blainey, B. and Schamschula, R.G. 1974. Associations Between Dental Plaque and Fluoride in Human Surface Enamel. Archs Oral Biol. 19:139-143.

3. Charlton, G., Schamschula, R.G. and Blainey, B. 1975. Relationship Between Volume and Streptococcal Population in Dental Plaque. J. Dent. Res. 54:1094.

4. Agus, H., Schamschula, R.G., Barmes, D.E. and Bunzel, M. 1976. Associations Between the Total Fluoride Content of Dental Plaque and Individual Caries Experience in Australian Children. Community Dent. Oral Epidemiol. 4:210-214.

5. Schamschula, R.G., Agus, H.M., Bunzel, M. Adkins, B.L. and Barmes, D.E. 1977. The Concentrations of Selected Major and Trace Elements in Human Dental Plaque. Archs. Oral Biol. In press.

6. Schamschula, R.G., Bunzel, M., Agus, H.M., Adkins, B.L., Barmes, D.E., and Charlton, G. Plaque Minerals and Caries Experience: Associations and Interrelationships. J. Dent. Res. Submitted for Publication.

7. Schamschula, R.G., Adkins, B.L., Barmes, D.E., Charlton, G. and Davey, B.G. 1977. A study of Caries Etiology in Papua New Guinea. World Health Organization. Monograph. In press.

8. Schamschula, R.G. 1974. Relationships Between Selected Intra-Oral Characteristics, Environmental Variables and Caries Experience of Primitive Peoples in New Guinea. D.D.Sc. Thesis, University of Sydney.

9. McClure, F.J. 1970. Water Fluoridation. The Search and the Victory, U.S. Department of Health, Education, and Welfare, National Institutes of Health, p. 302.

10. Hardwick, J.L. 1971. Fluorides and Dental Health. In: Forum Medici No.13, Caries and Dental Health, Zyma, Nyon, p.66.

Discussion of aspects of design and data evaluation in population studies

H.K. Lu

School of Dentistry, 611 S.W. Campus Drive, Portland, Oregon 97201

Dr. Schamschula has stated that (1) Longitudinal data are better for caries prediction studies than cross sectional ones because they afford the investigators opportunity to monitor the changes in time; (2) The best results of caries prediction studies may be expected from data based on homogeneous groups; (3) Conscientious and prudent choice of "causal" variables is a pre-requisite for success. Failure to do so will result in loss of information; and (4) The relative importance of any causal factor must be assessed in conjunction with others, otherwise attempts to evaluate it in isolation are unlikely to succeed. We shall discuss these points in the order listed.

Longitudinal Data: The advantages of longitudinal data over the cross-sectional is a well known and established fact, no further comment is necessary.

Homogeneity of Groups: In order to discuss the point of homogeneity of groups more precisely we must first define the purpose of the study. If it were to test the efficacy of a certain public health measure of a therapeutic agent against tooth decay, the situation would lend itself suitably to a class of experimental designs, known as the randomized complete blocks, in which one always seeks to minimize the within block variations (homogeneous groups) and maximize the variations between the blocks. The experimental error would be larger if one pools all blocks into one large hetergeneous block, in which case, it will be a completely randomized block design. However, the stress on within group homogeneity should not be construed as to mean that we confine our analysis to only within group analyses. To do so would result in a number of small analyses, each of which is from a different group. We would have detailed information about the peculiarities and idiosyncrasies of each group, but miss the over all picture of the population altogether. The proper way to handle this type of data is to separate the effects of the differences between blocks from that of the variables of interest by appropriate statistical analysis.

However, if our purpose were to investigate the cause-effect relationship between "background" factors and caries development (DMFT), one must allow variations among them. Heterogeneity among the population is a fact we must accept. We should take into consideration the heterogeneity of certain pertinent variables and make appropriate adjustment accordingly, but must accept the remaining heterogeneity as experimental error. There are inherent dangers in using groups, with all the pertinent factors being homogeneous for cause-effect system study.

Let us imagine that if we have some groups in which all the pertinent and important factors are homogeneously the same, then any difference observed would be the results of random variations or irrelevant factors. Thus defeating the original purpose completely.

Conscientious Choice and Relative Importance of Pertinent Causal Variables:

The discussion of these points may be carried out by means of the example offered by Prof. Schamschula. Conveniently, data obtained from the graph in Figure 1 of his paper is presented in table 1. Although the example is an idealized simplification, it well serves the purpose to illustrate the essential points of interest.

As Dr. Schamschula demonstrated, failure to include the fluoride level (FL $_1$ X $_2$) as a causal variable resulted in low correlation between plaque activity (PA$_1$ X $_1$) and DMFT (X_3). On the other hand, the inclusion of FL in the model is compellingly obvious. One only needs to examine the coefficients of determination, of the two variables, i.e., r^2_{13} = 33.5% for PA and r^2_{23} = 93.0% for FL. Most certainly, no one would choose to ignore FL as a factor. The point that in the absence of plaque, caries would simply not develop is well taken, therefore, the inclusion of PA is also obvious. In reality, the causal variables affecting the caries process seldom function in tandem or independently. Instead, they function simultaneously and jointly. Our task is to discern them, construct a working model which can sufficiently approximate the real process such that we may use it to explain or predict its future development.

The present case lends itself to a very simple linear model, considers the DMFT as a linear function of two variables, namely, the plaque activity and the fluoride level. The necessary statistics were calculated as in table 1.

Before we get into the substance of the results, a few words of explanation on the differences among the simple, partial and multiple correlations would seem to be helpful for those who are not familiar with these terms and I beg indulgence from those to whom these are commonplace. Let us consider the different correlations between the DMFT and PA, say,

(1) The simple correlation r_{13} denotes the linear association between DMFT and PA with the effects of all other variables simply ignored;

(2) The partial correlation, $r_{13.2}$ denotes the degree of linear associations between DMFT and PA with the effect of fluoride level FL held constant; and

(3) The multiple correlation, $R_{3.12}$ denotes the total linear association between DMFT and the variables PA and FL.

On occasions these correlations may have similar numerical values, they however, are distinctly different, each measures a different type of association.

Geometrically speaking, a simple perfect correlation implies that all data points are on the regression line and a perfect multiple correlation implies that all data points are on the plane (or hyperplane in higher dimensions) defined by the multiple regression equation. In such cases, the prediction is perfect without error. The relationships are graphed in figure 1.

In our present case, the computed model we have here is $X_3 = 8 + 5 X_1 - 2.25 X_2$, the multiple and both partial correlations are perfect, thus all 12 points are on the slanting plane and all 4 data points within each fluoride level are on a straight line with slope identically equal to 0.5. The inclusion of both variables yielded a perfect multiple correlation. It is not restoring a simple correlation r_{13} = .58 to perfection. The partial

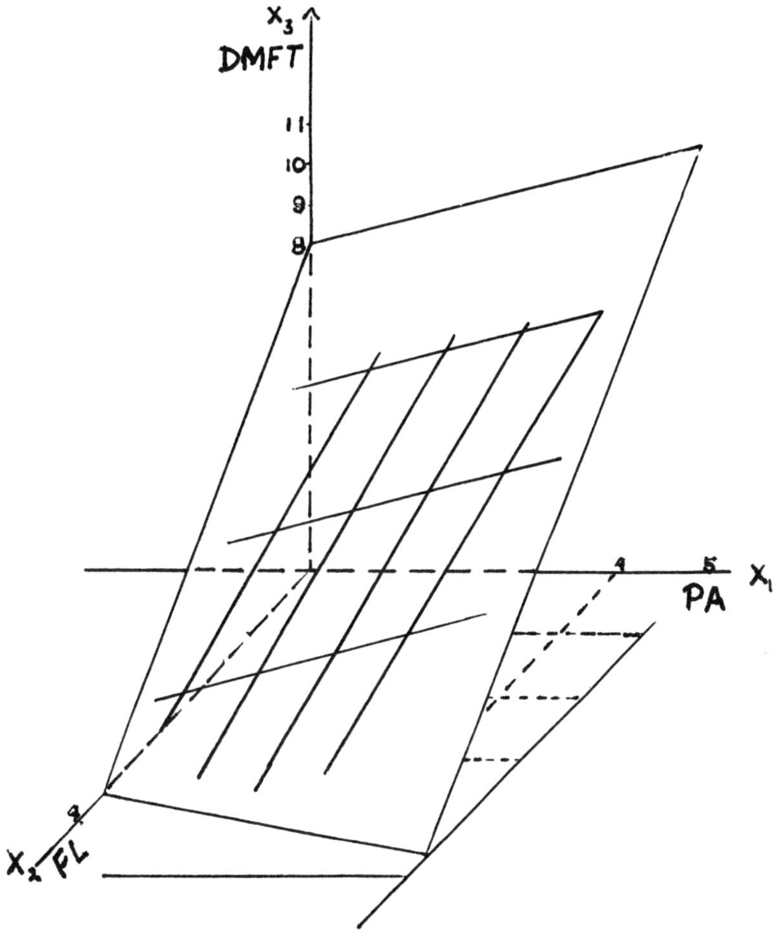

FIGURE 1

correlation $r_{13.2}$ has been perfect all the time in this case.

In general, the model being fitted is written as

$$X_3 = C + b_{13.2}\,X_1 + b_{23.1}\,X_2$$

and can be rewritten as,

$$Z_3 = P_1Z_1 + P_2Z_2$$

where the Z's are the standardized versions of X_1, X_2 and X_3 are where

$$P_1 = b_{13.2}\,\frac{S_1}{S_3} \qquad P_2 = b_{23.1}\,\frac{S_2}{S_3}$$

P_1 and P_2 are dimensionless coefficients, and are known as the path coefficients or beta coefficients. (Kemthorne and Leroy Folks 1971. Wright 1968, Mills 1955). They measure the direct effect of one variable on the other.

Table 1

Plaque Activity	(x_1)	2.50	1.24
Fluoride Level	(x_2)	2.00	0.85
Caries Experience	(x_3)	4.75	2.21

Regression and Correlation Coefficients

	b	R	R^2
simple	$b_{3.1}$ = 1.03	r_3 = .5789	r_3^2 = .3351
	$b_{3.2}$ = -2.50	r_{32} = -.9645	r_{32}^2 = .9303
		r_{12} = -.3430	r_{12}^2 = .1176
partial	$b_{31.2}$ = .50	$r_{31.2}$ = 1.00	$r_{31.2}^2$ = 1.00
	$b_{32.1}$ = -2.25	$r_{32.1}$ = -1.00	$r_{32.1}^2$ = 1.00
multiple		$r_{3.12}$ = 1.00	$r_{3.12}^2$ = 1.00

In the example, we have $P_1 = .2811$, $P_2 = .8680$, giving

$$Z_{3.1} = .2811\ Z_1 = .8680\ Z_2$$

It is well known the

$$R^2_{3.21} = P_1\, r_{13} + P_2\, r_{23}$$

The first term measures the total contribution to R^2 due to PA, and the second the contribution due to FL. Since

$$1 = R^2_{3.21} = .1628 + .8372$$

It is clear that fluoride level is more than 5 times as important as plaque when these variables are considered simultaneously. The moral of the above is that from the public health point of view, while diligent efforts should be directed toward good home care (removal of plaque), the single most effective measure against tooth decay is water fluoridation, Use of fluoride dentifrice is an effort incorporating both factors.

Other relationships can also be established between these path coefficients and the correlation coefficients.

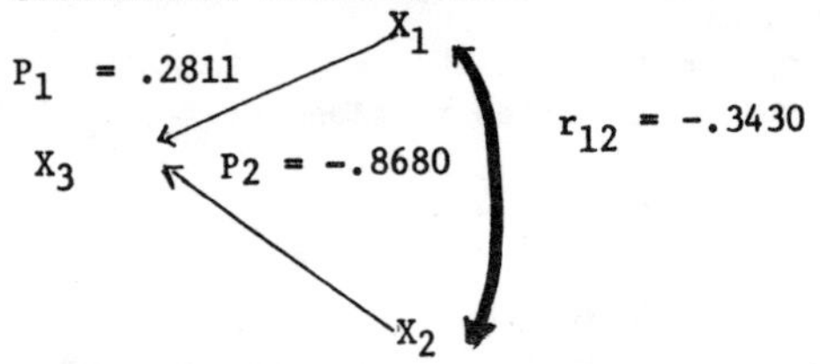

A word about linearity seems appropriate here. Indeed, many relationships in reality are not linear. For example the threshold effect;

below and above certain limits the factor simply ceases to function. However, it is also true that the behavior of variables outside these limits are as a rule not interesting. The behavior between these limits may indeed in many cases be approximated by a linear relationship.

The linear model is the simpliest, but most certainly not sacred. If patterns of behavior cannot be satisfactorily approximated, we will have to consider a non-linear model. Due to the limit of time and space, it should not be considered here.

Let us suppose that we agree to use DMFT as the measure of the caries process. The definition itself suggests the approach of a model which guarantees perfect linearity at least at the initial stages. Note that

$$X = DMFT$$
$$= D + M + F$$

We have a model

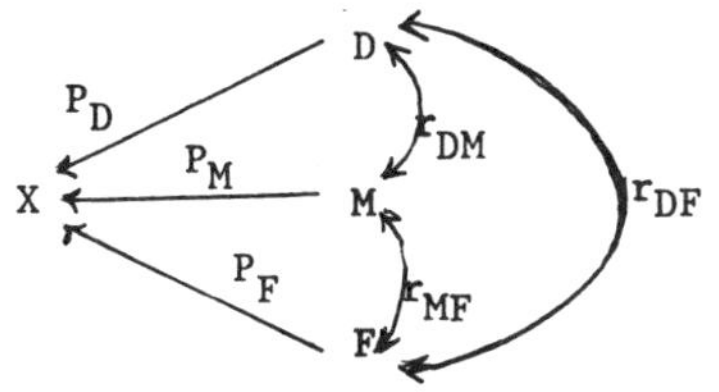

We know $R_{X.DMF} = 1$

Any variable affecting caries experience must exercise its influence through one or more of these components, and nothing else.

The model may go further as begin to bring in pertinent variables that affect one or more of the variable DMFT. While the exact magnitudes of each path coefficient are not known, we may have some prior knowledge about them.

Using data of an on-going experiment, which does not need to be described at this time, we have constructed a working model that purports to portray the relationship between caries experience x (DMFT), and a variety of affecting factors. As stated before, each affecting factor must exert its influence through one or more of the three components PA, FL or CHO. The positive or negative signs along the paths of the model serve to indicate whether the particular factor is promoting or inhibiting caries respectively.

References

Kempthorne, Oscar and Leroy Folks, 1971, Probability, Statistics, and Data Analysis, Iowa State University Press, Ames, Iowa, USA.

Mills, Frederick C. 1955, Statistical Methods, 3rd Edition, Henry Holt and Co., New York.

Wright, Sewall 1968, Evolution and the Genetics of Populations Vol. 1 Genetic and Biometric Foundations, University of Chicago Press, Chicago and London.

Discussion of the selection of study design and measurements used for predicting dental caries

R.J. Shern

National Institute of Dental Research, Auburn Building, Bethesda, Maryland 20014

Dr. Schamschula presented a systematic method for studying the association among factors that may be involved in the pathogenesis of dental caries using the multiple regression technique. He has shown the importance of correct selection of population and study design. He noted that the nature of the associations changed as caries progressed and suggested that factors related to the initiation of dental caries differ from factors involved in the progression of the lesions.

My comments will reiterate many points discussed by Dr. Schamschula and will supplement some of his observations with some of my own.

Study Strategy

A variety of strategies and approaches are available to study associations between dental caries and its possible determinants. Both inductive and deductive methods can be used to study the etiology of complex diseases such as caries. Initially, an inductive strategy is often useful because it can be used to postulate hypotheses. Statistical tools such as multiple regression can help an investigator select variables that deserve additional scrutiny. Dr. Schamschula used inductive strategy in the New Guinea prevalence studies. Specifically, he measured 80 variables on 292 subjects and noted many provocative associations. As he noted, interpretation of such data should be done cautiously because the nature of many of the associations might have been observed and explained *ex post facto* and some of the relationships might have been due to chance. As the pathogenesis becomes better understood, a deductive strategy should be used to test and cross-validate hypotheses. Dr. Schamschula (1) demonstrated the use of deductive strategy when he predicted that decreases in fluoride or increases in age would be associated with increases in dental caries in several populations.

The cross-sectional or prevalence study is only one approach for studying measurements that predict dental caries. Early in an investigation one should decide if an association is consistent with reason and with current knowledge. The validity of the association can often be strengthened by testing it in an animal study. Next, a retrospective study might be considered. For example, Krasse and co-workers (2) chose their populations on the basis of caries prevalence and noted the proportions of *S. mutans* associated with the groups experiencing high and low caries prevalence. Such retrospective studies should be interpreted with care because the observed association may have been due to other factors not considered; for example, sugar consumption. Recognizing this problem, Krasse and co-workers (2) subsequently conducted a cross-sectional and a longitudinal study.

Cross-sectional studies often precede longitudinal studies. In fact, a cross-sectional study can be designed to provide the baseline for a longitudinal study. In both types of studies we can select a sample, classify the sample on the basis of factors thought to be associated with caries, and then note the caries status. If the cross-sectional study suggests variables associated with caries prevalence, then we may want to know whether the biologic response being measured are antecedent and, therefore, are predictors of caries incidence. Longitudinal studies are necessary to establish antecedence; that is, did the bacteria cause the lesion or does the lesion harbor the bacteria? Once causal associations are noted, they should be strengthened by retesting in other populations. As Dr. Schamschula noted, "longitudinal data provide a more realistic basis for caries prediction than cross-sectional data."

Measurements

When predicting the outcome of various promotive and preventive forces on a disease process such as dental caries, we must consider the reliability and validity of the measures used in the assessment. The forces or independent variables involved in the pathogenesis of caries are dynamic, with the interplay of forces constantly changing. The forces may result in carious lesions that are reversible in incipient stage; however, if the forces continue unbated, the lesions progress and accumulate. The promotive and preventive effects are of different intensity within the mouth, among teeth and among tooth surfaces. Consequently, we should know whether the area from which we obtain microbiological and biochemical samples is representative of caries-susceptible areas. For example, if we are studying pit and fissure caries, we need to know whether pit and fissure areas were sampled for bacteria and we also need to know the variability of the bacterial population of the susceptible site over time.

Another important question should be asked: are we measuring what we purport to measure? For instance, what is our specificity and sensitivity for identifying S. mutans? Or, is tooth resistance more closely related to fluoride levels in the plaque and pellicle than to fluoride levels in the outer layer of enamel?

The measures selected for predicting caries outcome should represent different aspects of the caries challenge. Results from our laboratory and Dr. Schamschula's have indicated that the forces initiating caries differ from those which influence its progression (1,3,4). In 1970 we conducted a prevalence study on 36 boys, aged 12-14 years, who attended a correctional school in North Carolina. Table 1 summarizes the methods for measurement used in the study. Table 2 provides the means and standard deviations of the various measurements. Table 3 shows the associations between various independent variables with the two dependent variables -- incipient lesions and established lesions (DMFT). The major factors relating to DMFT were acid production by aciduric organisms (acid) and bacterial adherence in vitro (adherence). In contrast, incipient lesions were related to more advanced decay (DMFT) and to acid produced by a wide variety of bacteria (non-specific fermentation).

Ideally, predictive measures should be mutually exclusive and collectively exhaustive. Even though it is impossible to achieve this, redundancy of tests should be minimized. Interpretation of the data for the New Guinea study and the Australian study could be aided by a matrix showing correlations within clusters of independent variables (such as enamel properties) and between clusters (such as between enamel properties and plaque properties).

Table 1.
Summary of Methods Used for Measuring Dental Caries and Possible Promotive Factors in 36 Boys, 12-14 Years of Age, North Carolina, 1970

DMFT	=	Decayed Missing Filled Teeth excluding third molars on each individual (5)
Acid	=	pH value of swab test medium after 72 hours of incubation (6).
Non-specific fermentation	=	pH value of basal medium (7) containing 5% sucrose after 48 hours of incubation. Inocula for the microbiological procedures except the swab test were obtained from buccal, lingual and occlusal surfaces of the mandibular right second molar.
Adherence	=	Adherent bacterial deposits ranked 0-5.
S. mutans	=	Percentage of colony forming units growing on Mitis-Salivarius agar that were identified as S. mutans.
Plaque	=	The ratio of the plaque height to the tooth height measured midcoronally on the buccal-lingual surfaces of the mandibular right second molar.
Incipient lesions	=	Incipient and advanced lesions (grade 0) (9) on the buccal, occlusal and lingual surfaces of the mandibular right second molar.

Table 2.
Means and Standard Deviations of Measurements of Dental Caries and Possible Promotive Factors

	Mean (S.D.)
DMFT	6.06 (4.88)
Acid	3.74 (0.36)
Non-Specific fermentation	4.51 (0.42)
Adherence	2.17 (1.08)
S. mutans	4.24 (6.37)
Plaque	0.27 (0.18)
Incipient lesions	1.5 (1.00)

Table 3.
Correlation Coefficients (r) of Dental Caries with Measurements of Possible Promotive Factors in 36 Boys, 12-14 Years of Age, North Carolina, 1970.

	DMFT	Acid	Non-Specific Fermentation	Adherence	S. Mutans	Plaque	Incipient Lesions
DMFT	-						
Acid	-0.39**	-					
Non-specific fermentation	-0.14	0.04					
Adherence	0.32*	0.16	-0.23	-			
S. mutans	-0.03	-0.12	0.03	-0.09	-		
Plaque	0.06	-0.29	0.10	-0.06	0.10	-	
Incipient lesions	0.32*	- .10	-0.33**	0.13	-0.17	-0.03	-

**P < .05 *P < .10

Population Selection

Study of both primitive and advanced populations is useful. In initial studies, primitive populations, such as those in New Guinea, provide homogeneity of lifestyle and genetic background. This homogeneity may reduce sources of variability that otherwise could obscure the detection of associations. However, primitive populations may have habits such as betel nut chewing that are uncommon to other populations but that strongly affect dental caries. Definitive, longitudinal studies should be made on a sample of a more advanced population. Findings gained from such a sample may then more validly be extrapolated to the population in this country and in other westernized societies.

Dr. Schamschula reminded us of the value of selecting a homogeneous population. This is consistent with the epidemiological principles of avoiding factors which could confound a correlation, keeping constant as many variables as possible and trying to randomize the remaining ones. Statistical methods can also aid in controlling the influence of confounding variables.

In our North Carolina study, we tried to select a homogeneous population representative of a larger population. The fluoride history of each individual was not taken because most of the boys had resided in more than one town. The school water supply contained fluoride (1µg/ml). The diets the boys consumed before coming to the school were unknown. However, their diet during the study was rigidly controlled and contained no snacks between meals.

As Dr. Schamschula noted, statistical methods can be made adaptable to the biologic processes. For example, multiple regression methods can be used to model nonlinear or curvilinear relationships as well as linear ones. Also, he noted that interpretations of etiological studies are easier to make when the investigator specifies the number and nature of predictive variables prior to final data analysis. In the North Carolina study, both _in vitro_ plaque formation (measured by the adherence test) and acid production (measured by the swab or acid test) appeared to increase R^2 (Table 4) as we had anticipated. The joint association of acid and adherence is being investigated further despite the low "R". Grainger (6) has reported that the swab test has a high correlation with caries incidence in certain populations. The association between adherence and caries prevalence (r = 0.58) was also noted by Shern (4) in a primitive population. Recently Bowen (10) reported a similar association using a different method for measuring adherence.

We are initiating a cross-sectional study, hypothesizing that prediction will be increased if we add some measure of tooth resistance, such as tooth-associated fluoride. Fluoride biopsies of enamel have been unpredictive in past studies (11). However, recent work by Agus and coworkers suggests that fluoride analysis of plaque would give more meaningful data than analysis of enamel (12).

These considerations lead to the conclusion that many biologic factors are involved in the pathogenesis of caries. Therefore, several measurements will no doubt be necessary to predict caries prevalence and incidence. Statistical methods such as multiple regression can be used both for selecting the most effective predictive measures and for forming a predictive profile.

Table 4.
Analysis of Variance for Regression of Variables on DMFT

** P<.05
* P<.10

Source	D.F.	Sum of Square	Mean Square	Variance Ratio
Acid	1	124.204	124.204	5.967**
Residual	34	707.681	20.814	
Acid	1	124.204	124.204	
Added by Adherence	1	57.617	57.617	2.925*
Residual	33	650.064	19.699	
Acid and Adherence	2	181.821	90.911	
Added by others	3	45.816	15.272	0.758
Residual	30	604.249	20.142	
Total	35	831.886	Total R^2 = .274	

LITERATURE CITED

1. Schamschula, R.G., Adkins, B.L., Agus, H.M., Barmes, D.E. and Charlton, G. Caries prediction: aspects of design and data evaluation in population studies. Workshop Conference on Caries Prediction, Niagara Falls, New York, October 2-5, 1977.

2. Krasse, B., Jordan, H.V., Edwardsson, S., Svensson, I. and Trell, L. 1968. The occurrence of certain "caries-inducing" streptococci in human dental plaque material. Arch. Oral Biol. 13:911-918.

3. Shern, R.J. 1970. Development of a caries activity profile. M.S. thesis, University of North Carolina.

4. Shern, R.J. and Crawford, J.J. 1971. Development of a caries activity profile. J. Dent. Res. IADR Abstract #643.

5. Klein, H., Palmer, C.E. and Knutson, J.W. 1938. Studies on dental caries. I. Dental status and dental needs of elementary school children. Public Health Reports 53:751-760.

6. Grainger, R.M., Jarret, M. and Honey, S.L. 1965. Swab test for dental caries activity: and epidemiological study. Canad. Dent. J. 31:515-526.

7. Jordan, H.V., Fitzgerald, R.J. and Bowler, A.E. 1960. Inhibition of experimental caries by sodium metabisulfite and its effect on growth and metabolism of selected bacteria. J. Dent. Res. 39:116-123

8. McCabe, R.M., Keyes, P.H. and Howell, A., Jr. 1967. An in vitro method for assessing the plaque-forming ability of oral bacteria. Arch. Oral Biol. 12:1653-1656.

9. Marthaler, T.M. 1965. The caries-inhibiting effect of amine fluoride dentrifices in children during three years of unsupervised use. Brit. Dent. J. 119:153-163.

10. Bowen, W.H., Velez, H., Aguila, M., Velasquez, H., Sierra, L.I. and Gillespie, G. 1977. The microbiology and biochemistry of plaque, saliva and drinking water from two communities with contrasting levels of caries in Columbia, S.A. J. Dent. Res. 56: in press.

11. Shern, R.J., Driscoll, W.S. and Korts, D.C. 1977. Enamel biopsy results of children receiving fluoride tablets. J.A.D.A. 95:310-314.

12. Agus, H.M., Schamschula, R.G., Barmes, D.E. and Bunzel, M. 1976. Associations between total fluoride content of dental plaque and individual caries experience in Australian school children. Community Dentistry and Oral Epidemiol. 4:210-214.

TOPIC VIII

TASK FORCE REPORTS

Moderator:

Irwin D. Mandel
Columbia University
630 West 168th Street, New York
New York 10032

Report of task force I. Use of clinical data for caries prediction

R.M. Grainger, Moderator, S.B. Heifetz, Recorder

Prescott, Ontario, Canada

The group's discussion on the use of clinical data for the prediction of dental caries centered on three areas: selection of dependent variables, identification of predictor variables, and statistical methods for analyzing possible functional relationships between predictor and dependent variables. Common to all three areas was the emphasis given to the need for developing and improving technics of measurement and more sharply defining criteria.

Dependent variables: While evidence of frank cavitation is still the most widely recognized criterion for the diagnosis of a carious lesion, it would be desirable to utilize earlier signs of the developing condition, such as visually detectable white spot or demineralized areas, or areas of altered tooth structure that can be demarcated by ultra-violet or polarized light, fluorescent dyes, conductivity measurements, ultra-sound technics, etc. Methods for the early diagnosis of a carious lesion would materially shorten the time required for clinical studies. However, the "pre-carious" conditions that are detectable by these new technics must be validated as true precursors of the eventual overt lesion. For example, the type of longitudinal studies carried out by Dr. Marthaler in following the eventual clinical fate of white spot areas on smooth surfaces should be encouraged.

Concerning the early detection of fissure caries, we support the approach taken by Dr. White and his co-workers in measuring the electrical conductivity of tooth structure because histologic evidence of decay was used as the validating criterion. At present, our efforts should be directed to demonstrating the validity and reliability of these new technics in detecting the early carious lesion. However, we should not forget that a principle aim of preventive dentistry is to reverse or remineralize the same early lesion that we are so interested in detecting.

In order to attain efficient predictive capability, reproducible observations of the dependent variable are essential. In identifying lesions at any stage of development, efforts should be made to keep diagnostic errors of measurement to a minimum. Investigators should conduct standardized and replicate examinations, and should report their reversal rates along with their findings.

In trials involving the use of radiographs, examiners should strive for closer agreement in the extent of radiolucency that is required for the detection of early proximal lesions. In short, poorly reproducible observations inflate the variance of the dependent variable and cause a loss in predictive efficiency.

Predictor variables: It was generally agreed that prior caries experience, number of surfaces at risk, and possibly some expression of their product or powers, can be considered as fundamental indicators of future caries experience. Other epidemiologic parameters that appear interesting as predictor variables are: dental age or period of exposure of teeth to the oral environment, pattern of caries attack with respect to dental age, level of dental care, caries experience, particularly that of the mother. Oral hygiene status is a predictor of some interest, but the condition may be too transitory and subject to bias because of a subject's tendency to "scrub up" before an examination. The status of oral cleanliness may be better implied from measurements of other oral conditions such as gingival health. Also identified were several etiologic factors associated with dental caries that show promise as predictor variables. Included among them were: microbiologic correlates, plaque and salivary factors, dietary composition and practices and morphologic and chemical structure of teeth. All of these factors deserve serious attention and further study, but the difficulty of measuring them in the field must be weighed in relation to their potential value as predictors. Of further value would be the identification of some predictor variables that can shed light on the tendency for remineralization of early lesions. Based on Dr. Schamschula's findings, it appears to be necessary to consider predictors of the initiation of the carious lesion as separate from those influencing the progression of the lesion. Similarly, forecasting fissure caries may require somewhat different predictors than can be used for smooth surface caries.

Statistical Methodology: Extensive use of regression and correlation statistics has been made to analyze the relation between predictor and dependent variables. When numerous correlations are made from one set of data, chance relationships often emerge that may have little, if any, clinical meaning. Caution must be exercised in interpreting such findings. Moreover, relationships found in one study should be corroborated by other sets of data. In a clinical trial, predictor variables that prove satisfactory in estimating new decay in the control group may differ in value when considering the findings in the treatment group because of interaction with the therapeutic agent. For example, in a fluoride dentifrice trial, the sex of subjects can be a factor bearing on the treatment response because girls may better adhere to a regime of toothbrushing than boys. Finally, caution must also be exercised in using arbitrary or empirical scoring methods in that they will affect the appropriateness of the statistical analysis to follow. For example, a simple classification scheme should not be treated as an ordinal scale of measurement.

Report of taskforce II. Microbiological and biochemical aspects of caries prediction

I. Kleinberg, Moderator, R.G. Schamschula, Recorder

State University of New York, School of Dental Medicine, Stony Brook, New York 11790

On the question of which bacteria should be considered for microbiological tests of caries prediction, there was general agreement that whether sampled from saliva, pooled plaque, or specific sites, no procedure was entirely satisfactory. Using a test which included both *S. mutans* and lactobacilli as indicator organisms was better than studying either alone. Because the species within the lactobacillus genus have not been as well defined as has been *S. mutans* within the genus streptococcus, it was felt that it would be useful to make such a sharper definition of the lactobacilli.

It was suggested that in order to identify microbial parameters which might precede or correlate with caries lesion development longitudinal studies should be carried out relating changes in microbial flora to changes in caries activity. In this way additional microbial predictors might be identified. The density of the total bacterial population should also be investigated.

A number of biochemical tests are available. However because of inconvenience, low correlation, or need for further development, they are not entirely suitable for caries prediction. These are pH measurements of plaque in situ in response to a standardised carbohydrate challenge, determinations of buffer capacity of saliva, and quantitation of plaque calcium, phosphorus and possibly fluoride.

It was proposed that caries-active and caries-free plaques should be studied to identify other parameters such as plaque enzymes, matrix components, and other minerals than calcium, phosphorus, and fluoride. Plaque fluid offers a new area of research that should be explored. To identify differences in properties or constituents of saliva that could be predictors, the saliva of caries-free and caries-active individuals should be re-examined.

It was felt that a multi-component test which included both microbial and biochemical parts was more likely to produce a high degree of prediction than either alone. There was a consensus that recent research presents encouraging possibilities for caries prediction.

Report of taskforce III. Tooth morphology and chemistry as caries indicators

W.W. Briner, Moderator, L. Silverstone, Recorder

Proctor & Gamble Company, 6110 Center Hill Road, Cincinnati, Ohio 45224

It was agreed that certain macromorphological characteristics of teeth are related to their caries susceptibility. The fissures of young teeth are most prone to caries and will develop lesions within one year of their eruption. Smaller teeth such as those found in low caries areas makes it seem likely that they are less susceptible to caries than teeth with larger mesio-distal dimensions. However, the size of the dental arch and closeness of the teeth play a part. Flatness of fissure slopes and size reduction have been noted in fluoride areas. Consequently the interdependence of eruption time, tooth size and fluoride background is worth investigation.

Whether morphological features of the Mongoloid dentition are responsible for its low caries prevalence or whether it is the result of dietary influences should also be clarified. Enamel hardness or softness was not believed to affect the caries susceptibility of teeth.

The development of caries on a tooth on one side of the mouth was accepted as an important indicator of caries development on the contra-lateral tooth. The greater porosity, lower mineral content and thinner enamel and dentin of deciduous teeth was believed to predispose them to caries but their heavier covering of exogenous organic material may decrease their susceptibility. These variables may have potential as caries predictors. Questions that need to be answered include: does caries in the primary dentition predicate caries in the permanent teeth; does occlusal caries relate to development of smooth surface caries in the same patient; do changes in contact resulting from placement of a filling in an approximal surface predispose to caries, and although surfaces under continuous abrasion are not caries susceptible, what happens when abrasion ceases?

There was agreement that chemical variations in tooth composition have much potential as indicators of future caries but consideration of the fluoride levels in enamel has almost monopolized attention. It was decided that, except on a population basis, neither the acid etch or abra-sion technique for estimating the fluoride content were usable as caries predictors. Questions regarding the effect of the pellicle or organic layers on fluoride activity still need to be answered. However, enamel biopsies do provide information on enamel composition and could be used to compare the fluoride content of accessible buccal sites with that of caries susceptible interproximal areas. They could also supply information on chemical changes in the enamel from time of eruption through enamel maturation during post eruptive years. Investigations should be made on the fluoride content of pellicle and plaque to determine whether they might be caries predictors. The chemistry of the pellicle itself should be stud-ied to find out what effects it has on caries. Other basic studies on caries interactions should also be encouraged.

Methods for earlier diagnosing of clinical caries should be developed thereby opening the way for using enamel changes that now require histological identification, as caries predictors. Relevant information could be obtained by developing different degrees of artificial caries lesions *in vitro* and testing them by various methods (ultrasonic, electrical conduction, etc.) to establish what stages of "histological" (sub clinical) caries could be detected.

Report of task force IV. Dietary information as a means of caries prediction

F.M. Parkins, Moderator, K.O. Madsen, Recorder

University of Iowa, College of Dentistry, Iowa City, Iowa 52242

The task force charge was interpreted as asking for the identification of dietary factors which would be of value in predicting caries activity. Despite agreement that dietary factors are of unquestioned importance in caries causation, the group experienced frustrations in naming specific predictive tests. Therefore, the question was approached by discussing the relative cariogenicity of food components.

The presence of sucrose-containing foods was ranked as the greatest caries threat. Habitual use of non-food items containing sucrose, such as cough medicines and tonics was also regarded as contributing to its onset. It was noted that the timing or manner in which sucrose-containing items are used by an individual influences their cariogenicity. It was agreed that since sugars, other than sucrose, are readily fermentable in the mouth they will contribute to caries, but probably less actively. Nevertheless, the predictive value of known exposures to lactose, fructose, or other sugars in foods, requires further study. Such study should recognise that very low concentrations of some sugars could be highly cariogenic, and efforts should be made to determine the exact types of exposures needed for producing caries and the effects of raising the concentrations of sugars on caries activity.

The role played by starches was discussed. It was noted that caries occurs in animals on diets containing starches and no known sugar. Variable cariogenicity could result from exposure to different starches or to changes produced in them during food processing and preparation. Starch foods such as breads and cereals may contain a variety of additives, including sugars that could modify their cariogenicity.

The role of food acids in cariogenesis was considered. While the erosion caused by some fruit juices or acid drinks is well known, a definite conclusion could not be reached as to what they might contribute to caries. It was felt that further investigation might be fruitful.

After considering caries-promoting food components, attention was given to caries-protective factors in the diet. Although special diets in which fermentable foods are replaced by unprocessed foods, high fiber foods, high protein foods, etc. were agreed to be conducive to lower cariogenicity, this result can be attributed to concomitant sugar reduction rather than a positive caries-protective effect. Specific food components such as phosphates, buffers, and other inorganic constituents such as trace elements were recognised as potentially protective factors. These along with organic protective agents could be present in unprocessed foods. Organic factors such as organic phosphates, proteins or cross reacting antigens that might occur in milk need further investigation.

The mere presence of certain foods and their constituents was not considered to be adequately predictive of caries. The history of total fluoride intake was thought to be of importance in anticipating caries increments. Humanistic factors influencing food selection and ingestion patterns were also recognized as critical to caries prediction.

There was unanimous belief that the duration of exposure of teeth to cariogenic food was crucial. The concept of clearance times for substances which were fermentable and therefore sustained a lowered intra-oral pH was agreed to be a basic consideration in evaluating cariogenic challenges. A high frequency of eating was agreed to be of special importance in prolonging the cariogenic exposure. Its effect would be modified according to: (a) the retentive nature or stickiness of foods, (b) the rate at which fermentable components are released from ingested foods, (c) the method of food use, such as sipping, holding in the mouth, etc. Caries activity could be predicted, it was agreed, whenever the eating frequency of cariogenic foods was closely spaced during the day so that inadequate time was allowed between cariogenic exposures for enamel remineralization. The work of Edgar and Jenkins was cited to support the conclusion that the ingestion sequence of certain cariogenic substances could either decrease or increase their overall cariogenic impact.

Besides frequency factors, other behavioural traits that determine cariogenicity were suggested. These included evaluations not only of personal habits, such as those influencing the oral clearance of caries inducive substances, but also personal reactions to societal influences, such as excessive anxiety.

Cultural and ethnic habits were observed to be important in the selection of subjects for clinical trials because of their influence on the adoption of non-cariogenic behavioural patterns. It was noted that an environmental change can occur even during the course of study that could have a wide effect on a test population. Altered local oral environmental influences may change caries activity. The over-use of sorbitol sweetened foods was reported to induce bacteriological mutants which can metabolise this substance.

It was proposed that the current large epidemiological studies, such as the Framingham Study, which are considering dietary factors in heart and other diseases, be examined for guidelines applicable to the study of the multiple factors contributing to dental caries.

It was particularly noticable that the dietary factors associated with caries have been so inadequately studied that there are no unquestioned caries prediction tests for the evaluation of foods use on either an individual or group basis. This was considered especially noteworthy in comparison to the greater efforts being expended on other possibly less directly related caries factors.

Summary of general discussion

Irwin D. Mandel, Moderator

Columbia University, 630 West 168th Street, New York, New York 10032

During the open discussion of Task Force Reports it was suggested that one approach to shortening the time needed for obtaining results from clinical tests would be to study changes occurring on single tooth surfaces of high caries susceptibility rather than dealing with pooled results from teeth with widely divergent caries susceptibility. Attention was directed to the need for more critical detection of the first or white spot stages of caries. It was stated that in spite of its limitation dental xrays provide the most objective assessment of caries and that it is possible to reduce radiation exposure greatly without loss of diagnostic sensitivity. The need for more information regarding clinically precarious lesions or white spots was pointed out and it was proposed that in order to determine the extent to which they remineralized or advanced to clinical caries it was necessary to observe them for a period of a year or more in a population group receiving no dental care beyond prophylactic cleanings. The opinion was offered that because some plaques might be caries protective prophylaxis should not be given during the sutdy period. Any disturbance of plaque might change a harmless association of bacteria into a harmful one.

Several speakers endorsed the concept that all plaques should not be regarded as cariogenic and attention was redirected onto the variations in plaque composition that occur from area to area even on the same tooth. It was noted that plaque composition was dynamic and changed from time to time in response to factors such as hygiene or diet. The study of the Strep mutans or other bacterial components of interproximal areas on high and low caries subjects was proposed as a way of determining plaque relationships to caries. This was questioned because several bacterial types have properties that predicate cariogenicity. It would be better to make correlations with several types of organisms in plaques rather than with any single type. It was noted that gingival exudates, particularly in cases of gingivitis, could modify plaque function. This could be significant in white spot formation on erupting teeth where some gingivitis is a normal occurrence.

During the discussion of effects of tooth structure it was noted that while the morphology of fissures had been studied in relation to caries there was inadequate information on other morphological variations such as those on the approximal areas. It was suggested that small depressions in the tooth surface could provide protected areas for bacteria that could be important for regrowth of plaques. Emphasis was placed on the fact that defects of the enamel which cannot be distinguished clinically may have very different liability to caries. For instance polarized light studies of experimental caries show that opacities resulting from fluoride break down much less rapidly than those of yet unknown causation. The fact that both types of enamel defects are freely permiable to imbibing agents indicates that permiability cannot by itself be used to determine caries susceptibility of teeth. It was proposed that the needed information on the relationship between the fluoride content of enamel and dental decay should be established by making analyses of a large collection of teeth from persons with known caries histories.

While the importance of the frequency of eating on caries activity was not questioned it was felt that fuller documentation was needed, particularly as it related to the use of specific types of foods. It was suggested that some such information could be obtained by making critical dietary-caries surveys, one of which had already shown a relationship between caries and the use of chewing gum or chocolates both of which were related to the amount of money children had to spend. The need for more data on the relative cariogenicity of individual foods was emphasized. In view of the impossibility of carrying out extensive clinical studies the use of semi-clinical tests of the sort described by Koulourides and Bibby was proposed.

In response to the question of whether his intra-oral pH measurements could be used to develop a scale of relative cariogenicity, Dr. Mühlemann said that at this time all he would claim for his method was that foods that formed no acid in the intra-oral test would not cause caries. In response to the same question regarding his procedures Dr. Bibby stated that he agreed with Dr. Mühlemann regarding non acid forming foods but believed that with a further decade or so of research relatively simple methods could be developed that would give a measurement of the relative cariogenicity of individual foods.

The point was made that the hoped for low cariogenic foods would have to be price competitive or, like what happened to low cariogenic calcium-sucrose phosphate products in Australia, they wouldn't be purchased and would be withdrawn from the market.

List of Participants

John Alman
Dept. of Statistics
Boston University
Boston, Massachusetts 02111

Basil G. Bibby
Eastman Dental Center
800 Main Street East
Rochester, New York 14605

George H. Bowden
London Hospital Medical College
London, England

William H. Bowen
National Institutes of
Dental Research
Bethesda, Maryland 20014

William W. Briner
Proctor & Gamble Company
6110 Center Hill Road
Cincinnati, Ohio 45224

John P. Brown
Dental School
University of Brisbane
Brisbane, Australia

Finn Brudevold
Biochemistry & Preventive Med.
Forsyth Dental Center
140 The Fenway
Boston, Massachusetts 02115

Janet Brunelle
National Institute of
Dental Research
Westwood Building
Bethesda, Maryland 20014

James P. Carlos
National Institute of
Dental Research
Westwood Building
Bethesda, Maryland 20014

Sebastian Ciancio
Dental School
N.Y. State University3435 Main Street
Buffalo, New York 14214

Martin E.J. Curzon
Eastman Dental Center
800 Main Street East
Rochester, New York 14605

Colin Dawes
University of Manitoba
780 Bannatyne Avenue
Winnipeg, Manitoba

Martin C. Downer
University of Manchester
Manchester, England

Paul F. De Paolo
Forsyth Dental Center
140 The Fenway
Boston, Massachusetts 02115

W. Michael Edgar
University of Newcastle on Tyne
Newcastle, England

Frederick F. Feagin
University of Alabama
College of Dentistry
Birmingham, Alabama 35294

Michael L. Freedman
University of Connecticut
Health Center
Farmington, Connecticut 06032

Robert M. Grainger
Prescott, Ontario
Canada

John A. Gray
Proctor & Gamble Company
6110 Center Hill Road
Cincinnati, Ohio 45224

John Hefferen
American Dental Association
Health Foundation
Chicago, Illinois 60611

Stanley B. Heifetz
National Institute of
Dental Research
Westwood Building
Bethesda, Maryland 20014

Herschel S. Horowitz
National Institute of
Dental Research
Westwood Building
Bethesda, Maryland 20014

H. Gordon Huxley
National Institute of
Dental Research
Auburn Building
Bethesda, Maryland 20014

Harold B. Jordan
Forsyth Dental Center
140 The Fenway
Boston, Massachusetts 02115

Simon Katz
Indiana University
1121 W. Michigan Street
Indianapolis, Indiana 46202

Albert Kingman
National Institute of
Dental Research
Westwood Building
Bethesda, Maryland 20014

Israel Kleinberg
State University of New York
School of Dental Medicine
Stony Brook, New York 11790

Bjorn Klock
Faculty of Odontology
University of Göteborg
Göteborg, Sweden

Robert A. Kolstad
Baylor College of Dentistry
3802 Gaston Avenue
Dallas, Texas 75246

David C. Korts
Department of Statistics
Mount Sinai School of Medicine
5th Avenue & 100 Street
New York, New York 10026

Theodore Koulourides
University of Alabama
School of Dentistry
Birmingham, Alabama 35294

Bo Krasse
Faculty of Odontology
University of Göteborg
Göteborg, Sweden

Rachel H. Larson
9310 Fernwood Avenue
Bethesda, Maryland 20034

Sidney Lees
Forsyth Dental Center
140 The Fenway
Boston, Massachusetts 02115

Kuo H. Lu
School of Dentistry
611 S.W. Campus Drive
Portland, Oregon 97201

Kenneth O. Madsen
University of Texas
6516 John Freeman Avenue
Houston, Texas 77025

Irwin D. Mandel
Columbia University
630 West 168th Street
New York, New York 10032

Thomas M. Marthaler
Dental Research Institute
Zurich, Switzerland

Frans H.M. Mikx
Institute Preventive &
Community Dentistry
Nijmegen, The Netherlands

Hans R. Mühlemann
Dental Research Institute
Zurich, Switzerland

Abraham Nizel
Tufts University
School of Dental Medicine
Boston, Massachusetts 02111

Dennis M. O'Mullane
Turner Dental School
Bridgeford Street
Manchester, England

Carl A. Ostrom
University of Alabama
School of Dentistry
Birmingham, Alabama 35294

Frederick M. Parkins
University of Iowa
College of Dentistry
Iowa City, Iowa 52242

Henry R. Rawls
Louisiana State University
Dental School
New Orleans, Louisiana 70119

Rudi G. Schamschula
Dental Research Institute
2 Chalmers Street
Sydney, Australia

Ira L. Shannon
University of Texas
6516 John Freeman Avenue
Houston, Texas 77025

Roald J. Shern
National Institute of
Dental Research
Auburn Building
Bethesda, Maryland 20014

Francis E. Shovlin
College of Medicine & Dentistry
100 Bergen Street
Newark, New Jersey 07103

Leon M. Silverstone
University of Iowa
College of Dentistry
Iowa City, Iowa 52242

Jason M. Tanzer
University of Connecticut
Health Center
Farmington, Connecticut 06032

John Townsley
National Institute of
Dental Research
Westwood Building
Bethesda, Maryland 20014

J.S. van der Hoeven
University of Nymegen
Nijmegen, The Netherlands

Stephen H.Y. Wei
University of Iowa
College of Dentistry
Iowa City, Iowa 52242

George E. White
Tufts University
School of Dental Medicine
1 Kneeland Street
Boston, Massachusetts 02111

Samuel J. Wycoff
University of California
Division of General Dentistry
San Francisco, California 94143

Stuart O. Zimmerman
Anderson Hospital
Department of Biomathematics
Houston, Texas